European Surgical Research

Clinical and Experimental Surgery

Founded 1969

KARGER

Appears bimonthly:
1 volume per year
(6 issues)

Guidelines for Authors

European Surgical Research

Submission: Only original papers written in English are considered and should be sent to:

Prof. Dr. K. Messmer
Institute for Surgical Research
University of Munich
Marchioninistrasse 15
D–81366 München (Germany)
Tel. +49 89 7095 4400
Fax +49 89 7095 8897
E-mail messmer@icf.med.uni-muenchen.de

The manuscript, together with a disk, should be submitted in triplicate with three sets of illustrations, typewritten double-spaced on one side of the paper with a wide margin. **The manuscript should match the file on disk exactly.** For details refer to 'Disk Submission' or www.karger.com/journals/disksub.htm. Editorial work and copy-editing will be executed from the disk version of your manuscript. Authors are requested to keep their manuscripts as succinct as possible.

Conditions
All manuscripts are subject to editorial review. Manuscripts are received with the explicit understanding that they are not under simultaneous consideration by any other publication. Submission of an article for publication implies the transfer of the copyright from the author to the publisher upon acceptance. Accepted papers become the permanent property of 'European Surgical Research' and may not be reproduced by any means, in whole or in part, without the written consent of the publisher. It is the author's responsibility to obtain permission to reproduce illustrations, tables, etc. from other publications.

Arrangement
Title page: The first page of each paper should indicate the title, the authors' names, and the institute where the work was conducted. A short title for use as running head as well as the full address of the author to whom correspondence should be sent are also required.

Full address: The exact postal address complete with postal code must be given at the bottom of the title page. Please also supply phone and fax numbers, as well as your e-mail address.

Key words: For indexing purposes, a list of 3–10 key words in English is essential.

Abstract: Each paper needs an abstract of up to 10 lines.

Small type: Paragraphs which can or must be set in smaller type (case histories, test methods, etc.) should be indicated with a 'p' (petit) in the margin on the left-hand side.

Footnotes: Avoid footnotes. When essential, they are numbered consecutively and typed at the foot of the appropriate page.

Tables and illustrations: Tables and illustrations (both numbered in Arabic numerals) should be prepared on separate sheets. Tables require a heading and figures a legend, also prepared on a separate sheet. For the reproduction of illustrations, only good drawings and original photographs can be accepted; negatives or photocopies cannot be used. Due to technical reasons, figures with a screen background should not be submitted. When possible, group several illustrations on one block for reproduction (max. size 181 × 223 mm) or provide crop marks. On the back of each illustration, indicate its number, the author's name, and 'top' with a soft pencil.

Color illustrations: Up to 6 color illustrations per page can be integrated within the text at the reduced price of CHF 660.–/USD 545.00 per page. Color illustrations are reproduced at the author's expense.

References: In the text identify references by Arabic numerals [in square brackets]. Material submitted for publication but not yet accepted should be noted as 'unpublished data' and not be included in the reference list. The list of references should include only those publications which are cited in the text. Do not alphabetize; number references in the order in which they are first mentioned in the text. The surnames of the authors followed by initials should be given. There should be no punctuation other than a comma to separate the authors. Cite all authors, 'et al' is not sufficient. Abbreviate journal names according to the Index Medicus system. (Also see International Committee of Medical Journal Editors: Uniform requirements for manuscripts submitted to biomedical journals. N Engl J Med 1997;336:309–315.)

Examples
(a) Papers published in periodicals: Sun J, Koto H, Chung KF: Interaction of ozone and allergen challenges on bronchial responsiveness and inflammation in sensitised guinea pigs. Int Arch Allergy Immunol 1997;112:191–195.
(b) Monographs: Matthews DE, Fare-well VT: Using and Understanding Medical Statistics, ed 3, revised. Basel, Karger, 1996.
(c) Edited books: Parren PWHI, Burton DR: Antibodies against HIV-1 from phage display libraries: Mapping of an immune response and progress towards antiviral immunotherapy; in Capra JD (ed): Antibody Engineering. Chem Immunol. Basel, Karger, 1997, vol 65, pp 18–56.
(d) Papers published in electronic format: Black CA: Delayed type hypersensitivity: Current theories with a historic perspective. Dermatol Online J 1999;5:7. http://dermatology.cdlib.org/DOJvol5num1.

Page Charges
A charge of CHF 125.–/USD 98.00 per page will be levied for the first 4 printed pages of an article. Any additional page will be charged to the author at CHF 275.–/USD 196.00. The allotted size of a paper is equal to approx. 12 manuscript pages (including tables, illustrations and references).

Galley Proofs
Unless indicated otherwise, galley proofs are sent to the first-named author and should be returned with the least possible delay. Alterations made in galley proofs, other than the correction of printer's errors, are charged to the author. No page proofs are supplied.

Reprints
Order forms and a price list are sent with the galley proofs. Orders submitted after the issue is printed are subject to considerably higher prices.

KARGER

Fax +41 61 306 12 34
E-Mail karger@karger.ch
www.karger.com

The Guidelines for Authors are available at:
www.karger.com/journals/esr/esr_gl.htm

European Surgical Research

General Information

Publication data: 'European Surgical Research' is published 6 times a year. Volume 34 with 6 issues appears in 2002.

Subscription rates: Subscriptions run for a full calendar year. Prices are given per volume.
Personal subscription:
Subscription + postage and handling
CHF 460.– + CHF 28.80 Europe
CHF 460.– + CHF 42.70 Overseas
USD 354.00 + USD 28.80
+ online subscription per volume:
CHF 39.–/USD 30.00
(Must be in the name of, billed to, and paid by an individual. Order must be marked 'personal subscription'.)
Institutional subscription:
Subscription + postage and handling
CHF 920.– + CHF 36.– Europe
CHF 920.– + CHF 53.40 Overseas
USD 708.00 + USD 36.00
+ online subscription per volume:
CHF 58.–/USD 45.00
Airmail postage: CHF 36.–, USD 30.00.
(Extra per volume.)

Microforms: Please direct all enquiries and orders to: University Microfilms Inc.
300 North Zeeb Road, P.O. Box 1346
Ann Arbor, MI 48106-1346 (USA)

Advertising: Correspondence and rate requests should be addressed to the Publisher.
Subscription orders: Orders can be placed at agencies, bookstores, directly with the
Publisher S. Karger AG, P.O. Box,
CH–4009 Basel (Switzerland)
or with any of the following distributors:
Deutschland: S. Karger GmbH, Postfach
D–79095 Freiburg
France: Librairie Luginbühl
36, bd de Latour-Maubourg
F–75007 Paris
Great Britain, Ireland: S. Karger Publishers
58 Grove Hill Road
Tunbridge Wells, Kent TN1 1SP, UK
USA: S. Karger Publishers, Inc.
26 West Avon Road, P.O. Box 529
Farmington, CT 06085, USA
India, Bangladesh, Sri Lanka:
Panther Publishers Private Ltd.
39, 6th Cross
Wilson Gardens
Bangalore 560 027, India
Japan: Katakura Libri, Inc.
2F, Marushima Bldg, 4-6-17, Yushima,
Bunkyo-ku, Tokyo 113-0034, Japan

Change of address: Both old and new address should be sent to the subscription source.

Single issues: Information can be obtained through the Publisher.

Bibliographic indices: This journal is regularly listed in bibliographic services, including *Current Contents®*.

Copying: This journal has been registered with the Copyright Clearance Center (CCC), as indicated by the code appearing on the first page of each article.
For readers in the US, this code signals consent for copying of articles for personal or internal use, or for the personal or internal use of specific clients, provided that the stated fee is paid per copy directly to
Copyright Clearance Center Inc.
222 Rosewood Drive
Danvers, MA 01923 (USA).
A copy of the first page of the article must accompany payment. Consent does not extend to copying for general distribution, for promotion, for creating new works, or for resale. In these cases, specific written permission must be obtained from the copyright owner,
S. Karger AG, P.O. Box,
CH–4009 Basel (Switzerland).

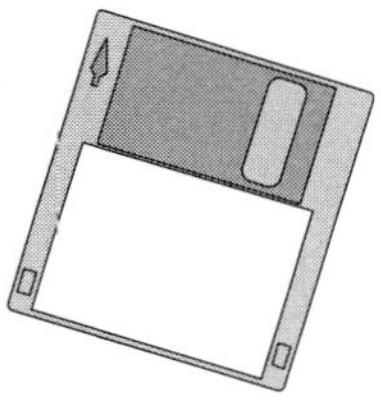

Disk Submission

A **comprehensive version** of these guidelines for the **submission of manuscripts and illustrations on disk** can be accessed online under **www.karger.com/journals/disksub.htm** or requested as a leaflet from the editorial department.

Please follow the general rules on style and arrangement in the **'Guidelines for Authors'** of the journal. Submit a **double-spaced printout** of your manuscript matching the file on disk exactly.

Technical Information

Store only data pertinent to this manuscript. Include your fonts (screen and printer fonts for Macintosh).
For a **text only** manuscript, use a 3.5-inch disk.
For **text and illustrations,** use 3.5 or 5.25 Magneto Optical Disc; CD-ROM (DOS or hybrid); iomage Zip/DOS (100 MB), or 44 MB, 88 MB or 200 MB SyQuest. Compress extensive data using ZIP format.

Data Description

Label your disk with the **title of the journal or book** for which it is submitted; a **short version** of the paper's title; your **name,** postal and e-mail address, fax and phone number; **hards and software** used, including the version; and the **complete list of the file names.** File names consist of eight characters before the dot identifying the file and three characters after the dot identifying the application.

Text and Format

The **preferred word-processing package is MS-Word.** Other commonly used PC text programs and ASCII formats are accepted.
Update your data when you revise subsequent to the reviewer's or editor's decision and mark revisions clearly. Manuscripts accepted for publication are subject to **copy editing:** changes and/or questions will be marked in the manuscript, which will be returned to you with your disk and the galley proofs for checking.
Enter your text continuously flush left. Do not use any layout functions. Do not split words at the end of a line. **Do not use indentations.** Use a blank line before and a hard return at the end of paragraphs. **Arrange headings flush left.** Insert only **one space after punctuation marks.** Insert Greek letters, mathematical symbols etc. with your word-processing program. Use **boldface and italics** as well as sub- and superscript where appropriate. **Tables are part of the text** and should be placed at the end of the text file. Separate the individual parts of a table by lines. Use the tabulator instead of spaces. Format operation data on one line in the same column. **Legends to illustrations are part of the text** and should also be listed at the end of the text file.

Illustrations

Store illustrations as separate files: do not integrate them in your text. Export **line drawings/vector graphics** as TIF, EPS or WMF format. Use Photoshop for processing and retouching **scanned half-tone images.** Save the original scan and the processed version. Export **black and white or color images** as TIF or EPS format in their anticipated size in print.
For detailed information on how to submit illustration data on disk please consult the leaflet or **www.karger.com/journals/disksub.htm.**

KARGER

Fax+41 61 306 12 34
E-Mail karger@karger.ch
www.karger.com

The Journal Home Page is available at:
www.karger.com/journals/esr

KI 98 DISK

European
Surgical Research

37th Congress of the European Society for Surgical Research (ESSR)

Szeged, Hungary, May 23–25, 2002

Abstracts

Guest Editors
M. Boros, Szeged, Hungary
A. Szabó, Szeged, Hungary
J. Kaszaki, Szeged, Hungary
T. Jánossy, Szeged, Hungary

KARGER
Basel · Freiburg · Paris · London · New York ·
New Delhi · Bangkok · Singapore · Tokyo · Sydney

S. Karger
Medical and Scientific Publishers
Basel · Freiburg · Paris · London
New York · New Delhi · Bangkok
Singapore · Tokyo · Sydney

Drug Dosage
The authors and the publisher have exerted every effort to ensure that drug selection and dosage set forth in this text are in accord with current recommendations and practice at the time of publication. However, in view of ongoing research, changes in government regulations, and the constant flow of information relating to drug therapy and drug reactions, the reader is urged to check the package insert for each drug for any change in indications and dosage and for added warnings and precautions. This is particularly important when the recommended agent is a new and/or infrequently employed drug.

P.O. Box, CH–4009 Basel (Switzerland)
Printed in Hungary by J. Nyomda, Szeged
ISBN 3–8055–7450–9

KARGER

Fax + 41 61 306 12 34
E-Mail karger@karger.ch
www.karger.com

European Surgical Research

Contents Vol. 34, Suppl 1, 2002

Oral Presentations

Walter Brendel Session

1 **1 Continuous Monitoring of Cerebrospinal Fluid Oxygen Tension in Relation to Motor Evoked Potentials During Spinal Cord Ischemia in a Porcine Model of TAAA Surgery**
J. Lips, P. de Haan, M.J. Jacobs, T.M. van Gulik, C.J. Kalkman (The Netherlands)

1 **2 Suppression of Kupffer Cell Function and Administration of Protease Inhibitor are Keys for Successful Liver TX in Non-Heart-Beating Donor**
N. Ohkohchi, K. Oikawa, S. Tsukamoto, M. Sato, S. Miyagi, S. Satomi (Japan)

2 **3 Three Percent Relapse after Five Years Follow-up of 200 Patients with Ventral Abdominal Wall Hernia Treated by Carbajo Laparoscopic Technique**
M.A. Carbajo, M. García-Caballero, J.I. Martin, J.I. Blanco, M. Delacuesta, F. Martin, M. Toledano (Spain)

2 **4 The Role of Neuronal Nitric Oxide in the Mechanism of Intestinal Preconditioning**
S. Varga, V. Krishnan, L. Balázs, P. Gál, J. Kaszaki, M. Boros (Hungary)

3 **5 The Regenerative Effect of Hepatocyte Growth Factor (HGF) on Severe Ischemic Acute Tubular Necrosis (ATN) in Rats Improves Survival in Kidney Transplantation**
T. Karatzas, S. Santiago, A. Tsamandas, W. DeFaria, C. Gandia, S. Salgar, A.G. Tzakis (Greece and USA)

3 **6 Long-Term Survival of *Macaca Fascicularis* in a Life-Supporting hDAF Pig-to-Primate Renal Xenotransplantation Model With Triple Maintenance Therapy and Without Splenectomy**
A. Dedja, R. Cadrobbi, N. Baldan, C. Vinanzi, A. Taglioni, F. Calabrese, M.C. Varagnolo, R. Busetto, M. Castagnaro, P. Rigotti, E. Cozzi, E. Ancona (Italy)

4 **7 Brain Plasticity Following Hand Transplantation**
M. Vossen, D. Molfese, A. Fonaryova-Key, S. Kelly, C. Maldonado, M. Kon, J.H. Barker (The Netherlands and USA)

4 **8 Expression and Function of L-Type Calcium Channels in Human Colon Cancer Cells**
A. Zawadzki, Q. Liu, Y. Wang, A. Melander, B. Jeppsson, H. Thorlacius (Sweden)

Microcirculation

5 **9 Analysis of Angiogenesis, Microcirculation, and Growth of Primary and Secondary Bone Tumors: An Experimental Study in Mice**
A. Sckell, F. Klenke, T. Merkle, M.M. Gebhard, V. Ewerbeck (Germany)

5 **10 Generalized and Local Circulatory Disorders Differentially Affect the Microcirculation of the Different Layers of the Rat Small Intestine**
K. Vajda, A. Szabó, A. Sárkány, K. Kucsa, A. Thoman, M. Boros (Hungary)

6 **11 Improvement of Hepatic Microcirculation by ROCK Inhibitor Y-27632 in Hepatic Ischemia/Reperfusion Model in Rat**
F. Ikeda, H. Terajima, Y. Simahara, Y. Yamaoka (Japan)

6 **12 Improvement of Microcirculation in Severe Experimental Pancreatitis Enhances Hepatic Capillary Blood Flow and RES Function**
B. Forgács, E. Wudel, J. Franke, G. Eibl, H.J. Buhr, T. Foitzik (Hungary and Germany)

7 **13 A New Model for Fluorescence Video Microscopy of Coronary Terminal Arterioles *in situ:* Effects of Perfusion Pressure**
S. Goebel, W.M. Kuebler, A.R. Pries, H. Kuppe, H. Habazettl (Germany)

7 **14 The Role of Nitric Oxide in the Pathomechanism of Biliary Gastro-Esophageal Reflux**
G. Erős, J. Kaszaki, K. Szentpáli, M. Boros (Hungary)

Gastrointestinal Surgery

8 **15 Enhanced Anti-tumor Efficacy by Combining Conventional Chemotherapy with Angiostatin or Endostatin in a Murine Liver Metastasis Model**
E.A. te Velde, J.M. Vogten, M.F.B.G. Gebbink, E.E. Voest, I.H.M. Borel Rinkes (The Netherlands)

8 **16 Local Tumor Recurrence Influenced by Systemic Factors**
W.M.U. van Grevenstein, J. Jeekel, C.H.J. van Eijck (The Netherlands)

9 **17 Adhesion of Human Colon Carcinoma Cells to the Extracellular Matrix**
M. ten Kate, W.M.U. van Grevenstein, R.L. Marquet, J. Jeekel, C.H.J. van Eijck (The Netherlands)

9 **18 FAK Expression in Colon Carcinoma and Correlation with Survival**
S. Theoharis, G. Kouraklis, D. Mantas, A. Margeli, A. Glinavou, G. Karatzas, A. Koutselinis (Greece)

9 19 **PPAR-γ Expression in Colon Cancer Patients and Correlation with Cell Cycle-Related Molecules**
S. Theoharis, G. Kouraklis, D. Mantas, A. Margeli, A. Glinavou, G. Karatzas, A. Koutselinis (Greece)

10 20 **Analysis of 426 Cases of Gastrectomy for Primary Gastric Cancer in a Single Institution: The Feasibility of Proximal Gastrectomy**
S. Okamoto, S. Yokoyama, T. Kamigaito, M. Shimoda, W. Sato, S. Yagi, F. Nishizawa, S. Uyama, H. Utsunomiya, H. Kato (Japan)

10 21 **Immediate Postoperative Immune Response in Histamine H1 and H2 C57BL/6J Knockout Mice**
M. García-Caballero, K. Nakano, H. Suzuki, J.M. Martínez-Moreno, Y. Takagawa, I. Nakashima (Spain)

Organ and Tissue Transplantation I

11 22 **The Effect of FR167653 on Warm Ischemia/Reperfusion Injury of the Liver Graft from NHBD**
S. Miyagi, N. Ohkohchi, K. Oikawa, M. Satoh, S. Tsukamoto, S. Satomi (Japan)

11 23 **Transplantation of Hepatocytes - Elimination of Granulocytes and Monocytes Prevents Early Loss of Grafted Cells**
W.L. Olszewski, A. Rudowska, M. Durlik (Poland)

12 24 **Impact of Graft Rearterialization after Auxiliary Partial Orthotopic Liver Transplantation (APOLT) in the Treatment of Acute Liver Failure**
J.P. Hölzen, D. Palmes, T. Budny, K.H. Dietl, H. Herbst, H.U. Spiegel (Germany)

12 25 **Synergistic Value of Fibrinolysis and Hypothermic Aerobic Preservation with O_2 in the Protection of Livers from Non Heart Beating donors**
R.H. Tolba, S. Akbar, M. Sitzia, T. Minor (Germany)

12 26 **Effect of a Novel Potent Cytokine Suppressor on Toxic Liver Syndrome in the Pig Treated by Auxiliary Partial Orthotopic Liver Transplantation for Fatal Fulminant Hepatic Failure**
S. Ishiguro, Y. Takada, K. Seino, H. Taniguchi, T. Kawamoto, K. Yuzawa, M. Otsuka, T. Todoroki, K. Fukao (Japan)

13 27 **Can we Guarantee the Safety of Donor Operation in Living Donor Liver Transplantation? Analysis of 52 Donors**
N. Ohkohchi, M. Shoji, K. Fujimori, N. Kawagishi, S. Tsukamoto, S. Satomi (Japan)

Organ and Tissue Transplantation II

13 28 **Sensitivity, Specificity and Prognostic Value of E-Cadherin During Preservation of the Porcine Pancreas with Histidine-Tryptophan-Ketoglutarate Solution or University of Wisconsin Solution**
P. Demetter, R. Troisi, C. van den Broecke, C.A. Cuverlier, U.J. Hesse (Belgium)

14 29 **Functional and Immunogenic Changes of Human Fetal Pancreatic Islet Following Long-Term Cultivation**
G. Farkas, J. Csanády, Y. Mándi, A. Pál (Hungary)

14 30 **Successful Islet Xenotransplantation Following Macrophage Blockade Induced by Repeated Gadolinium Chloride Injections in Rats**
A. Paszt, G. Farkas, Z. Szász, G. Lázár Jr., J. Csanády, G. Lázár (Hungary)

15 31 **The Use of Octreotide in Pancreatic Transplants with Enteric Drainage Results of a Prospective Randomised Single Centre Trial**
H. van der Bracht, D. Meester, R. Troisi, B. Jacobs, B. de Hemptinne, N. Lameire, U.J. Hesse (Belgium)

15 32 **The Incidence of Rejection with Quadruple Immunosuppression, Including ATG or IL2 Antibodies and Mycophenolate Mofetil (MMF) Following Simultaneous Pancreas and Kidney (SPK) Transplantation**
U.J. Hesse, B. Jacobs, R. Troisi, B. van Vlem, B. de Hemptinne, R. van Holder, F. Vermassen, J. de Roose, N. Lameire (Belgium)

16 33 **Acute Small Bowel Rejection and Mucosal Perfusion in CD4, CD40 and CD28 Knock-out Mice**
G. Dindelegan, H. Liden, G. Kurlberg, O. Nilsson, A. Aneman, N. Lycke, M. Olausson (Sweden)

16 34 **Moderating of Oxidative Stress by Ischemic Preconditioning: Role of Cellular Signal Mechanisms in Small Bowel**
A. Ferencz, B. Borsiczky, Z. Szántó, K. Kiss, J. Szeberényi, K. Kalmár-Nagy, Ö.P. Horváth, E. Rőth (Hungary)

17 35 **Effects of Ischemic Preconditioning on the Graft Microcirculation During Small Bowel Transplantation**
A. Wolfárd, J. Kaszaki, L. Szalay, S. Varga, Á. Balogh, M. Boros (Hungary)

17 36 **Protective Effects of Exogenous Fructose-1,6-biphosphate Added to University of Wisconsin Preservation Solution in Rat Intestinal Transplantation**
A. Sola, J. de Oca, V. Alfaro, C. Xaus, G. Hotter (Spain)

17 37 **Xanthine/Adenosine and NO Modifications During Rat Intestinal Cold Perservation Modulates the Apoptotic Response**
M. Genesca, A. Sola, L. Palacios, F. Pi, G. Hotter (Spain)

Organ and Tissue Transplantation III

18 38 **Different Pictures of Autogenous Infection and Rejection in Human Skin Allografts**
W.L. Olszewski, M. Moscicka, D. Zolich (Poland)

18 39 **The Mechanisms Involved in Initiation of Skin Allograft Rejection - Inhibition of Antigen Presentation by CsA and Prograf**
J. Mijal, H. Galkowska, W.L. Olszewski (Poland)

19 40 **Damage of Graft by Ischemia and Rejection Results in Release of DNA and its Accumulation in Recipient Tissues**
B. Interewicz, W.L. Olszewski, J. Stanislawska, E. Szyper, M. Maksymowicz (Poland)

19 41 **Experimental Model of Heterotopic Uterus Transplantation in Rat**
P.L. Jiga, C.M. Lupu, B.S. Zoica, M. Ionac (Romania)

20 42 **Elastic Properties of Bone in Composite Tissue Allotransplantation**
M. Vossen, G. Perez-Abadia, C. Maldonado, M.J. Voor, V.S. Gorantla, C. Francois, P.C.R. Brouha, L. Perez-Laurentin, J.H. Barker, M. Kon (The Netherlands and USA)

20 43 **CK-MB/CK Serum Values after Heart Transplantation Do Not Correlate with Cardiac Damage.**
J.H. Fischer, S. Jeschkeit, F. Kuhn-Régnier, R. Switkowski (Germany)

21 44 **Preserved Endothelial Function of Large and Small Coronary Vessels After Prolonged Storage Including Coronary Oxygen Persufflation**
M. Bosse, S. Dahnken, J.H. Fischer (Germany)

Traumatology and Orthopedics

21 45 **Long-Term Preservation with UW Solution Improves Revascularization and Viability of Transplanted Bone Versus LPD and EC at 4 °C**
M.H. Kirschner, L. Suess, A. Wanders, G.O. Hofmann, K. Messmer (Germany)

22 46 **MedEdit: Computer-Assisted Orthopedic-Trauma Surgery Planner System**
K. Ollé, A. Kuba, E. Varga (Hungary)

22 47 **Trauma of Soft Tissues and Bones Evokes Local Inflammatory Reaction Expressed in the Lymphatic System**
G. Szczesny, W.L. Olszewski, M. Zaleska (Poland)

22 48 **Intraarticular Leukocyte Activation During Acute Clinical Haemarthrosis**
B. Borsiczky, B. Fodor, J. Lantos, G. Jancsó, E. Rőth, J. Nyárády (Hungary)

23 49 **DYNASTAB-T external stabilizer for open femoral and tibial shaft fractures**
G. Szczesny, J. Deszczynski, J. Karpinski, A. Stolarczyk (Poland)

23 50 **External Stabilization for Articular Fractures of Knee, Ankle and Elbow Joints Using DYNASTAB Stabilizers**
J. Deszczynski, J. Karpinski, G. Szczesny, M. Ziólkowski (Poland)

23 51 **Intramedullary Nailing in Ankle Arthrodesis: Anterograde vs Retrograde**
M. Goebel, M.H. Kirschner, M. Militz (Germany)

24 52 **Vascular Tunnel Concept in the Surgical Treatment of Brain Swelling**
A. Csókay (Hungary)

24 53 **Surgical Consequences of the Polytrauma Equivalent Syndrome (PES) to the Spleen Injuries Treatment**
G. Ács, A. Furka, T. Lesznyák, Z. Záborszky, I. Furka, I. Mikó (Hungary)

25 54 **A New Pressure-Free Intramedullary Reamer for Reducing Fat Intravasation: An Experimental Study in Sheep**
H.U. Spiegel, A. Kröpfl, H. Redl, U. Frerichmann, C. Ortmann, A. Joist (Germany)

Shock and Ischemia-Reperfusion I

25 55 **Regulation of the Ischemia-Reperfusion-Syndrome in Liver Ischemia by Transcription Factors - A Clinical Trial**
S. Kersting, T. Zimmermann, G. von Gagern, D. Ratayczak, S. Albrecht, D. Ockert, H.D. Saeger (Germany)

26 56 **Role of Pyrrolidine Dithiocarbamate in the Induction of Ischemic Tolerance of the Liver: Heme Oxygenase 1 Induction and Sinusoidal Dilatation**
K. Hata, Y. Yamamoto, K. Yonezawa, K. Taura, A. Nakajima, H. Uchinami, Y. Yamaoka (Japan)

26 57 **Heat Shock Preconditioning Enhances JNK/AP-1 Cascade Following Hepatic Ischemia-Reperfusion**
H. Uchinami, Y. Yamamoto, K. Hata, K. Taura, A. Nakajima, K. Yonezawa, Y. Yamaoka (Japan)

27 58 **Involvement of ELR (-) CXC and CC Chemokines in Hepatic Ischemia/Reperfusion Injury in Mice**
D. Takeuchi, H. Yoshidome, Y. Morita, H. Ito, F. Kimura, H. Shimizu, A. Togawa, Y. Shimizu, M. Ohtsuka, A. Kato, M. Miyazaki (Japan)

27 59 **Role of Selective COX-2 Inhibition by Meloxicam in the Ischemia/Reperfusion Injury of the Liver**
R.H. Tolba, K. Yonezawa, Y. Yamamoto, K. Taura, A. Nakajima, K. Hata, H. Uchinami, T. Minor, Y. Yamaoka (Germany and Japan)

28 60 **The Influence of Phosphodiestherase-Inhibition on the Ischaemia-Reperfusion Injury of the Liver**
A. Zaránd, R. Banafsche, M. Kume, H. Uchinami, M. M. Gebhard, T. Gondos, F. Perner, E. Klar (Hungary and Japan)

Shock and Ischemia-Reperfusion II

28 61 **Local Intravascular Coagulation and Inhibition of Fibrinolysis with Subsequent Fibrin Deposition due to Intestinal Ischemia and Reperfusion in Rats**
E.H.P. Roossink, I.G. Schoots, P.B. Bijlsma, M. Levi, T.M. van Gulik (The Netherlands)

29 62 **Antithrombin III Substitution Inhibits Local Intravascular Coagulation and Fibrin Deposition after Intestinal Ischemia in Rats.**
I.G. Schoots, E.H.P. Roossink, P.B. Bijlsma, M. Levi, T.M. van Gulik (The Netherlands)

29 63 **Antioxidants and Ischemia-Reperfusion of the Rat Intestine in the Absence of Leucocytes**
I. García-Alonso, I. Goicoechea, J. Caramés, B. Otero, J. Bilbao (Spain)

30 64 **Changes of the Red Blood Cells Deformability Caused by Mesenteric Ischemia-Reperfusion Injury. An Experimental Animal Study**
E. Bráth, I. Furka, G. Szabó, K. Pető, G. Ács, N. Németh, T. Lesznyák, T. Cserni, J. Papp Szekeres, I. Mikó (Hungary)

30 65 **Ischemia / Reperfusion-Induced Leukocyte-Endothelium Interactions in the Colon: Importance of P-Selectin, Lymphocyte Function Antigen-1 and CXC Chemokines**
A.A. Riaz (Sweden)

31 66 ***In Vivo* Neuronal Nitric Oxide Synthase Stimulation Protects Intestinal Ischemic Injury**
A. Sola, M.A. Peinado, E. Martínez-Lara, A. Jiménez, E. Gelpí, G. Hotter (Spain)

31 67 **Hemodynamic Effect of Intestinal Nitrite under Normoxic and Hypoxic Conditions**
L. Szalay, F. Umar, A. Kozlov, H. Redl, S. Bahrami (Hungary and Austria)

31 68 **Adenosine/Xanthine Level Modulates NO Generation and Tissue Injury in Renal Ischemia**
J. López-Martí, A. Sola, F. Pi, V. Alfaro, G. Hotter (Spain)

32 69 **Thromboxane Release in Ischemia and Reperfusion Injury Studied by Microdialysis**
M. Ionac, D. Bordos (Romania)

32 70 **Gender Differences in Neutrophil Priming and Oxidative Injury Following Trauma and Hemorrhagic Shock**
B. Toth, J.F. Kuebler, M. Schwacha, J. Hamar, K.I. Bland, P. Wang, I.H. Chaudry (USA)

Sepsis and Inflammation

33 71 ***Lactobacillus Plantarum 299v* Reduces Endotoxin-Induced Bacterial Translocation in Rats**
P. Mangell, M. Wang, S. Ahrné, G. Molin, H. Thorlacius, B. Jeppsson (Sweden)

33 72 **The Effect of Epidermal Growth Factor, *Lactobacillus Plantarum 299v* and Oat Fiber on Dextran Sulfate Sodium-Induced Colitis Model**
C. Trably, D. Adawi, R. Ehrnström, B. Veress, M. Eklund, B. Jeppsson (Sweden)

34 73 **Regulation of the Inflammatory Response on the Molecular Level in Mononuclear Blood Cells in Patients with Sepsis**
T. Zimmermann, G. von Gagern, S. Albrecht, S. Kersting, H. D. Saeger (Germany)

34 74 **The Role of IκBa on Regulation of Inflammatory Response in Septic Patients**
T. Zimmermann, G. v. Gagern, H. Schikore, I. Alldinger, S. Kersting, S. Albrecht, H.D. Saeger (Germany)

34 75 **With or Without? Role of FAS in Sepsis**
U. Glatzel, R.H. Tolba, M. Tinelli, M. Lysson, A. Wentzensen, T. Minor (Germany)

35 76 **Antibiotic Prophylaxis in Clean Surgery. A Spanish Inquiry**
M. Caínzos, F. Lozano, J.L. Balibrea, J. Culebras, D. Dávil, A.A. Gomez, I. Iturburo, S. Morales, B. Oller, J. Potel, L.M. Sánchez-Ortega, J.M. Tellado (Spain)

35 77 **The Soluble Tumor Necrosis Factor Receptor I (STNFRI) is an Early Predictor of Local Infective Complications after Colorectal Surgery**
R. Slotwinski, W.L. Olszewski, A. Chaber, M. Slodkowski, M. Zaleska, I.W. Krasnodebski (Poland)

Vascular and Cardiac Surgery

36 78 **Correlation Between Plasma Homocysteine, Aortic Aneurysms and Vitamins**
A.A. Warsi, D. Hullin, B. Davies, M.H. Lewis (Wales, UK)

36 79 **Topical Wall Shear Stress and Intimal Hyperplasia at End-to-Side Anastomosis**
H. Ishibashi, Y. Kiyota, H. Ikeda, M. Ojha (Japan)

36 80 **Extracellular Matrix Substance Coating on Culture Dish Inhibits Vascular Wall Cell Growth for Tissue Engineering**
T. Miyake, T. Shinoka, J. Kashiwagi, M. Watanabe, T. Konuma, N. Hibino, A. Murata, Y. Nation, K. Nakajima, H. Kurosawa (Japan)

37 81 **Titanium Clips and Bioglue in Vascular Surgery**
T. Kotsis, A. Pafiti, K. Katsenis, P. Dimakakos (Greece)

37 82 **Long-Term Result of Crossover Bypass to the Lower Limb**
Y. Hamada, A. Otaki, T. Ogata, Y. Morishita (Japan)

38 83 **Ventricular Rate Control during Atrial Fibrillation with Stimulation of the AV-Nodal Parasympathetic Plexus**
P. Soós, P. Horváth, P. Schauerte, E. Zima, A. Juhász-Nagy, B. Merkely (Germany)

Hepatobiliary and Pancreatic Surgery

38 84 **The CD14+ Class II+ Blood Cells Reveal Predilection to Liver Adenocarcinoma Metastases**
M. Stanczyk, W.L. Olszewski, A. Wesolowska, M. Maruszynski (Poland)

39 85 **Effect of Cyclophosphamide and Retinoic Acid on Hepatic Metastasis Following Liver Resection**
J. Caramés, T. Palomares, A. Alonso, B. Castro, A. Pineda, I. García-Alonso (Spain)

39 86 **The Survival Benefit of Surgical Treatment for Recurrence of the Remnant Liver and Lung after Hepatic Resection for Colorectal Metastases**
H. Yoshidome, H. Ito, F. Kimura, H. Shimizu, A. Togawa, Y. Shimizu, M. Ohtsuka, F. Shimamura, D. Takeuchi, M. Miyazaki (Japan)

40 87 **Pringle Maneuver Improves Lesion Size in Radiofrequency Application. Experimental Study in Porcine *In Vivo* Model**
F. Burdío, A. Güemes, A.C. Navarro, R. Sousa, T. Castiella, I. Cruz, O. Burzaco, S. Strassmann, J. Torcal, R. Lozano (Spain)

40 88 **Angiostatin Inhibits Experimental Liver Fibrosis**
J.M. Vogten, T.A. Drixler, E.A. te Velde, M.F.B.G. Gebbink, E.E. Voest, I.H.M. Borel Rinkes (The Netherlands)

41 89 **Receptor-Mediated Acceleration of Hepatocellular Transport System as Measured by Near-Infrared Spectroscopy**
A. Tanaka, H. Shinohara, Y. Yamaoka (Japan)

41 90 **Estrogen has a Potential Role in the Development of Hepatopulmonary Syndrome in Rats**
S. Yol, S. Toprak, A. Kartal, L. Tavli, M. Sahin (Turkey)

42 91 **The Effect of Tamoxifen and Oophorectomy in Preventing the Development of Hepatopulmonary Syndrome in Cirrhotic Rats**
S. Yol, S. Toprak, C. Vatansev, L. Tavli, M. Belviranli, A. Karta (Turkey)

42 92 **Importance of Cytokines, NO and Apoptosis in the Pathological Process of Necrotising Pancreatitis in Rats**
L. Leindler, G. Farkas, Á. Morschul, F. László Jr., Y. Mándi, J. Fejős, T. Takács, K. Jármai (Hungary)

42 93 **Changes of Quality of Life and Nutritional State in Surgically Treated Patients with Chronic Pancreatitis**
B. Tihanyi, I. Farkas, Z. Csapó, R. Schwab, Á. Pap, T. Tihanyi (Hungary)

Molecular Biology, Gene Therapy in Surgical Diseases

43 94 **Effect of Cycloprodigiosin on the Induction of Inducible Nitric Oxide Synthase by Interleukin-1β in Primary Cultured Hepatocytes**
S. Teshima, H. Nakanishi, M. Kaibori, H. Toyokawa, A.H. Kwon, Y. Kamiyama, T. Okumura (Japan)

43 95 **Effect of Pirfenidone on the Induction of Inducible Nitric Oxide Synthase by Inflammatory Cytokine in Hepatocytes**
H. Nakanishi, M. Kaibori, S. Teshima, H. Tsuchiya, A.H. Kwon, Y. Kamiyama, T. Okumura (Japan)

44 96 **Stromal Interaction Upregulates Gelatinase Activity in Pancreatic Tumours *In Vitro***
S.T. Ivanova, P.F. Ridgway, P. Ziprin, D.H. Peck, A.W. Darzi (United Kingdom)

44 97 **Cepharanthine Conquers P-Glycoprotein-Associated Drug Resistance in Hepatocellular Carcinoma Cells**
A. Nakajima, Y. Yamamoto, K. Hata, K. Taura, H. Uchinami, K. Yonezawa, Y. Yamaoka (Japan)

45 98 **The Prognostic Significance of Proliferating Cell Nuclear Antigen in Colorectal Cancer. A Prospective Study with Clinical Correlation**
R. Harisi, J. Dudás, G. Bodoky, T. Winternitz, L. Flautner, J. Weltner (Hungary)

45 99 **Identification and Validation of Candidate Genes in Pancreatic Cancer**
R. Grützmann, I. Alldinger, M. Foerder, M. Peiper, R. Jesenofsky, D. Ockert, A. Rosenthal, C. Pilarsky, H.D. Saeger (Germany)

45 100 **Detection of Occult Tumour Cells in Bone Marrow by Reverse Transcriptase-Polymerase Chain Reaction (RT-PCR) in Breast Cancer Patients**
S. Dubecz, O. Csuka, K. Tóth, I. Köves, G. Péley, I. Láng (Hungary)

46 101 **Differential Gene Expression Profile in Monocytes (M) from Multiple Injured Patients**
P. Biberthaler, B. Bach, V. Mayer, T. Mussack, W. Mutschler, M. Jochum (Germany)

46 102 **Liver Regeneration-Biochemistry-Insulin Uptake-PCNA Marking**
T. Kotsis, A. Fotopoulos, I. Chondroudaki, A. Pafiti, M. Frangou, S. Kotsovolou, F. Nikolopoulou, K. Chondros, D. Rizos, B. Smyrniotis, J. Papadimitriou (Greece)

New Surgical Techniques

47 103 **A Systematic Approach to the Surgical Treatment of Gynaecomastia**
B. Fruhstorfer, C.M. Malata (United Kingdom)

47 104 **An Experimental Model for Alternative Blood Supply of the Kidney in the Aspect of Renal Function**
T. Lesznyák, N. Németh, G. Ács, I. Mikó, I. Furka (Hungary)

47 105 **A Combination of Endoscopic Laser Surgery and Segment Resection for the Treatment of Cricotracheal Stenoses**
Z. Bella, L. Rovó, M. Brzózka, L. Tiszlavicz, J. Czigner (Hungary)

48 106 **Laryngeal Reinnervation in Animal Experiments**
A. Tóth, A. Szűcs, K. Matesz, C. Harasztosi, I. Furka, I. Mikó, I. Sziklai (Hungary)

48 107 **A New, Minimally Invasive Treatment Concept for the Bilateral Vocal Cord Paralysis - A Prospective Study**
L. Rovó, J. Jóri, M. Brzózka, J. Czigner (Hungary)

49 108 **The Experimental Examination of the Healing Process of Telescopic Anastomosis**
G. Szűcs, I. Tóth, T. Barna, E. Bráth, K. Gyáni, I. Mikó (Hungary)

Immunology

49 **109 Chimerism and Tolerance through Vascularized Bone Marrow Transplantation: Fact or Fiction?**
M. Vossen, V.S. Gorantla, G. Perez-Abadia, C.G. Francois, P.C.R. Brouha, L.A. Laurentin-Perez, D. Pidwell, C. Maldonado, M. Kon, J.H. Barker (The Netherlands and USA)

50 **110 Mast Cell-Dependent Neutrophil Recruitment in the Skin is Importantly Mediated by KC and LFA-1: Inhibitory Mechanisms of Action of Dexamethasone**
R. Schramm, T. Schaefer, M.D. Menger, H. Thorlacius (Germany)

50 **111 Conditioning of Donor Graft with Recipient Bone Marrow Cells Predisposes for Acute Rejection**
M. Maksymowicz, E. Cybulska, W.L. Olszewski (Norway)

51 **112 Studies on the Role of T Cells and T Cell Subclasses in Graft Rejection**
T. Jánossy, G.A. Ceepil, C. Vizler, I. Ocsovszki, R. Benner, P. Végh (Hungary and The Netherlands)

51 **113 Studies on the Prevention of Graft-versus-Host Disease (GVHD) by *in vitro* Pretreatment of Donor Cells with Anti-T Cell Antibodies**
L. Szalai, M. Laurinyecz, G.A. Ceepil, C. Vizler, I. Ocsovszki, R. Benner, T. Jánossy (Hungary and The Netherlands)

52 **114 Physiological Roles of Kupffer Cells in Liver Injury**
G. Lázár, E. Husztik, E. Duda, G. Lázár Jr. (Hungary)

52 **115 Changes in Immune Defence and Heat-Shock Protein 70 Level in the Various Stages of Tuberculosis**
J. Furák, I. Troján, T. Szőke, L. Tiszlavicz, Á. Balogh (Hungary)

52 **116 Methotrexate as an Immunosuppressive Agent in a Life-Supporting hDAF Pig-to-Primate Xenotransplantation Model**
R. Cadrobbi, A. Dedja, N. Baldan, F. Calabrese, M. Boldrin, F. Fante, M. Castagnaro, P. Carraro, F.M. Cancellotti, P. Rigotti, E. Cozzi, E. Ancona (Italy)

Thoracic and Esophageal Surgery

53 **117 Telescopic Esophageal Anastomosis: Clinical Results and Data of Animal Experiments**
G. Szűcs, I. Tóth, T. Barna, E. Bráth, K. Gyáni, I. Mikó (Hungary)

53 **118 Effect of Thoracic Epidural Anaesthesia During Experimental Gastric Tube Formation**
G. Lázár, J. Kaszaki, S. Ábrahám, G. Horváth, K. Szentpáli, A. Wolfárd, A. Paszt, Á. Balogh, M. Boros (Hungary)

54 **119 Usefulness of Phreno-Mediastinal Approach in Thoracoscopic Radical Esophagectomy**
T. Kawano, K. Nagai, T. Nishikage, K. Ami, Y. Nakajima, K. Kawada, T. Iwai (Japan)

54 **120 The Role of the VATS in the Treatment of Hydrothorax**
K. Kovács, G. Boross, M. Svébis, C. Oláh (Hungary)

55 **121 Isolated Lung Perfusion with Gemcitabine in the Rat: Pharmacokinetics and Survival**
B. van Putte, J. Hendriks, S. Romijn, B. Pauwels, G. Friedel, G. Guetens, P. van Schil (Belgium and Germany)

55 **122 Variations in Flow, Duration and Concentration Do Not Change the Final Lung Concentrations of Melphalan after Isolated Lung Perfusion in The Rat**
S. Romijn, J. Hendriks, B. van Putte, E. de Bruijn, P. van Schil (Belgium)

Surgical Pathophysiology

55 **123 How Do Redox-Sensitive Transcription Factors Influence the Inflammatory Reaction in Sepsis and Polytrauma?**
G. v. Gagern, T. Zimmermann, S. Albrecht, S. Kersting, H. Schikore, H. Zwipp, H.D. Saeger (Germany)

56 **124 Evaluation of Phagocytic Function of Spleen after Splenic Artery Ligation in Secondary Hypersplenism**
C. Vatansev, S. Tekin, M. Sahin, M. Avunduk, M. Serdengecti (Turkey)

56 **125 Endothelin-1 Upsets Homeostatic Equilibrium in the Coronary Bed**
A. Juhász-Nagy, V. Kékesi (Hungary)

57 **126 Increased Concentrations of Pericardial Cathecholamines Affect Cardiac and Circulatory Function and Pericardial Levels of Endothelin-1**
V. Kékesi, A. Nagy, I. Toma, L. Losonczi, M. Rusvai, A. Juhász-Nagy (Hungary)

57 **127 Role of Endothelin-1 in Tachyarrhythmias Developed during Myocardial Ischemia and Reperfusion**
H. Vágó, G. Szűcs, P. Soós, E. Zima, T. Andrási, L. Gellér, A. Szűcs, V. Kékesi, A. Juhász-Nagy, B. Merkely (Hungary)

58 **128 The Effect of Intestinal Lengthening on Adaptation in a Piglet SBS-model: A Pilot Study**
G.I. Koffeman, I.G. Schoots, D.C. Aronson, J.A.J.M. Taminiau, P.B. Bijlsma, T.M. van Gulik, H.A. Heij, W.G. van Gemert (The Netherlands)

58 **129 The Effects of Selective Neuronal NOS Inhibition during Acute Experimental Colonic Obstruction**
Z. Palásthy, J. Kaszaki, L. Szalay, Á. Balogh, M. Boros (Hungary)

59 **130 Effect of Cholic and Deoxycholic Acid Treatment on Colonic Mucosa in Rats**
P. Sipos, K. Hagymási, E. Fehér, A. Blázovics, P. Ondrejka (Hungary)

59 **131 Effect of Colloid Solution Ladpulin on the Blood Coagulation System during Hemorrhagic Shock in Dogs**
I.V. Kremenevskiy, V.N. Gapanovich, N.I. Melnova, A.L. Uss, P.T. Petrov, V.M. Tsarenkov, O.K. Kuzuk, A.S. Cheholskiy (Belarus)

59 132 ***In Vitro* Antineoplastic Activity of a Novel Steroidal Ester of Chlorambucil in Breast Cancer Cells**
M. Kontos, P. Karamanakos, D. Trafalis, C. Menenakos, M. Nikolopoulou, C. Camoutsis, E. Bastounis (Greece)

New Techniques

60 133 **Sonodynamic Treatment of Cancer Cell Lines - A New Method in Tumor Therapy?**
R. Grützmann, T. Zimmermann, S. Albrecht, H.D. Saeger (Germany)

60 134 **Effects of Different Physical Barriers in Prevention of Adhesions to Intraperitoneally Placed Polypropylene Mesh in Rabbits**
S.G. Sajjadi, G. Wéber , J. Baracs, I. Takács, M. Vajda, G.M. Giorgion (Hungary)

61 135 **The Use of a Suturing Task As a Measure of Technical Competence**
M.S. Khan, S.D. Bann, A. Darzi, P.E.M. Butler (United Kingdom)

61 136 **Heart Rate Variability Analysis as a Tool for Quantifying the Stress of the Surgical Team During Laparoscopic Versus Open Surgeries**
L. Hejjel, I. Gál (Hungary)

Nutrition/Glutamine

62 137 **Enteral Glutamine Reverses Th1/Th2 Shift In Severe Trauma Patients. A Randomised Double-Blind Controlled Study**
P.G. Boelens, A.P.J. Houdijk, J.C.M. Fonk, B.M.E. Blomberg, S. Meijer, H.J.T.M. Haarman, P.A.M. van Leeuwen (The Netherlands)

62 138 **Butyrate and Glutamate Mucosal Metabolic Substrate Utilization in Normal Colon and Colon Cancer Tissue**
D. Adawi, B. Jeppsson (Sweden)

62 139 **Comparison of the Effects of a Glutamine-Rich and Glutamine-Free Diet in Patients with Esophagectomy**
J. Hallay, G. Kovács, Gy. Kovács, S. Sz. Kiss, Z. Szentkereszty, P .Sápy, G. Lakos, S. Sipka (Hungary)

63 140 **Does the Addition of Glutamine to Total Parenteral Nutrition Have Beneficial Effect on The Healing of Colon Anastomosis and Bacterial Translocation after Preoperative Radiotherapy?**
M. El-Malt, W. Ceelen, T. Boterberg, G. Claeys, B. de Hemptinne, W. de Neve, P. Pattyn (Belgium)

Tissue Repair

63 141 **Phospholipids Reduce Adhesions in the Uterine-Horn-Model**
S.A. Mueller, K.H. Treutner, L. Tietze, M. Anurov, J. Conze, A.P. Oettinger, V. Schumpelick (Germany)

64 142 **Diphenhydramine and Hyaluronic Acid Derivatives Reduce Adnexial Adhesions and Prevent Tubal Obstruction Following Pelvic Operations**
F. Avsar, F. Avsar, M. Sahin, H. Vatansev (Turkey)

64 143 **Expression of Apoptosis and Cell Cycle-Related Proteins in Epidermis**
H. Galkowska, W.L. Olszewski, U. Wojewodzka, J. Mijal, E. Filipiuk (Poland)

65 144 **Increased Keratinocyte Motility in Hypoxic Wounds is Via an Integrin-Dependent Up-Regulation of MMPs**
P.F. Ridgway, P. Ziprin, D.H. Peck, A.W. Darzi (United Kingdom)

65 145 **The Effect of a Thermoreversible Gelatin Polymer (TGP) on Liver Regeneration in Experimental Hepatic Wound**
M. Nagaya, S. Kubota, A. Isogai, K. Akashi (Japan)

Video Presentations

66 VP1 **A New Technique for Radical Esophagectomy: Hand-Assisted Thoracoscopic Esophagectomy Using an Anterior Phreno-Mediastinal Approach**
T. Nishikage, T. Kawano, K. Nagai, K. Ami, Y. Nakajima, K. Kawada (Japan)

66 VP2 **Kidney Transplantation in Rats. How I Do It**
T. Karatzas, S. Santiago, C. Vagianos, W. DeFaria, C. Gandia, S. Salgar, A.G. Tzakis (Greece and USA)

66 VP3 **A New Method of Appendectomy for Complicated Acute Appendicitis**
M. Farima, V. Saban, A. Gorea (Republic of Moldova)

67 VP4 **New Organ-Preserving Pancreatic Head Resection in Chronic Pancreatitis**
G. Farkas, L. Leindler (Hungary)

67 VP5 **Endoscopic Ultrasonography Using Sonoprobe for Early Esophageal Carcinoma**
K. Kawada, T. Kawano, K. Nagai, T. Nishikage, K. Ami, Y. Nakajima (Japan)

68 VP6 **Analysis of the Quality and Efficiency in Learning Laparoscopic Skills**
D. Bordos, F. Lazar, F. Miculit, C. Duta, M. Miclaus, M. Ionac, S. Pantea, S. Vascu, M. Groza (Romania)

Poster Sessions

Gastrointestinal Surgery

69 PP1 **Evaluation of Usefulness of Enteral Nutrition for Three-Field Radical Surgery and Palliative Surgery of Esophageal Carcinoma**
M. Ohara, M. Ishizaka, N. Iwashiro, K. Saito, H. Hashida (Japan)

69 **PP2 Roux-Y Reconstruction after Distal Gastrectomy Reduces IL-8 in the Gastric Remnant**
K. Fukuhara, H. Osugi, N. Takada, M. Takemura, S. Lee, M. Ueno, Y. Tanaka, Y. Fujiwara, S. Nishizawa, Y. Hashimoto, H. Kinoshita (Japan)

69 **PP3 Etiology and Prevention of Stomal Prolapse in Loop Stoma**
K. Maeda, M. Maruta, T. Utsumi, H. Sato, H. Aoyama (Japan)

70 **PP4 Treatment of Fecal Incontinence and Defecatory Disturbances**
K. Maeda, M. Maruta, T. Utsumi, H. Sato, Y. Koide (Japan)

70 **PP5 Contrast Radiography for Anastomotic Integrity Prior to Reversal of Defunctioning Stoma - Does it Change Management?**
A.A. Warsi, A. Woodward, M.E. Foster (United Kingdom)

70 **PP6 Prevention of Permanent Colostomy**
V. Sulyma (Ukraine)

Surgical Pathophysiology

71 **PP7 Progenitor-Like Cells of Islets from Pancreatic Ductal Tissue Fragments in Three-Dimensional Culture System**
A. Isogai, M. Nagaya, K. Akashi, S. Kubota (Japan)

71 **PP8 The Effect of Mycophenolate Mofetil on Liver Fibrosis in an Experimental Model**
N. Sikas, K. Patsiaoura, G. Imvrios, F. Karasavidou, I. Antoniadis, S. Papaemanouil, A. Antoniadis (Greece)

72 **PP9 The Mid-Term Effectiveness of Branched Chain Amino Acid Supplement in Cirrhosis**
H. Nozaki, T. Inoau, T. Takano, Y. Kuroki (Japan)

72 **PP10 The Role of Predicting Factors in Progression and Response of Patients with Oesophageal Cancer Undergoing Neoadjuvant Therapy (An Immunohistochemical Study)**
G. Bognár, A. Imdahl, G. Ledniczky, G. István, P. Ondrejka (Hungary and Germany)

72 **PP11 Histochemical Appearance and Prognostic Significance of *Maackia amurensis* Leukoagglutinin-Positive Glycoconjugates in Human Gastric Cancer**
W. Tang, M. Nakata, K. Mafune, T. Konishi, N. Kokudo, M. Usuda, N. Kojima, T. Mizuochi, M. Makuuchi (Japan)

73 **PP12 Expression of Cell Cycle Control Proteins in Colon Cancer and Their Correlation in Prognosis**
G. Kouraklis, D. Mantas, S. Theoharis, A. Glinavou, C. Vagianos, G. Karatzas (Greece)

73 **PP13 Analysis of K-Ras and P53 Gene Mutations in Human Colorectal Carcinoma: Relationship to Clinicopathological Variables**
L. Zajac, J. Polanski, J. Dluzniewska, B. Interewicz, J. Stanislawska, E. Szyter (Poland)

74 **PP14 Copper-Transporting P-Type Adenosine Triphosphatase (ATP7B) is Expressed in Human Gastric Carcinoma**
K. Ogawa (Japan)

Hepatobiliary and Pancreatic Surgery

74 **PP15 Consideration of Detection of *Helicobacter Pylori* in the Gastric Mucosa as a Respective Factor for Occurrence of Acute Attack of Cholecystitis at a Glance of Asymptomatic Cholecystolithiasis**
N. Ueno, H. Haranomura, S. Matsuoka, M. Terada, Y. Makino, M. Fujikura, Y. Fujio (Japan)

74 **PP16 Liver Regeneration and Angiogenesis in Mice Deficient for Plasminogen**
J.M. Vogten, T.A. Drixler, I.H.M. Borel Rinkes (The Netherlands)

75 **PP17 Anterior Liver Resections for Surgical Treatment of Primary and Secondary Liver Tumours**
I. Takács, A. Vágvölgyi, M.G. Boland, P. Sápy (Hungary)

75 **PP18 Surgical Impact of Liver Resections with Microwave Tissue Coagulator**
S. Satoi, Y. Matsui, H. Kitade, M. Kaibori, H. Yamada, T. Hijikawa, N. Terakawa, S. Takai, A.H. Kwon, Y. Kamiyama (Japan)

76 **PP19 Experimental Model of Intraoperative Radiotherapy on Ischemic Rat Liver**
O. Hahn, A. Szijártó, P. Kupcsulik (Hungary)

76 **PP20 Pattern and Risk of Postoperative Recurrence in Solitary Hepatocellular Carcinoma**
Y. Takada, M. Otsuka, T. Todoroki, K. Fukao (Japan)

76 **PP21 Hepatocyte Growth Factor Level in Liver and Blood and Post-Operative Liver Cell Proliferation in Patients with Benign and Malignant Liver Tumors Underwent Partial Hepatectomy**
B. Lukomska, J. Dluzniewska, J. Polanski, L. Zajac, D. Sitkiewicz (Poland)

77 **PP22 Antireflux Effectivity of Various Porto-Enterostomas**
T. Cserni, I. Csízy, I. Furka, T. Józsa, J. Papp Szekeres, T. Lesznyák, I. Mikó (Hungary)

77 **PP23 The Effect of Intraductal Corticosteroid Treatment on the Experimental Acute Pancreatitis of Dogs**
L. Kerekes, S. Sipka Jr., B. Dezső, A. Furka, K. Pető, E. Bráth, I. Mikó, I. Furka, P. Sápy (Hungary)

78 **PP24 Clinicopathological Evaluation of Long and Short-Term Survivors Treated for Pancreatic Carcinoma**
S. Takai, S. Satoi, H. Yanagimoto, Y. Koike, H. Toyokawa, H. Araki, A.H. Kwon, Y. Kamiyama (Japan)

Sepsis and Inflammation

78 **PP25 The Effects of Dimethylsulfoxide and Pentoxifylline on Plasma Malondialdehyde Levels and Tissue Damage in Sepsis**
S. Tekin, M. Sahin, H. Alptekin, M. Avunduk, M. Gürbilek (Turkey)

78 **PP26 The Effects of Selective iNOS Inhibitory Aminoguanidine on Plasma NO Levels, Tissue Damage and Organ Function in Sepsis**
M. Sahin, M. Belviranli, M. Gölcük, F. Avsar, H. Pasaoglu, S. Hücümenoglu (Turkey)

79 **PP27 Pirfenidone Ameliorates Endotoxin-Induced Liver Injury after Partial Hepatectomy in Rats**
H. Tsuchiya, M. Kaibori, N. Yokoigawa, A.H. Kwon, T. Okumura, Y. Kamiyama (Japan)

79 **PP28 The Influence of Probiotics in Bacterial Translocation**
K. Kotzampassi, E. Tsiakiri, D. Paramythiotis, N. Charlaftis, G. Metaxas, A. Zatagias, E. Eleftheriadis (Greece)

79 **PP29 Diagnostic Value of Urine "Biopyrrins" (Bilirubin Oxidative Products) in Severity of Acute Abdomen**
Y. Tsuji, M. Misumi, T. Takahashi, K. Kaai, R. Hirayama (Japan)

80 **PP30 Effect of Octreotide on the Oxidative Stress of Acute Experimental Pancreatitis**
K. Kotzampassi, A. Makedou, D. Paramythiotis, G. Metaxas, K. Kourti, E. Eleftheriadis (Greece)

80 **PP31 Tissue Factor in the Pathophysiology of Patients with Major Trauma - Role of NF-κB and AP-1**
G. von Gagern, T. Zimmermann, M. Kotzsch, H. Zwipp, H.D. Saeger (Germany)

80 **PP32 ATP Synthase and Keratinocyte Growth Factor Gene Expression in Experimental Gastroesophageal Reflux Disease**
K. Szentpáli, M. Széll, J. Kaszaki, G. Lázár, L. Kemény, A. Dobozy, Á. Balogh, M. Boros (Hungary)

81 **PP33 Pathophysiology of Decrease in Erythrocyte Deformability in Acute Pancreatitis**
B. Chmiel, R. Grabowska-Bochenek, L. Cierpka, K. Zagalski (Poland)

Shock and Ischemia-Reperfusion Injury

81 **PP34 Formation of Peroxynitrite as a Result of Nitric Oxide-Superoxide Interaction in Ischemia and Reperfusion - A Clinical Trial**
D. Ockert, T. Zimmermann, S. Kersting, S. Albrecht, H.D. Saeger (Germany)

82 **PP35 The Antioxidative Effect of DHEA-S *In Vitro* and *In Vivo* - Chemiluminometric Determination of Hydroperoxy-groups in Lipoproteins**
T. Zimmermann, S. Albrecht, H.D. Saeger, W. Distler (Germany)

82 **PP36 Characterization of a Hemorrhagic/Traumatic Shock Model in Rats Mimicking Clinical Settings**
L. Szalay, F. Umar, A. Khadem, C. Weber, M. Jafarmadar, H. Gasser, W. Fürst, H. Redl, S. Bahrami (Hungary)

82 **PP37 Comparison of Granulocyte Activation and Leukocyte Adhesion Molecule Expression Through Acute Ischemia and Prolonged Reperfusion in Open and Closed Chest Dog Model**
J. Lantos, G. Jancsó, M.T. Jaberansari, E. Rőth (Hungary)

83 **PP38 Relative Antioxidant Activity in Relation with Renal Ischemia-Reperfusion Injury**
K. Pető, V.A. Oláh, E. Bráth, I. Furka, I. Mikó (Hungary)

83 **PP39 Follow-Up of Red Blood Cell Deformability after Short Hindlimb Ischemia in Rat**
N. Németh, T. Lesznyák, G. Ács, E. Bráth, I. Furka, I. Mikó (Hungary)

84 **PP40 Special Adaptation of Different Measuring Methods on Experimental Animals in the Aspect of Ischemia-Reperfusion Injuries**
N. Németh, G. Ács, T. Lesznyák, G. Szabó, E. Bráth, K. Pető, A. Dán, J. Tumpek, I. Furka, I. Mikó (Hungary)

84 **PP41 Endothelin-A Receptor Antagonism Reduces Torsion-Induced Aspermatogenesis and Microcirculatory Failure in the Rat**
R. Varga, A. Szabó1, M. Pákáski, Z. Bajory, L. Pajor, M. Boros (Hungary)

85 **PP42 Akt Activation Protects Rat Liver from Ischemia-Reperfusion Injury**
N. Harada, E. Hatano, N. Koizumi, T. Nitta, M. Yoshida, N. Yamamoto, Y. Yamaoka (Japan)

85 **PP43 Lower Limb Ischaemia-Reperfusion Induced Remote Hepatic Injury Is Not Altered by Kupffer Cell Depletion**
A. Lewis, D.W. Harkin, M. Hoper, F.C. Campbell, A.A.B. Barros D'Sa (Northen Ireland)

Organ Transplantation

85 **PP44 Urinary Trypsin Inhibitor (UTI) Exerts Protective Effects on the Hepatic Microvasculature in Hypotensive Brain-Dead Rats**
T. Takahashi, K. Itabashi, Y. Ito, K. Sato, A. Kakita (Japan)

86 **PP45 Diagnosis and Treatment for the Late Vascular and Biliary Complications after Living Donor Liver Transplantation**
N. Kawagishi, N. Ohkohchi, S. Satomi (Japan)

86 **PP46 Indication and Efficacy of Apheresis for the Liver Transplant Recipients - Experiences of 22 Cases in 52 LDLTx**
N. Kawagishi, N. Ohkohchi, N. Koyamada, S. Sekiguchi, S. Tsukamoto, S. Satomi (Japan)

87 **PP47 Experimental Study on Hepatic Reinnervation after Orthotopic Liver Transplantation in Rats**
I. Sakamoto, T. Takahashi, A. Kakita, I. Hayashi, M. Majima, S. Yamashina (Japan)

87 **PP48 Dual Kidney Transplantation in the Use of Marginal Donors** R. Cadrobbi, N. Baldan, M.L. Valente, S. Scapin, F. Marchini, L. Dall'Olmo, E. Ancona, P. Rigotti (Italy)

87 **PP49 Omental Flap Harvesting for Free Transplantation. Preliminary Data on the Operative Technique in Dogs**
J. Pap Szekeres, I. Furka, M. Svébis, T. Cserni, E. Bráth, N. Németh, I. Mikó (Hungary)

88 **PP50 Histologic Findings in Small Bowel Tissue Following Pancreatico-Duodenal Allotransplantation with Venous Drainage into the Portal or Systemic Circulation**
U.J. Hesse, D. Meester, R. Troisi, B. de Hemptinne, P. Pattyn, H. van Vlierberghe, M. De Vos, N. Lameire, C. Cuverlier (Belgium)

Circulation

88 **PP51 Pharmacological and Ischemic Preconditioning of Pig Hearts in the Working Heart Model**
W. Beierlein, A.M. Scheule, J. Haas, D. Jost, H.P. Wendel, G. Ziemer (Germany)

89 **PP52 Selective and Immediate Neuronal Injury during Cardiac Surgery in Domestic Pig**
Z. Tóth, I. Győrimolnár, Á. Hevesi, L. Papp (Hungary)

89 **PP53 Microcirculatory Changes in Ischemia-Reperfusion-Induced Cystitis in Rats**
Z. Bajory, J. Hutter, F. Krombach, K. Messmer (Germany and Hungary)

90 **PP54 Strain and Physical Activity: Determinants of Lymph Drainage in Murines**
M. Ionac, D. Bordos (Romania)

90 **PP55 Effects of Extracellular Magnesium Concentration on Inflammatory Stimulus Induced Enhancement of Granulocyte MAC-1 Avidity and Affinity**
H. Habazettl, A. Vogel, S. May, M. Gründel, W.M. Kuebler, H. Kuppe (Germany)

90 **PP56 Effects of Celecoxib on the Synovial Microcirculation in Mouse Antigen-Induced Arthritis**
H. Gebhard, H. J. Refior, K. Messmer, A. Veihelmann (Germany)

91 **PP57 Comparison of the Circulatory Effects of Different Hypertonic Colloid Volume Expanders**
E. Eszlári, E. Csonka, J. Kaszaki, G. Molnár, A. Szabó, M. Boros (Hungary)

91 **PP58 Co-Localization of the Vanilloid VR1 and Trka Receptors and Substance P in Neurons of the Cochlear and Vertebro-Basilar Arteries**
Z. Vass, P.S. Steyger, D.R. Trune, A.L. Nuttall (Hungary and USA)

Traumatology and Tissue Repair

92 **PP59 Promotive Effects of Far-infra Red Ray on Full-Thickness Skin Wound Healing**
H. Toyokawa, Y. Masui, H. Tsuchiya, S. Teshima, H. Nakanishi, A.H. Kwon, Y. Azuma, T. Nagaoka, Y. Ogawa, Y. Kamiyama (Japan)

92 **PP60 Therapeutic and Prophylactic Management of Silicone Gel Sheeting (Epiderm) in Hypertrophic and Keloid Scarring**
O. Kelemen, L. Kollár, K. Szilágyi (Hungary)

92 **PP61 Prospective Trial Comparing the Prolene and Dacron Mesh in the Lichtenstein Tension-Free Inguinal Hernia Repair**
G. Antsaklis, I. Karanikas, A. Fotopoulos, A. Karkaletsis, S. Lamprou, E. Konstantinidou, I. Sahin, C. Alexiou, D. Zogas (Greece)

93 **PP62 Vascular Tunnel Concept in the Acute Surgical Treatment of Severe T-L1 Fractures**
A. Csókay, L. Együd, L. Nagy (Hungary)

93 **PP63 The Treatment of Polytraumatic Patient's Diaphragm Injuries**
C. Oláh, K. Kovács, P. Frölich, M. Svébis, G. Boross, A. Száz (Hungary)

93 **PP64 Surgical Security by Limb Replantation: an Experimental Amputat Model**
M. Szokoly, G. Ács, E. Bráth, N. Németh, T. Lesznyák, I. Mikó, I. Furka (Hungary)

94 **PP65 Evaluation of Monopolar and Bipolar Electrocoagulation in Normal and Abnormal Coagulation Status**
M. Kontos, T. Diamantis, A. Arvelakis, D. Koronarchis, S. Syroukis, E. Agapitos, E. Felekouras, E. Bastounis (Greece)

New Techniques

94 **PP66 Minimal Invasive Adrenal Gland Surgery - Chance and Option**
T. Jacobi, U. Wehrmann, T. Zimmermann, H.D. Saeger (Germany)

95 **PP67 Anaesthesiological Management for Swine Laparoscopic Experimental Surgery**
O. Toma, C. Balasa, C. Plavat, M. Papurica, D. Sandesc, M. Ionac (Romania)

95 **PP68 First Results of the Inguinal Hernia Repair with the Prolene Hernia System**
G. Antsaklis, N. Economou, C. Alexiou, A. Karkaletsis, E. Kefalogiannis, N. Fotopoulos, P. Karydakis, E. Bobotis, I. Karanikas (Greece)

95 **PP69 The Electric Oscillating Brush Dissection Instrument: Evaluation of Vascular Trauma and Clinical Applications for Laparoscopic Cholecystecomy and Colectomy**
M. Kakihara, Z. Szabó, Y. Kagata, K. Hatsuse, T. Aihara, H. Mochizuki (USA)

96 **PP70 Comparison of Different Anastomotic Techniques in Tracheal Replacement**
Z. Szántó, A. Ferencz, G. Jancsó, Á. Boronkai, E. Rőth, Ö.P. Horváth, T.F. Molnár (Hungary)

96 **PP71 Experiences with the Retrograde Percutaneous Translaryngeal Tracheotomy (Fantoni) on a Surgical Intensive Care Unit**
R. Konopke, T. Zimmermann, S. Kersting, H. Schikore, G. von Gagern, D. Ockert, H.D. Saeger (Germany)

96 **PP72 Validation of a Skills Course Using Objective Measures of Technical Ability**
M.S. Khan, S.D. Bann, A. Darzi, P.E.M. Butler (United Kingdom)

Molecular Biology and Immunology

97 **PP73 Bioluminometric TC-Assay in Cases of Gynaecology Malignancies - Useful as Pretherapeutical Factor?**
S. Albrecht, T. Zimmermann. T. Köppen1, B. Richter, W. Distler (Germany)

97 **PP74 Suppression of Proliferative Cholangitis by E2F Decoy Oligodeoxynucleotide**
M. Yoshida, N. Yamamoto, T. Nitta, T. Uehara, R. Terao, E. Hatano, Y. Iimuro, Y. Yamaoka (Japan)

98 **PP75 Participation of ERCC1 in Resistance against Cisplatin for Human Esophageal Cancer Cell Lines**
T. Miyahara, K. Yanagibashi, T. Kajiwara, M. Akaboshi, A. Kawabe, J-I. Kaganoi (Japan)

98 **PP76 Severe Tissue Injury Alters Self-Regulation of Neutrophil Phagocytosis**
G. Pap, J. Fűrész, L. Nagy, J. Hamar (Hungary)

98 **PP77 Enhancement of Circulating Dendritic Cell Activity by Immunomodulators (OK432 and KP-40)**
H. Yanagimoto, H. Toyokawa, M. Inaba, S. Takai, S. Satoi, J. Beuth (Japan)

99 **PP78 Activation of RET Tyrosine Kinase Modulates IL-8 Production**
N. Iwahashi, M. Takahashi, Y. Nimura (Japan)

99 **PP79 Modification of the Endotoxin-Induced Inflammatory Cell Response by Glucocorticoids**
J. Szakács, G. Lázár, G. Lázár Jr., E. Husztik (Hungary)

European
Surgical Research

Oral Presentations

Eur Surg Res 2002;34(suppl 1):1-99

Walter Brendel Session

1

Continuous Monitoring of Cerebrospinal Fluid Oxygen Tension in Relation to Motor Evoked Potentials During Spinal Cord Ischemia in a Porcine Model of TAAA Surgery

J. Lips, P. de Haan, M.J. Jacobs, T.M. van Gulik, C.J. Kalkman

Academic Medical Center, Amsterdam, The Netherlands

Introduction: Lower limb paralysis after resection of thoracoabdominal aneurysms (TAAA) is a major complication. Assessment of spinal cord oxygenation might guide measures to prevent neurological deficits during TAAA surgery. Although cerebrospinal fluid (CSF)-pO_2 measurement has been used to detect spinal cord ischemia (SCI), the diagnostic value and the spatiotemporal resolution of CSF-pO_2 measurement compared to functional assessment of the spinal cord is presently unknown. This study compared CSF-pO_2 with transcranial motor evoked potentials (tcMEP) for detection of experimental SCI. Because tcMEP responds slowly to ischemia that remains confined to the thoracic spinal cord, the characteristics of the techniques were examined both during selective thoracic and selective lumbar SCI.
Methods: The aorta and segmental arteries (SAs) were exposed in ten sufentanil/ketamine-anesthetized pigs (40-50 kg). Myogenic tcMEP were recorded from the upper and lower limbs, and continuous assessment of CSF-pO_2 was provided by two Clark type microcatheters inserted in the lumbar and thoracic intrathecal space. In a randomised order, ischemia that remained confined to the thoracic and the lumbar spinal cord was produced by sequential clamping of SAs. The relationship between CSF-pO_2 and tcMEP during graded SCI was determined using linear regression. The critical threshold and diagnostic properties of CSF-pO_2 during lumbar and thoracic SCI were determined. The time between onset of progressive SCI and reduction to below the critical threshold was compared for both monitoring techniques.
Results: The median lumbar and thoracic CSF-pO_2 during critical tcMEP values was 11 mmHg (4-29) and 23 mmHg (18-37) during lumbar and thoracic SCI, respectively. Optimal sensitivity and predictive values of CSF-pO_2 measurement for SCI were between the critical thresholds 40-60% of baseline. Time to reduction of thoracic CSF-pO_2 was shorter (40.2±20.9 min) compared to clinical tcMEP loss (25% of baseline, 53.8±26.0 min, $p<0.01$) during thoracic SCI.
Discussion: To evaluate the diagnostic properties of CSF-pO_2 for detection of SCI, tcMEP was used as the independent variable because the latter monitoring technique allows for direct functional assessment of the spinal cord. Critical reduction of CSF-pO_2 was linearly related to loss of tcMEP amplitude in all animals. CSF-pO_2 monitoring does not carry the risks of sudden patient movements as introduced by tcMEP application, and detects thoracic SCI in an early stage.
Conclusions: The data indicate that intrathecal pO_2 measurement is a sensitive monitoring technique to track real-time changes in local spinal cord oxygenation. A 40% reduction of local CSF-pO_2 precedes clinical tcMEP loss during ischemia that is confined to thoracic spinal cord segments. Continuous monitoring of CSF- pO_2 might be applied in addition to classical tcMEP monitoring for the evaluation of patients who are at risk for spinal cord ischemia.

2

Suppression of Kupffer Cell Function and Administration of Protease Inhibitor are Keys for Successful Liver TX in Non-Heart-Beating Donor

N. Ohkohchi, K. Oikawa, S. Tsukamoto, M. Sato, S. Miyagi, S. Satomi

Division of Advanced Surgical Science and Technology, Graduated School of Medicine Tohoku University, Sendai, Japan

Introduction: Microcirculatory disturbance, which is induced by warm ischemia during agonal condition of the donor and by the reperfusion, is a main obstacle to liver transplantation (LTx) from non-heart-beating donors (NHBD). It is attributed to activation of Kupffer cells and a deterioration of sinusoidal endothelial cells (SEC). We investigated role of Kupffer cells (KC) in the sinusoidal microcirculation of the graft of NHBD, focusing on expression of transcriptional factors and release of cytokines and eicosanoids. We also investigated effects of KC elimination and rinse with protease inhibitor and cytokine suppression in LTx from NHBD.
Materials and Methods: Experiment A) Role of Kupffer cells on expression of transcriptional factors, cytokine release and eicosanoid production: Livers of Wistar rat were retrieved and perfused for 60 minutes with Krebs-Henseleit bicarbonate buffer. Agonal condition of the NHBD was induced thoracotomy under general anesthesia. Animals were divided into 4 groups (n=6): I) control group, liver was perfused without preservation; II) HB group, livers were retrieved under heart beating and perfused after 6 hr cold preservation; III) NHB group, liver from NHBD was perfused after preservation; IV) KE group, donor were administered chlodronate to eliminate KC of the liver and retrieved liver was perfused after preservation. Examination items: transcriptional factors (NF-κB, AP-1, NFIL-6), cytokines (TNF-α, IL-1ß, IL-6), eicosanoids (TXA_2, 6-keto-PGF-α, LTB_4), and histological findings were measured. Experiment B) LTx of the graft from NHBD: Pigs were allocated to 5 groups (n=6): I) NHB group, liver graft from NHBD was transplanted; II) NM group, graft from NHBD was rinsed with nafamostat mesilate (NM) solution, which contains serine protease inhibitor, and transplanted; III) KC eliminated group, KC eliminated graft of NHBD was transplant-

ed; IV) KC eliminated+NM rinse group, KC eliminated graft from NHBD was transplanted with rinsing with NM rinse solution; V) cytokine suppression group, FR167653, which suppresses the release of TNF-α and IL-1ß was administered before and after LTx. Survival rate, TEM findings and energy charge were investigated.
Results: A) NF-κB activity of the NHB group was significantly higher but in KE group, it was suppressed as the same level in control group. Expression of AP-1 and NFIL-6 were the same as those of NF-κB. TNF-α, IL-1ß, and LTB4 were significantly higher and sinusoidal structure was severely destroyed in NHB group. However, in KE group cytokines and eicosanoid levels were completely suppressed and sinusoidal structures were well preserved as same as HB group. In histological findings the structure of sinusoid was well maintained in KE group. B) In NHB and KC eliminated groups all recipients died within a day. On the other hand, both in KC eliminated+NM rinse and cytokine suppression groups, 4 of 5 recipients survived. In TEM findings after reperfusion elimination of Kupffer cells prevented SEC deterioration and NM rinse prevented sinusoidal narrowing. Energy charge of liver tissue recovered in all groups except NHB group.
Conclusion: KC activities have an important role in the disturbance of sinusoidal microcirculation in LTx from NHBD. Suppression of KC activities and prevention of sinusoidal narrowing in the liver grafts are keys for the success on LTx from NHBD.

3

Three Percent Relapse after Five Years Follow-up of 200 Patients with Ventral Abdominal Wall Hernia Treated by Carbajo Laparoscopic Technique

M.A. Carbajo, M. García-Caballero, J.I. Martin, J.I. Blanco, M. Delacuesta, F. Martin, M. Toledano

Dept. Surgery, Medical Faculty, University of Malaga, Spain

Introduction: The treatment of incisional and other abdominal wall hernia by open surgery is unsatisfactory due to the necessary large incisions and wide tissue dissection, non-acceptable higher relapse rates with single closure techniques but even high after using prosthetic materials that furthermore have the risk of infection and/or rejection. All that provoke a prolonged hospital stay with increasing costs and the consequent loose of work hours never well enough evaluated. Trying to find a solution to this surgical problem, M.A. Carbajo and coworkers developed and tested in the past seven years a laparoscopic technique whose fundamental is to identify the hernia hole (after emptying the hernia content) and to close it with a PTFE mesh (Dual Mesh PlusR Gore) fixed by helicoidal staples (ProTackR Tyco).
Objective: We present the results of a prospective protocolized observational study including 200 patients operated by the above mentioned technique and follow-up each three months during a mean of five years (36 to 92 months).
Patients and Methods: All patients with ventral abdominal wall hernia were included without exclusions due to surgical reasons. The mean age was 61 years (range 22 to 89). There were 33 cases of primary ventral hernia, 102 incisional hernia and 65 multi-relapsed incisional large hernia. Seventy eight percent of the patients were epigastric, umbilical or ventral large hernia, and the other 32% have several other localisations. Following the size we classify the defect minor (10 cm^2) in 8 cases.
Results: Mean operation time was 64 minutes (20 to 180) and hospital stay 28 hours (10 to 72). In one case we converted to open procedure (0.5%). Average of hernia defect were 4.3/patient (1 to 14). Mean surface area of the defect was 138 cm^2 (20 to 480 cm^2). The hernia sac content was in 72 cases only epiploon and in 93 cases epiploon+small or large bowel. To close these defects we used in 187 cases a 19x15 cm mesh, in 8 cases 24x18 cm, and in 3 cases 30x20 cm. In 61 cases it was necessary to use more than one mesh (1 to 3 pieces). The most frequent minor complications were seroma (14%) and as major complications presented an intestinal incarceration (0.5%) and 6 cases of hernia relapse (3%).
Conclusions: The treatment of incisional and primary ventral hernias is an indication for laparoscopic surgery. There are few objective limitations (non-anaesthetic) for applying the Carbajo laparoscopic technique. This technique reduces the operative time and hospital stay, improves the postoperative comfort and recovery of the patient, and decreases immediate complications and long term relapse to a minimum improving high significantly the open procedures.

4

The Role of Neuronal Nitric Oxide in the Mechanism of Intestinal Preconditioning

S. Varga, V. Krishnan, L. Balázs, P. Gál, J. Kaszaki, M. Boros

Institute of Surgical Research, University of Szeged, Hungary

Introduction: Ischemic preconditioning (IPC) refers to a mechanism when brief periods of ischemia and reperfusion (I/R) render a tissue relatively resistant to the harmful effects of a subsequent prolonged period of ischemia. I/R of the intestine occurs in several clinical conditions. Nitric oxide (NO) has been implicated in the triggering mechanism of intestinal preconditioning. It has been demonstrated that the isoforms of nitric oxide synthase (NOS) are constitutively expressed in the gastrointestinal tract and the predominant form is neuronal NOS (nNOS). Our aims were to investigate the effects of selective nNOS inhibition on the IPC-induced protection in the small intestine.
Methods: Na-pentobarbital anesthetized dogs were randomly allocated to 3 groups. In group 1 the animals were exposed to 60 min of superior mesenteric artery (SMA) occlusion and 120 min reperfusion (n=5). In group 2 (n=6), preconditioning was performed (3 times 5 min SMA occlusion) 30 min prior to ischemia. Group 3 (n=5) was pretreated with the selective nNOS inhibitor 7-nitroindazol (7-NI; 5 mg/kg, i.v.) before preconditioning. Systemic and local hemodynamics, intramucosal pH (pHi by indirect tonometry) and small bowel motility index (strain-gauge technique) were measured and analysed with computerised data acquisition system. Blood samples were taken from the mesenteric vein and plasma nitrite/nitrate (NOx) levels were determined by the Gries method. At the beginning and end of the reperfusion period intestinal biopsies were taken to quantify granulocyte accumulation with myeloperoxidase (MPO) assay.
Results: 60 min mesenteric ischemia followed by 120-min reperfusion significantly decreased the pHi, and increased intestinal motility and tissue MPO activity (by 90% compared to baseline). IPC prior to mesenteric I/R resulted in a significantly improved pHi, and low-

ered MPO activity to the control level at the end of observation period. Pretreatment with 7-NI prior to IPC decreased the motility index during the reperfusion phase, caused a 3-fold elevation in plasma NOx level and increased MPO activity by 120% as compared to the baseline.

Discussion: Our results demonstrate that IPC may offer a possibility to reduce functional damage and local accumulation of granulocytes in the postischemic intestine. Inhibition of nNOS reduced further the IPC-induced decrease in local granulocyte accumulation.

Conclusion: NO produced by nNOS may play an important role in the mechanism of intestinal preconditioning by inhibiting the leukocyte-mediated inflammatory processes. Supported by research grant OTKA T035275.

5

The Regenerative Effect of Hepatocyte Growth Factor (HGF) on Severe Ischemic Acute Tubular Necrosis (ATN) in Rats Improves Survival in Kidney Transplantation

T. Karatzas[1], S. Santiago[3], A. Tsamandas[2], W. DeFaria[3], C. Gandia[3], S. Salgar[3], A.G. Tzakis[3]

Department of Surgery[1], Department of Pathology[2], University Hospital of Rion-Patras School of Medicine, Patras, Greece; Department of Surgery, Division of Liver/GI Transplantation[3], University of Miami, Jackson Memorial Hospital, Miami-FL, USA

Introduction: Acute tubular necrosis induced either by ischemia or by various drugs elicits a process of increased cell turnover in the renal tubular epithelium (tubular regeneration). Tubular cells are the major source of many growth factors, that play an important role in maintaining the histological structure and functions of renal tubules. HGF is the most potent among growth factors, proven to stimulate DNA synthesis of many epithelial cells including renal tubular cells, stimulates cell motility and induces tubule formation. Despite considerable evidence that HGF is involved in renal tissue repair in animals, no data are available on the outcome of transplanted kidneys recovered from severe ATN following HGF administration.

Objectives: 1) To establish a model of severe ischemic ATN, 2) to confirm the regenerative effect of HGF on severely injured kidney grafts, and 3) to assess graft survival in kidney transplantation using severely damaged kidneys from ATN and treated with and without HGF.

Methods: Induction of ATN. Severe ischemic ATN was induced by clamping the vascular pedicle of the left kidney for 1 hour. ATN was confirmed by histological and immunohistochemical staining and graded as minimal (0-25%), mild (26-50%), moderate (51-75%) and severe (76-100%). Administration of HGF. HGF was administered as one-time dose of 50 µg i.v., through a tail vein, 30 min after reperfusion of the kidney. Kidney transplantation. Allografts were taken from DA to Lewis rats. Donor surgery and kidney transplant were performed. Cyclosporine was used for immunosuppression.

Design of the Study: Phase A. Groups: A1. Sham-operated rats (n=7). A2. Rats underwent severe ischemic ATN and sacrificed on days 2 (n=7), 4 (n=7) and 7 (n=7). A3. Rats underwent severe ischemic ATN (n=7) followed by HGF administration. Phase B. Kidney transplantation. Groups: B1. Recipient rats (n=5) received kidney grafts from donors that were subjected to ATN and treated with HGF. B2. Recipient rats (n=5) received kidneys as group B1 and also got a second dose of HGF iv. at the end of transplantation. C. Recipient rats (n=5) received kidneys from donors that were subjected to ATN, but not treated with HGF. All transplanted rats underwent nephrectomy of native kidneys one week after transplant and were sacrificed the following week.

Results: ATN: HGF administration reversed ischemic ATN from severe (>80%) to minimal (~25%). Kidney transplantation: Following native kidneys nephrectomies, rats survival was as follows: in group C, all rats died of renal failure, within the first 48 hours; in group B1, rats died of renal failure, between 4th and 6th day. In group B2, 3 rats survived for 7 days with moderately affected renal function, and 2 rats died on day 6.

Conclusions: HGF improves significantly the regenerative process of severe ischemic ATN in rat kidney. Double dose of HGF affects considerably graft survival of transplanted kidneys that are severely damaged from ATN.

6

Long-Term Survival of *Macaca Fascicularis* in a Life-Supporting hDAF Pig-to-Primate Renal Xenotransplantation Model With Triple Maintenance Therapy and Without Splenectomy

A. Dedja, R. Cadrobbi, N. Baldan, C. Vinanzi, A. Taglioni, F. Calabrese, M.C. Varagnolo, R. Busetto, M. Castagnaro, P. Rigotti, E. Cozzi, E. Ancona

Department of Medical and Surgical Sciences; Padua General Hospital; Institute of Pathology; Veterinary Clinical Sciences Department, University of Padua, Italy

Introduction: Pig organs are currently being investigated as a possible solution to the worldwide organ shortage. To date, the best results with this model have been achieved when kidneys from pigs transgenic for human Decay Accelerating Factor (hDAF) were transplanted in splenectomized recipients, exposed to a maintenance immunosuppression with cyclophosphamide (CyP), cyclosporine A (CyA) (Neoral, Novartis) and steroids. In this series, the potential effect of maintenance immunosuppression with CyA, mycophenolate sodium (MPS) (ERL080, Novartis) and steroids on the survival of hDAF kidney xenografts transplanted into non-human primates was investigated.

Materials and Methods: Five Macaca fascicularis underwent bilateral nephrectomy and heterotopic renal xenotransplantation. HDAF transgenic pigs (Imutran/Novartis) were used as the source of organs. Each recipient was treated with an induction of 4 peri-operative doses of intravenous CyP and a maintenance therapy with oral MPS (aiming for trough levels of 3-6 µg/ml), CyA (trough levels: 300-500 µg/l) and steroids. No splenectomy was performed in this trial. All primates were closely monitored for levels of hemolytic anti-pig antibodies (APA), serum biochemistry and full blood count.

Results: One xenograft underwent hyperacute rejection in the first few hours after transplantation. The remaining 4 animals survived 20, 40, 48, and 90 days (median 44 days). Postoperatively, the creatinine in each of these animals reached a nadir between 50 to 60 µmol/l. The mean preoperative APA levels were 1138 arbitrary units (AU) (range: 427-1540) and dropped to less then 4 AU on the first postoperative day. The clinical parameters related to graft function remained within normal range for most of the life span. All animals were sacrificed due to kidney failure, in the presence of grade II or III acute humoral xenograft rejection (AHXR).

Conclusions: These results confirm that hDAF porcine renal xenografts enable long-term survival of non-human primates. Here we report the longest survival time (90 days) described to date in the medical literature of a primate receiving a life-supporting porcine renal xenograft. The organ maintained a valid function and fluid balance for most of the postoperative period. These findings also indicate that splenectomy may not be essential for a prolonged survival of non-human primates receiving porcine kidney xenografts. Finally, AHXR remains the main cause for xenograft loss in long-term survivors of this pig-to-primate xenotransplantation model.

7

Brain Plasticity Following Hand Transplantation

M. Vossen, D. Molfese, A. Fonaryova-Key, S. Kelly, C. Maldonado, M. Kon, J.H. Barker

Department of Plastic, Reconstructive and Hand Surgery at the University Medical Center in Utrecht, The Netherlands and the Division of Plastic and Reconstructive Surgery and the Department of Psychological and Brain Sciences at the University of Louisville, USA

Introduction: Over the past three years sixteen hands have been transplanted in 12 human recipients and the outcomes are promising. While the majority of clinical and scientific focus has been directed towards toxic side effects of the immunotherapy and the functional return of the transplanted hands, a wealth of information exists regarding changes occurring in the brain of the hand recipients. It has been documented that in the months following limb amputation the cortical area of the brain responsible for controlling hand function is lost to adjacent areas in the motor cortex. We have repeatedly measured the cortical reorganization in the brain of a hand transplant recipient. In this study we investigated whether the cortical area of the brain, lost following amputation, regains its functional control of the transplanted hand.

Methods: The participant, was a Caucasian male, 36 years of age, who received a hand transplant. Five years earlier (July 6, 1996) he lost his non-dominant, left hand at the wrist as a result of a fireworks accident. Prior to receiving the transplant, he used a cable hook prosthesis. Electrophysiological brain profiles were obtained using auditory evoked responses to tones during sensory and motor ideation tasks to track changes in brain organization for sensory and motor processing across 5 subsequent test dates over a 10 week period following the transplant.

Results: The time course of changes in topographic maps of electrical brain activity based on auditory brain responses showed clear, linear changes in brain organization for sensory and motor inputs in both the transplanted and non-transplanted hand. Furthermore, the neural substrate supporting unrelated functions such as tone perception also changed markedly, indicating that brain reorganization following hand transplantation extends well beyond the cortices that immediately subserve hand functions.

Conclusion: These findings note for the first time in humans that there are significant organizational changes in the brain following the gain of a body part. Functional return to the hand following transplantation, while dependent on neural regrowth in the allotransplant, clearly leads to cortical reorganization of the brain, even in brain areas not involved in hand sensory or motor functions. This knowledge could be useful to create new approaches for rehabilitation, such as biofeedback mechanisms, and to help in the development of new myoprosthetic devices. Furthermore, this information opens new pathways to understand the complexities of phenomena such as phantom pain and the impact of nerve regeneration and brain reorganization following surgery.

8

Expression and Function of L-Type Calcium Channels in Human Colon Cancer Cells

A. Zawadzki, Q. Liu*, Y. Wang*, A. Melander**, B. Jeppsson*, H. Thorlacius**

Department of Surgery* and Community Medicine**, and NEPI Foundation**; Malmö University Hospital, Lund University, SE-20502 Malmö, Sweden.

Introduction: Epidemiological studies have suggested that use of calcium channel antagonists is associated with an increased incidence in colon cancer. However, there is no biologic data supporting the concept that calcium channel antagonists may promote colon carcinogenesis and it is not known whether colon cancer cells express functional calcium channels. In the present study, we examined the expression of calcium channels in human colon cancer cells. Moreover, the effect of calcium channel agonists and antagonists on calcium influx and apoptosis in colon carcinoma cells were examined.

Methods: A primary (AZ-97) and established (HT-29) human colon cancer cell line were used. Apoptosis was quantified with flow cytometric analysis of Annexin V binding. Fluorimetric detection of Fluo-4-AM was used to measure intracellular calcium. Total cellular RNA was extracted using an acid guanidinium-phenol-chloroform method and RT-PCR was performed with SuperScrip One-Step system. Tumor cells were incubated with different concentrations of three different calcium channel antagonists (verapamil, diltiazem or nifedipine) and one agonist (BayK 8644).

Results: AZ-97 and HT-29 cells expressed L-type calcium channel mRNA whereas these cells were negative for N- and P-type channels. The L-type calcium channels in AZ-97 and HT-29 cancer cells were both composed of a1D and b3-subunits. Challenge with a specific L-type calcium channel agonist (BayK 8644) markedly increased calcium influx and apoptosis in colon cancer cells. Indeed, pretreatment with calcium channel antagonists (verapamil, diltiazem or nifedipine) alone did not change the level of apoptosis in colon cancer cells. However, pretreatment with verapamil abolished BayK 8644-provoked calcium influx and apoptosis.

Discussion: These data demonstrate that human colon cancer cells express L-type calcium channels (a1D and b3-subunits). Activation of this L-type channel triggers calcium influx and causes apoptosis in colon cancer cells. The calcium channel antagonist verapamil inhibited calcium channel agonist-induced calcium influx and apoptosis, suggesting that there is a biological basis for the observed association

between the use of calcium antagonists and colon cancer in epidemiological studies.
Conclusion: Human colon cancer cells contain functional L-type calcium channels with the capacity to increase intracellular calcium and apoptosis.

Microcirculation

9

Analysis of Angiogenesis, Microcirculation, and Growth of Primary and Secondary Bone Tumors: An Experimental Study in Mice

A. Sckell, F. Klenke, T. Merkle, M.M. Gebhard[1], V. Ewerbeck

Departments of Orthopaedic Surgery and Experimental Surgery[1] of the University of Heidelberg, 69118 Heidelberg, Germany

Introduction: In the treatment of solid tumors, established procedures such as surgery, chemotherapy, and radiation often fail. Due to the knowledge that the growth of solid tumors is angiogenesis dependent, the idea of anti-angiogenesis as a therapeutic strategy is very promising. For the lack of an appropriate experimental model to investigate this strategy in primary and secondary bone tumors, the aim of the study was to develop an animal model to characterize angiogenesis, microcirculation, and growth of primary and secondary bone tumors with a high temporal and spatial resolution using intravital microscopy.
Methods: Chunks (volume 0.5 to 1.0 mm^3) of solid tumors (osteosarcoma, SAOS II, n=6; prostatic carcinoma, PC-3, n=3; glioblastoma, U87, n=3) were implanted in a newly developed cranial window preparation where the calvaria of adult male severe combined immunodeficient (SCID) mice serves as site for implantation, each. To determine the first appearance of newly formed vessels (V) and the onset of perfusion in these vessels, tumors were investigated daily with intravital microscopy. FITC-Dextran as a plasma marker and Rhodamine 6G to stain leukocytes *in vivo* enabled investigation of microcirculation and leukocyte-endothelium interaction.
Results: Data are presented as mean±SD. In all tumors the onset of perfusion in newly formed vessels occurred within 24 hours after the first appearance of the latter (V: 104±12 h in SAOS II, 84±14 h in PC-3, 60±16 h in U87). Due to an extremely rapid tumor growth, animals with PC-3 and U87 had to be killed on days 16±0 and 18.5±3.5, respectively, while SAOS II reached a two-dimensional tumor surface of 20.4±0.9 mm^2 on day 28 after implantation. On day 28 versus day 7 after implantation, in SAOS II, there was a significant (t-test, χ^2), rolling leukocytes (27.9±2.2 vs. 19.5±2.7%), and sticking leukocytes (513±44 vs. 362±105 cells/mm^2) while there were no differences in vessel diameters and hemodynamics such as erythrocyte velocity, leukocyte flux, blood flow and shear rate.
Discussion and Conclusion: Our model allows continuous quantitative and qualitative analysis of angiogenesis, microcirculation, and growth of primary and secondary bone tumors over several weeks. The data obtained provide an important basis for further studies investigating the mechanism of action and therapeutic potency of newly developed anti-angiogenic agents in addition to established procedures such as surgery, chemotherapy, and radiation.

10

Generalized and Local Circulatory Disorders Differentially Affect the Microcirculation of the Different Layers of the Rat Small Intestine

K. Vajda, A. Szabó**, A. Sárkány**, K. Kucsa**, A. Thoman**, M. Boros***

Department of Surgery*, Bács-Kiskun County Teaching Hospital, Kecskemét, Hungary Institute of Surgical Research**, University of Szeged, Hungary

Introduction: Microcirculatory parameters (capillary red blood cell velocity/RBCV; functional capillary density/FCD) were determined in different layers of the rat small intestine using the orthogonal polarization spectral imaging (OPS) technique. The aim was to identify the significance of local compensatory factors that may influence the intramural flow responses after various circulatory disturbances. Perfusion characteristics were determined in the mucosa and in the Peyer's patches during systemic circulatory failure (various types of endotoxemia, hemorrhagic shock and inhibition of nitric oxide synthesis) or after splanchnic ischemia/reperfusion.
Methods: Mucosal villi were exposed by enterotomy and the mucosal and serosal orientations of two ileal segments were examined simultaneously. Ischemia/reperfusion was elicited by occluding the superior mesenteric artery (SMA) for 30 min followed by 180 min of reperfusion (Group 1). The microcirculatory effects of endotoxemia were examined in Group 2 (6 hr after 10 mg/kg intraperitoneally injected LPS), Group 3 (for 2 hr after 10 mg/kg intravenous bolus LPS) and Group 4 (during 10 mg/kg/h continuous LPS infusion for 2 hr), respectively. In Groups 5 and 6 the animals were bled to a mean arterial pressure of 45 mmHg which was followed by resuscitation with saline (200% of the shed blood volume over 10 min) or hyperosmotic/hyperoncotic saline solution (7.2% NaCl-10% hydroxyethylstarch HES 200/0.5; Osmohes; 4 ml/kg) followed by 10ml/kg/h of Ringer's lactate infusion. In Group 7 inhibition of nitric oxide synthesis was achieved by 10 mg/kg of L-NAME administration.
Results: Reperfusion of the small intestine after a 30-min SMA occlusion resulted in a progressive fall in RBCV values and villus FCD over the course of the examination period. LPS in i.v. bolus (Group 3) caused a transient deterioration of the microcirculation of the villi which was less severe than after continuous LPS infusion (Group 4) as evidenced by capillary flow and FCD data. However, mucosal villus perfusion was maintained in both cases and muscle microcirculation was significantly deteriorated. Later phases of prolonged endotoxemia (Group 2) were accompanied by moderate fall in muscle and villus capillary flow without considerable changes in villus FCD. Hypovolemia and the late phase of resuscitation induced characteristic capillary flow motion in the villi, hence resuscitation resulted only in a transient reestablishment of the continuous flow pattern. Blood loss caused an almost complete stasis in the muscle which could only partially eliminated by saline and the heterogeneity of tissue perfusion persisted. Osmohes increased the duration of con-

tinuous flow period at the onset of resuscitation in the villi and ameliorated the loss of tissue perfusion in the muscle layer. The most severe microcirculatory disturbances were induced by inhibition of NO synthesis as shown by significant reduction in capillary flow and FCD in all tissue layers.

Conclusion: Generalized circulatory disorders are characterized by a redistribution of blood flow within the different layers of the intestine allowing the preservation of villus perfusion. Local circulatory insults such as arterial occlusion/reperfusion severely affect the efficacy of tissue perfusion in all layers of the small intestine. In this respect, the consequences of modulation of endothelium-derived regulatory mediator release (NO synthesis inhibition) are similar to that observed after ischemia-reperfusion and intramural flow redistribution can not be observed in this condition. Supported by ETT grants (to A.S. and M.B.)

11

Improvement of Hepatic Microcirculation by ROCK Inhibitor Y-27632 in Hepatic Ischemia/Reperfusion Model in Rat

F. Ikeda, H. Terajima, Y. Simahara, Y. Yamaoka

Department of Gastroenterological Surgery, Kyoto University Graduate School of Medicine, Kyoto, Japan

Introduction: The low molecular weight GTPase Rho is known to regulate various signal transduction. ROCK/Rho kinase transmits the signal as one of the effector molecules of Rho, and mediates cytoskeleton-dependent cell function by enhancing phosphorylation of the light chain of myosin. Recently Y-27632, a specific inhibitor of ROCK/Rho kinase, was reported to participate in the reduction of cell adhesion by suppressing the stress fiber formation, and to suppress the contraction of smooth muscle by inhibiting of calcium sensitization. By this function, Y-27632 is expected to reduce the ischemia/reperfusion(I/R)-induced injury through attenuation of microcirculatory disturbance. In this study, the effect of Y-27632 on hepatic microcirculatory disturbance was investigated during post ischemic period.

Methods: In male Sprague-Dawley rats, the left lobe of the liver was clamped for 90 minutes, followed by 120 minutes reperfusion. Before ischemia, 1mg Y-27632 /kg bw or 0.9% NaCl was intravenously given. Hepatic microvascular parameters were evaluated by using intravital fluorescence microscopy.

Results: During reperfusion period, the number of adherent leukocytes was significantly increased in postsinusoidal venules, and the diameter of postsinusoidal venule was decreased in the control group. On the contrary, in the group treated with Y-27632, the diameter of postsinusoidal venules was maintained at normal level and the number of adherent leukocytes was reduced as compared with the control.

Discussion and Conclusion: Y-27632 prevents the reduction of vascular diameter possibly by relaxation of vascular smooth muscle, and also leukocyte adherence in the postsinusoidal venules possibly by attenuation of the leukocyte-endothelial interaction. Thus, Y-27632 may be useful to reduce the hepatic I/R-induced injury through alleviation of microcirculatory disturbance.

12

Improvement of Microcirculation in Severe Experimental Pancreatitis Enhances Hepatic Capillary Blood Flow and RES Function

B. Forgács, E. Wudel**, J. Franke**, G. Eibl, H.J. Buhr, T. Foitzik*

Dept. of Surgery II*, Semmelweis Med. Univ. Budapest, Hungary and Depts. of Surgery and Nuclear Med.** Benjamin Franklin Medical Center, Freie Univ. Berlin, Germany

Background: Microcirculatory disorders in severe acute pancreatitis (AP) do not only affect the pancreas but can also be found in other organs including the lungs, colon and liver where they may contribute to AP-associated multiple organ dysfunction.

Aim: To investigate (1) whether improvement of microcirculation also stabilizes capillary blood flow in the liver and (2) whether enhanced hepatic microcirculation is associated with better liver RES phagocytic function.

Method: Severe acute pancreatitis (AP) was induced 24 rats by intraductal bile salt infusion and i.v. cerulein hyperstimulation. 24 sham operated rats (intraductal and i.v. saline infusion) served as controls (Contr). The animals were randomized to receive either specific endothelin-1 receptor antagonist LU-135252 (40 mg/kg) previously shown to increase capillary blood flow in various organs (Pancreas 1998;17:431) or saline. 6 hours after AP induction and treatment the phagocytic function of RES was evaluated in 6 animals per group by calculating the plasma clearance of 99mTc labelled Nanocoll (N-Clear.) from blood samples taken 10 and 30 min after injection. Hepatic capillary blood flow (H-CBF) was determined in the remaining 6 animals per group using intravital microscopy and computerized image analysis system.

Results:

	N-Clear. (ml/min)	H-CBF(nl/min)	(mean±SEM)
	Contr.+SAL:	3.1±0.4	1.4±0.05
	Contr.+LU:	2.9±0.4	1.3±0.005
	AP+SAL:	1.7±0.2*	0.9±0.04*
	AP+LU:	3.2±0.4**	1.3±0.04**

(*$p < 0.05$ AP+SAL vs Contr.+SAL, **$p < 0.05$ AP+LU vs AP+SAL).

Summary: Suppressed liver phagocytic activity early in severe acute pancreatitis is associated with impaired hepatic capillary blood flow. As previously shown in other organs, endothelin receptor blockade also improves capillary blood flow in the liver.

Conclusion: The present findings suggest that liver microcirculation is an important factor for RES function and that therapy aimed at improving disturbed hepatic microcirculation in severe AP stabilizes RES function.

13

A New Model for Fluorescence Video Microscopy of Coronary Terminal Arterioles *in situ*: Effects of Perfusion Pressure

S. Goebel, W.M. Kuebler, A.R. Pries, H. Kuppe, H. Habazettl

Dept. of Physiology, Freie Universität Berlin and Dept. of Anesthesiology, Deutsches Herzzentrum Berlin, Germany

Introduction: To date, investigation of coronary arteriole vasomotor activity has been limited to arterioles ≥ 30-40 μm due to methodological problems. However, terminal arterioles, i.e. < 25 μm, may considerably contribute to microvascular control of blood flow distribution. We, therefore, established a new experimental model to study regulatory mechanisms of coronary terminal arterioles by *in situ* video microscopy of the isolated heart.

Methods: Isolated, Langendorff-perfused rat hearts were arrested by tetrodotoxin (TTX). The closed loop perfusion system (filling volume 20 ml) was placed on a computer-controlled microscope stage. Tilting of the microscope by 90° allowed access to the ventricular surface. The 20x objective was optically coupled to the heart by a cover-glass and contact-gel. Images were generated by a CCD-camera (Kappa CF8/1FMC), recorded on tape, and arteriole diameters were measured offline. Isolation of the heart was followed by a 30 min non-recirculating stabilization period. With the onset of recirculation via the closed loop system, FITC-dextran was added. TTX (50 μM) induced electromechanical arrest of the myocardium and maintained oxygen demand at basal levels. Constant perfusate pH, pO_2, pCO_2, and temperature were maintained. Arterioles were identified by their characteristic morphology, confirmed by recording the flow direction of fluorescent beads (1 μm). Myogenic responses of arterioles (≤ 25μm) were investigated. Responses of terminal arterioles (<25 μm) to changes in perfusion pressure (PP, 60, 40, 100, 120, 140 mmHg) after baseline recordings at PP of 80 mmHg were investigated.

Results: Diameters of the smallest arterioles (<10 μm, n=22) changed by, respectively, +31.7±6.5, +18.4±4.8, 0.0±5.1, -7.7±6.3, and +4.5±7.8 at 40, 60, 100, 120, and 140 mmHg as compared to 80 mmHg PP. In arterioles >10 μm (n=19) diameters changed by +13.0±2.9, +9.7±2.3, -0.9±2.7, -10.7±3.0, and -11.9±3.6%. Thus, smallest arterioles dilated more prominently at low PP, while larger arterioles showed a more sustained constriction after an increase in PP.

Discussion: These data indicate that, consistent with transmural pressure distribution, the pressure range for effective myogenic control is lower in the smallest arterioles than in upstream larger vessels. Our results also confirm maintained vasomotor reactivity of coronary arterioles in the TTX arrested heart.

Conclusion: Our data indicate a substantial contribution of terminal coronary arterioles to PP induced microvascular regulatory responses. Supported by DFG Ha 1651/8-1 and by Medtronic GmbH

14

The Role of Nitric Oxide in the Pathomechanism of Biliary Gastro-Esophageal Reflux

G. Erős, J. Kaszaki, K. Szentpáli, M. Boros*

Institute of Surgical Research, Department of Surgery*, University of Szeged, Hungary

Introduction: Esophagitis is a frequent complication in gastroesophageal reflux disease (GERD) patients treated with acid-suppressive drugs or after total gastrectomy. The presence of regurgitated material could conceivably contribute to mucosal inflammation and injury in patients with GERD. Our previous study reported that reflux containing bile is more harmful than gastric juice alone. However, the exact pathomechanism of bile-induced inflammation is still unknown. It has been demonstrated that the isoforms of nitric oxide synthase (NOS) are constitutively expressed in the gastrointestinal tract and the predominant form is neuronal NOS (nNOS). This present study was designed to identify the effects of nitric oxide (NO) on the esophageal microcirculation and the changes in the activity of NOS isoforms under exposure to bile in a large animal model.

Methods: Na-pentobarbital anesthetized dogs were randomly allocated into 3 groups. A part of the collar esophagus was dissected free and filled-up with test solutions for 3 hr. Group 1 (n=5) served as saline-treated control, groups 2 (n=6) and 3 (n=5) were treated with bile (pH 6.5). Group 3 was pretreated with the selective nNOS inhibitor 7-nitroindazol (7-NI) (5 mg/kg, i.v.). During the experiments mucosal microcirculation was continuously monitored by using orthogonal polarization spectral imaging intravital videomicroscopy technique (Cytoscan A/R, Cytometrics, PA, USA). The capillary flow rate in submucosal vessels and the relative vessel area (RVA - ratio of perfused vessel area/mucosal area) were determined off-line. At the end of the experiments, tissue biopsy was taken to determine the constitutive and inducible NOS (cNOS; iNOS) activity (measured by the conversion of ^{3}H-arginine to ^{3}H-citrulline) and to quantify granulocyte accumulation (myeloperoxidase assay - MPO), respectively.

Results: There was a significant increase in the capillary flow rate and RVA in both bile-treated groups as compared to the baseline in Groups 2 and 3, respectively. However, the capillary flow rate was significantly higher after 7-NI pretreatment as compared to the data in Group 2. In the saline-treated group cNOS and iNOS activity were 94±11 and 18±5 fmol/protein/min, respectively. Exposure to bile decreased the cNOS activity by 54%; and in parallel caused a 6-fold increase in iNOS activity in the esophageal tissue. Bile treatment alone induced a 3-fold elevation in MPO activity whereas the 7-NI pretreatment triggered a 5-fold MPO activity increase as compared to the saline-treated group.

Discussion: Regurgitated bile induces local vasodilation and an increase in esophageal iNOS and MPO activity. Pretreatment with an nNOS inhibitor further increased the capillary flow rate and esophageal granulocyte accumulation.

Conclusion: NO produced by nNOS plays an important role in the pathophysiology of the bile-induced inflammatory process in the esophageal tissue during GERD. Supported by research grant ETT 172/2001

Gastrointestinal Surgery

15

Enhanced Anti-tumor Efficacy by Combining Conventional Chemotherapy with Angiostatin or Endostatin in a Murine Liver Metastasis Model

E.A. te Velde[1,2], J.M. Vogten[1,2], M.F.B.G. Gebbink[2], E.E. Voest[2], I.H.M. Borel Rinkes[1]

Department of Surgery[1] and Medical Oncology[2], University Medical Center Utrecht, Utrecht, The Netherlands

Introduction: Strategies targeting both tumor cells and vasculature have not been thoroughly investigated in models of early metastatic colorectal disease. We have studied the efficacy of combinations of conventional chemotherapy with endostatin or angiostatin (both currently tested in clinical trials) in a murine model of early colorectal liver metastases.
Methods: Control mice received solvent (PBS or citrate). Conventional chemotherapy consisted of adriablastin in a suboptimal dose of 10mg/kg iv. Angiostatin, generated from human plasma, was given continuously in high and low dose (HD-A 100mg/kg/d and LD-A 10mg/kg/d, respectively). Endostatin (Entremed) was given sc. (500 mg/d). Sixty-two mice were subjected to intrasplenic injection of C26 tumour cells to induce colorectal liver metastases. Treatment was initiated 6 hours postoperatively and consisted of single agent, or chemotherapy combined with either angiostatin or endostatin (n>5 per group). Clinical appearance was scored daily using a semi-quantitative scale. Liver weight, macroscopic and histological tumor involvement (hepatic replacement area, HRA) were measured upon sacrifice at day 12. ANOVA was performed to calculate the interaction effects between agents. A multiplicative effect was defined as an enhanced effect of anti-angiogenic therapy in the presence of chemotherapy, or vice-versa.
Results: Mice treated with either drug displayed significantly better clinical scores than controls, except for LD-A or its combination with chemotherapy. All single agent drugs were superior in anti-tumor efficacy compared to no treatment ($p<0.001$).The treatment of liver metastases with adriablastin mono-therapy resulted in a decrease in hepatic replacement area from 42.3±2.0% (non-treated controls) to 29.1%±0.9% ($p<0.001$). HD-A resulted in a HRA of 8.6±2.6% ($p<0.001$). LD-A resulted in a hepatic replacement area of 27.2±0.98% ($p<0.001$). The addition of HD-A and LD-A to the conventional chemotherapy resulted in HRA's of 3.3±1.4% and 8.7±0.7%, respectively. HD-A added to conventional chemotherapy was not significantly more effective than HD-A alone. However, LD-A combined with conventional chemotherapy significantly enhanced anti-tumor efficacy when compared to LD-A alone ($p<0.001$). When compared to chemotherapy alone the effect of addition of angiostatin was multiplicative. Endostatin mono-therapy resulted in a HRA of 12.4±1.4%. Addition to the conventional chemotherapy further reduced hepatic tumor load to a HRA of 3.8±1.1% ($p<0.001$). Again, the effect of co-administration of the anti-angiogenic agent and conventional chemotherapy was multiplicative ($p=0.017$).
Conclusion: The addition of angiostatin or endostatin to conventional chemotherapy enhances anti-tumoral efficacy in a multiplicative manner in a murine model of early colorectal liver metastases.

16

Local Tumor Recurrence Influenced by Systemic Factors

W.M.U. van Grevenstein, J. Jeekel, C.H.J. van Eijck

Laboratory of Experimental Surgery and Oncology, Erasmus MC, Rotterdam, The Netherlands

Introduction: Surgical handling of the peritoneum has a dual character regarding cancer. In case of massive tissue damage, the ensuing inflammatory reaction produces a potentially lethal cocktail of active mediators, including cytokines and growth factors. Beside the influence of these local factors we hypothesised that during surgery systemic produced mediators can be potential stimulators of the tumor cell adhesion as well. Therefore, the aim of this study was to investigate the influence of serum of 8 different time periods before, during and after surgery on the interaction between tumor cells and mesothelial cells.
Methods: To do so, serum was taken from a patient at 8 different periods (-24, 0, 2, 4, 8, 12, 24, 48 hours after surgery). From the same patient primary cultures of omentum derived mesothelial cells were used. An experimental human *in vitro* model was designed using Caco2 colon carcinoma cells. Tumor cell adhesion to a mesothelial monolayer was assessed after overnight pre-incubation of the mesothelium with RPMI 1640 culture medium enriched with 10% serum of the 8 different time periods.
Results: In the control situation the average adhesion of Caco2 cells to the mesothelial monolayers was 29%. Pre-incubation of the monolayer mesothelium with serum of 4, 8 and 12 hours after surgery resulted in an average of 25% enhanced tumor cell adhesion compared to the control situation ($p<0.05$).
Conclusion: Tumor recurrence will be influenced by substances of the cocktail of intra-abdominal produced mediators, which have conflicting demeanor regarding wound healing and local tumor recurrence. In addition to the influence of these locally produced factors, this study shows that systemic factors produced directly after surgery can influence local tumor recurrence as well. More than 12 hours after surgery the serum is not influencing the tumor cell adhesion anymore, probably caused by the decreasing activity of the reactive inflammatory response which causes less active mediators in the blood. More research is needed to investigate which factors in the blood are influencing local tumor recurrence, in order to unravel the process of local recurrences and block them in the end.

17

Adhesion of Human Colon Carcinoma Cells to the Extracellular Matrix

M. ten Kate, W.M.U. van Grevenstein, R.L. Marquet, J. Jeekel, C.H.J. van Eijck

Laboratory of Experimental Surgery and Oncology, Erasmus MC Rotterdam, The Netherlands

Introduction: An important step in metastasis formation is adhesion of tumour cells to the extracellular matrix (ECM) in which the integrins are thought to play an important role. In the case of a disrupted endo- or mesothelium tumour cells are able to adhere directly to the ECM leading to an increased chance of metastasis formation.
Aim of the study: To investigate the adhesion of human colon carcinoma cells to the ECM components *in vitro*. Furthermore we evaluate the role of integrins in this process.
Methods: Human colon carcinoma cell lines HT29 and Caco2 were labeled with calceine-AM and after 1 hr of incubation adhesion to various components of the ECM (collagen I, collagen IV, fibronectin and laminin) was measured by means of fluorescence. To study the role of the integrins in the process of adhesion, tumour cells were preincubated with the monoclonal antibodies anti-α1 till anti-α6 and anti-β1.
Results: HT29 cells particularly adhere to collagen I and laminin (resp. 59 and 50%). On the other hand, Caco2 cells exhibit firm adhesion to fibronectin (47%) and hardly adhere to laminin (15%). Anti-α2 significantly reduces the binding of HT29 and Caco2 cells to collagen I ($p<0.05$ and $p<0.01$ resp.) and of Caco2 cells to collagen IV ($p<0.05$). Anti- 6 inhibits the adhesion of HT29 cells to laminin ($p<0.01$), however this antibody does not reduce the binding of Caco2 cells to laminin. None of the antibodies used in this experiment significantly reduce the adhesion of the tumour cells to fibronectin. Antibodies to the integrins α1, α3, α4 and α5 did not influence the adhesion process.
Conclusions: We conclude that HT29 and Caco2 human colon carcinoma cells express a firm adhesion to components of the ECM. Furthermore these tumour cell lines exhibit an individual adhesion pattern to the ECM, probably because of a different pattern and activity of integrins expressed on the tumour cells. The integrins α2 and α6 play an important role in the attachment of these tumour cell lines to the ECM. Further studies will be needed to unravel the role of other adhesion molecules as well as the cooperation between these adhesion molecules.

18

FAK Expression in Colon Carcinoma and Correlation with Survival

S. Theoharis, G. Kouraklis, D. Mantas, A. Margeli, A. Glinavou, G. Karatzas, A. Koutselinis

2nd Department of Propedeutic Surgery, University of Athens, Greece

Introduction: Focal adhesion kinase (FAK) is an enzyme of the tyrosine kinase group linked to signaling pathways between cells and their extracellular matrix. It has previously been reported that FAK expression in tumor cells was correlated with their ability for invasion and metastasis.
Methods: In the present study, FAK expression was examined immunohistochemically in 80 cases of colon adenocarcinoma and was correlated with clinicopathological parameters, tumor proliferative capacity (reflected by Ki-67 protein expression) and patient's survival.
Results: All tumor samples were FAK positive compared with normal colonic mucosa, while FAK overexpression was evident in 32 out of 80 cases (40%). FAK overexpression was not correlated with tumor grade ($p=0.188$), or stage ($p=0.988$) or ki-67 positivity ($p=0.242$) or ki-67 overexpression ($p=0.066$) or patient's survival ($p=0.498$).
Conclusions: Up-regulation of FAK protein expression was noted in human colon carcinoma. As all cancerous tissue samples were FAK positive compared with the normal colonic mucosa, our data give evidence for participation of this protein at the early phases of malignant transformation. Although FAK overexpression was not correlated with any of the parameters examined and patient's survival, the aberrant expression of this molecule makes it a rational target for future cancer therapeutic approaches.

19

PPAR-γ Expression in Colon Cancer Patients and Correlation with Cell Cycle-Related Molecules

S. Theoharis, G. Kouraklis, D. Mantas, A. Margeli, A. Glinavou, G. Karatzas, A. Koutselinis

2nd Department of Propedeutic Surgery, University of Athens, Greece

Introduction: Peroxisome Proliferator Activated Receptor-gamma (PPAR-γ), a ligand-activated transcription factor, is a key regulator of adipogenic differentiation and glucose homeostasis. PPAR-γ ligands have recently been demonstrated to affect proliferation and differentiation in cancer cell lines.
Methods: In the present study, PPAR-γ expression was examined immunohistochemically in 89 cases of colon cancer and was correlated with clinicopathological parameters, tumor proliferative capacity, cell cycle related molecules and patient's survival.
Results: Positive PPAR-γ immunostaining was prominent in 47 out of 89 cases (56%) and negative in the rest. PPAR-γ positivity was not correlated with Duke's stage, histological grade of differentiation, lymph node and liver metastasis, venous invasion, tumor proliferative capacity and patient's survival. Statistically significant correlation was found between PPAR-γ expression and the cell cycle related molecules: pRb ($p=0.002$), cyclin D1 ($p=0.002$), p16 ($p=0.042$), p21 ($p=0.052$) and cyclin E ($p=0.009$). The pattern, intensity and extent of PPAR-γ positivity were not correlated to any of the examined variables.
Conclusions: Our findings support evidence for participation of this protein in the biological mechanisms underlying the carcinogenic evolution in the colon, suggesting also the importance of specific PPAR-γ ligands as cell cycle modulators for future therapeutic approach in colon cancer.

20

Analysis of 426 Cases of Gastrectomy for Primary Gastric Cancer in a Single Institution: The Feasibility of Proximal Gastrectomy

S. Okamoto, S. Yokoyama, T. Kamigaito, M. Shimoda, W. Sato, S. Yagi, F. Nishizawa, S. Uyama, H. Utsunomiya, H. Kato

First Department of Surgery, Japanese Red Cross Society Wakayama Medical Center, Wakayama, Japan

Introduction: A consecutive series of patients who underwent resection for primary gastric cancer were analysed retrospectively in order to elucidate the postoperative mortality, morbidity and survival with relation to the clinical stage and mode of operation. Furthermore, the feasibility of proximal gastrectomy with gastroesophagostomy was investigated.
Methods: Medical records of consecutive 426 patients who underwent resection for gastric cancer in the Japanese Red Cross Society Wakayama Medical Center between January 1996 and December 2000 were reviewed. The series consisted of 274 distal gastrectomy, 119 total gastrectomy and 33 proximal gastrectomy. Proximal gastrectomy was performed for the curative resection of primary gastric cancer in an early clinical stage located in the upper part of the stomach or for the palliative resection of advanced cancer with distant metastasis. Gastroesophagostomy using a double stapling technique was employed for the reconstruction.
Results: The mortality rates were 0.4%, 3% and 3% for distal, total and proximal gastrectomy, respectively. The postoperative hospital stay was 30±14 days (mean±SD), 42±21 days and 32±13 days for distal, total and proximal gastrectomy, respectively. As for postoperative complication the frequency of reflux esophagitis was significantly higher after proximal gastrectomy ($p<0.05$). Three year survival rates were 95%, 82%, 69%, 47%, 27% and 16% for stage IA, IB, II, IIIA, IIIB and IV (the Japanese classification of gastric carcinoma) after distal gastrectomy, 100%, 73%, 67%, 31%, 27% and 7% for stage IA, IB, II, IIIA, IIIB and IV after total gastrectomy, and 94% and 100% for stage IA and IB after proximal gastrectomy, respectively.
Discussion: Proximal gastrectomy was associated with higher incidence of reflux esophagitis, while total gastrectomy was related with longer hospital stay. For stage IA or IB cancer proximal gastrectomy provided comparable survival rate to distal and total gastrectomy.
Conclusion: Proximal gastrectomy for stage IA and IB cancer provided comparable survival to total gastrectomy and was associated with higher incidence of reflux esophagitis and shorter hospital stay compared with total gastrectomy. The postoperative nutritional advantage in proximal gastrectomy to total gastrectomy is to be evaluated.

21

Immediate Postoperative Immune Response in Histamine H1 and H2 C57BL/6J Knockout Mice

M. García-Caballero, K. Nakano, H. Suzuki, J.M. Martínez-Moreno, Y. Takagawa, I. Nakashima

Department of Surgery, University Malaga, Facultad de Medicina, 29080 Malaga, Spain

Introduction: Some evidences have clearly demonstrate that surgery induces suppression of cellular immunity. On the other hand, histamine exerts a variety immunoregulatory actions. These actions of histamine may be mediated by various lymphokines synthesized in the cells in response to histamine. The objective of this work is to study the effect of the administration of ranitidine to normal mice as well as the use of H1 and H2 gene knockout mice in the postoperative immune response after abdominal surgery.
Material and methods: We used 16 normal C57BL/6J both sexes mice, 8 C57BL/6J both sexes H1 gene knockout mice and 8 C57BL/6J both sexes H2 gene knockout mice. The animals aged 8 weeks and were approximately 25 g weight. The 32 animals were distributed in 8 groups (n=4): 1) Control; 2) Anaesthesia only; 3) Surgery 24 h; 4) Surgery 72 h; 5) Surgery in H1 KO 24 h; 6) Surgery in H1 KO 72 h; 7) Surgery in H2 KO 24 h; and 8) Surgery in H2 KO 72 h. In the operative groups, we performed a middle laparotomy followed by a right hemicolectomy. After experimental period, the animals were sacrified and spleen cells isolated for analysis. In these cells we determined CD4, CD8, CD4/CD8, CD90 and CD45R lymphocyte subsets in two millions spleen cells by flow cytometry. Three millions spleen cells per well were incubated without or with Concanavalin A during 24 h for determining the levels of IL-4, IL-10, IL-12 and IFN-gamma by ELISA. Statistical comparisons were performed by Mann-Whitney and Wilcoxon tests, and correlation analysis using Pearson test.
Results: After the induction of anaesthesia or 24 hours after surgery we measured a decrease in CD4 and an increase in CD8 T cells and CD4/CD8. This decrease in CD4 is even double more significant in H1 and H2 KO mice than in normal mice, although in these cases is accompanied by no increase or even decrease of CD8. Only in H2 KO we measured also a significant decrease in the total number of T and B cells. Surgery provoke an increase in IL-4, IL-10 and IFN-gamma and a decrease in IL-12 levels. These changes are 2 to 3 times greater in H2 and H1 KO mice in this order.
Conclusions: These first findings working with H1 and H2 knockout mice show the important role played by histamine in the differentiation, proliferation and activity of immune cells.

Organ and Tissue Transplantation I

22

The Effect of FR167653 on Warm Ischemia/Reperfusion Injury of the Liver Graft from NHBD

S. Miyagi, N. Ohkohchi, K. Oikawa, M. Satoh, S. Tsukamoto, S. Satomi

Division of Advanced Surgical Science and Technology, Tohoku University, Sendai, Japan

Introduction: Liver transplantation has become a standard therapy for end-stage liver diseases. But shortage of donor became big problem all over the world. Recently some institutes tried to carry out transplantation from non-heart-beating donor clinically, but the criteria and the retrieval procedure of the graft from non-heart beating donor (NHBD) are not established yet. The purpose of this study is a to investigate the cytoprotective effects of FR167653, which is a suppressant of the release of TNF-α and IL-1β, and protease inhibitor on warm ischemia/reperfusion injury and establish the procurement of the graft for successful liver transplantation from NHBD.
Methods: Male Wistar rat was used. Liver with/without agonal condition was retrieved and perfused for 60 minutes with Krebs-Henseleit bicarbonate buffer after 6 hr cold preservation. Animals were divided into four groups (n=5): HB group, liver was isolated from a heart beating donor and was perfused after 6 hr cold preservation; NHB group, liver was isolated from a non-heart beating donor and was perfused after 6 hr preservation; FR group, liver was isolated from non-heart beating donor pretreated with FR167653 (2 mg/kg) and was perfused 6 hr preservation; FR+NM group, liver was isolated from non-heart beating donor pretreated with FR167653 and liver graft was rinsed with nafamostat mesilate, which contained a strong serine protease inhibitor, and perfused after preservation. Examination items: bile production, flow volume, cytokines (TNF-α, IL-1β) products of arachidonic cascade (thromboxane B2, 6-keto prostaglandin-F1) in perfusate and transcriptional regulators (NF-κB, AP-1, STAT-3) of the tissue were measured. Histological findings were also investigated.
Results: Flow volume and bile production of NHB group decreased significantly compared with those in HB group, but those of FR and FR+NM groups were maintained as the same level of HB group. In NHB group, values of TNF-α, IL-1β, and thromboxane B_2, expressions of NF-κB, AP-1, and STAT-3 were significantly higher but those values of FR and FR+NM groups were low the same as in HB group. In NHB group sinusoidal endothelial cells were completely destroyed, hepatocytes were swollen. On the other hand, in both FR and FR+NM groups the structure of sinusoids was well preserved and sinusoidal lumen was maintained wide as same as those in HB group.
Conclusion: The suppression of TNF-α and IL-1β and administration of protease inhibitor was strongly associated with maintenance of sinusoidal microcirculatory structure in the liver graft from NHBD.

23

Transplantation of Hepatocytes - Elimination of Granulocytes and Monocytes Prevents Early Loss of Grafted Cells

W.L. Olszewski, A. Rudowska, M. Durlik

Dept. of Surgical Res. and Transplantation, Medical Research Center, Polish Academy of Sciences, Warsaw, Poland

Introduction: Only a few hepatocytes transplanted (HCtx) in suspension to tissues and body cavities survive compared to the large numbers of implanted cells. This untoward reaction of the recipient makes the method still of little use clinically. The destruction of both autologous and allogeneic HC takes place intravascularly as well as in spleen, liver, subcutis or peritoneal cavity. The question arises whether lysis of HC is an intrinsic property of leukocytes to scavenge isolated 'naked' organ cells with cadherin-exposed surface.
Aim: We investigated the *in vivo* and *in vitro* process of destruction of isolated HC by autologous polymorphonuclear (PMN) and mononuclear cells (PBM), and defined the phenotypes of cytolytic cells. Moreover, we depleted recipients of leukocytes by lethal irradiation, reconstituted with bone marrow cells (BMC) and followed the fate of txHC.
Methods: HC were isolated according to Seglen's method. *In vivo* loss of ^{51}Cr-labeled HC was measured in normal recipients and after pretreatment with Endoxan or sublethal irradiation. On histology, txHC and phenotypes of infiltrating leukocytes were evaluated in spleen, liver and subcutis. The *in vitro* PMN-HC and PBM-HC rosette formation rate and HC lysis in rosettes was measured. The phenotypes of PBM in rosettes with HC were determined by labeling with ED1, W3/13, W3/25, OX8 and OX6 moAbs. Chemotaxis of PMN and PBM to HC was measured in Boyden's chamber. LPS level in HC was estimated in a Limulus amebocyte lysis test. In other groups, depletion of blood leukocytes was obtained by 8Gy irradiation. On day 3, syngeneic BMC (10^7) were infused i.v. and 10^7 HC transplanted into spleen parenchyma. Histological evaluation was performed on day 14 and 21.
Results: Only around 10% of HC-bound radioactivity was recovered 6 h after i.v. tx in all lymphoid organs. In Endoxan-treated and irradiated rats radioactivity level was higher in spleen and livers, pointing to trapping non-lysed HC in these organs. Within 1 h 70% of HC were found in rosettes with PMN, 46% with PBM and below 20% with E. The percentage of lysed HC in rosettes with PMN was 70% and with PBM 55%. Lysis of control HC was below 10%. The main leukocyte phenotypes in rosettes were PMN and ED1 monocytes. The PMN and PBM were not attracted to HC in chemotaxis test and LPS level was negligible. On histology, PMN and ED1 were the most frequent infiltrating cells. Only few scattered HC could be identified in spleens on day 7 and 14. In contrast, in rats lethally irradiated and BMC-reconstituted dense foci of txHC could be shown in spleen and subcutis on day 14. In some cases, subcapsular liver tissue with glycogen-rich HC, Kupffer cells and portal triads could be seen.
Conclusion: Elimination of the initial attack of PMN and PBM on intrasplenic transplanted HC facilitates their take and proliferation.

24

Impact of Graft Rearterialization after Auxiliary Partial Orthotopic Liver Transplantation (APOLT) in the Treatment of Acute Liver Failure

J. P. Hölzen, D. Palmes, T. Budny, K.H. Dietl, H. Herbst, H.U. Spiegel

Surgical Research, Dept. of Surgery, Münster University Hospital, Münster, Germany

Introduction: The aim of this study was to investigate the impact of graft rearterialization after auxiliary partial orthotopic liver transplantation (APOLT) in the treatment of acute liver failure (ALF).
Methods: 35 Lewis rats were randomly divided into group I (ALF without therapy), group II (ALF treated by APOLT without graft rearterialization) and group III (ALF treated by APOLT with graft rearterialization). In all groups the ALF was induced by a 90% hepatectomy with only 50% of the quadrate lobe remaining. The left liver lobe of the donor rat served as auxiliary graft and was orthotopically implanted with graft rearterialization using an aortic segment (group III). Postoperatively, liver function and survival were observed until the 14th day (Kruskall-Wallis-test, $p<0.05$).
Results: Acute liver failure without therapy led to the death of all animals within 2 days. After APOLT, 80% of all animal survived until the 14th day showing significantly decreased liver enzymes. After 14 days the native liver was 5-fold enlarged showing signs of hyperplasia. The lack of graft rearterialization led to increased cholestatic parameters and a secondary biliary fibrosis 2-4° corresponding to Ruwart after 14 days. In contrast to this in group III the normal histoarchitecture of the graft could be preserved until the 14th day by graft rearterialization.
Conclusion: In this model the lack of graft rearterialization caused a progressive graft dysfunction. The consequences after APOLT depend on the regeneration and function of the native liver: in case of an insufficient native liver function an immediate retransplantation is required. In case of an advanced native liver regeneration the progressive failure of the auxiliary graft can be compensated by the native liver and furthermore avoid functional competition between the graft and the native liver after APOLT.

25

Synergistic Value of Fibrinolysis and Hypothermic Aerobic Preservation with O_2 in the Protection of Livers from Non Heart Beating donors

R.H. Tolba, S. Akbar, M. Sitzia, T. Minor

Division of Surgical Research, Dep. of Surgery, University of Bonn, Germany

Introduction: Chronic organ shortage has led to the reconsideration of marginal donor pools such as non heart beating donors (NHBD). The use of livers from this donors is limited due to the small tolerance of this organs during the hypothermic preservation. Aim of this study was to examine the combination of two different therapy strategies for the preservation of livers from NHBD to expand the donor pool.
Materials and Methods: Livers of male Wistar rats were harvested 30 or 90 min after the induction of cardiac arrest via phrenotomy in general anesthesia with Ketamin/Xylazin. All livers were perfused with 10 ml of UW solution (UW), followed by hypothermic preservation with or without insufflation of gaseous oxygen (O_2) via the vascular system. In one group a fibrinolytic pre-flush with 10 ml of Ringer's containing 7500 IU of streptokinase at 22°C was performed with subsequent preservation with O_2 (O_2+SK). All livers were stored for 24h at 4°C in UW. To assess the liver viability, all livers were reperfused *in vitro* at constant flow (3ml/g/min) with oxygenated Krebs-Henseleit-buffer at 37 °C for 45min. Livers, retrieved from heart beating donors with no warm ischemia served as controls (Con). To account for the period of rewarming during the surgical implantation, all livers were stored for 30 min at room temperature (22°C) prior to reperfusion.
Results: (n=5; Mean±SD. Statistics: ANOVA and SNK-Test)

	PVP (mmHg)	ALT (mU/g/l)
Con	4.1±0.5	683±152
30 min WI	7.4±0.2*	26819±513*
90 min WIO_2	4.8±0.8#	3204±549#
90 min WI+O_2+SK	3.8±0.65ns#	1623±432 ns#

	Bile-flow(µl/g/45min)	GLDH(mU/g/l)
Con	19.36±2.16	86±5
30 min WI	1.21±0.35*	399±14*
90 min WIO_2	7.15±1.33ns#	532±131ns#
90 min WI+O_2+SK	15.8±2.0 ns#	193±82 ns#

(* $p<0.05$ vs Con; # $p<0.05$ vs 30 min WI).
Discussion: These results show a serious disturbance of vascular perfusion (portal venous pressure, PVP) even after only 30 min of warm ischemia, associated with a 10 fold increase in enzyme release, which was in line with the significant depression of liver function (bile). However, these impairments could be prevented with O_2 after 30 min of WI and even after 90 min WI the function is significantly better by the use of aerobic preservation. With a supplementary fibrinolytic pre-flush we could preserve livers effectively after up to 90 min of WI with results comparable to livers from heart beating donors with no warm ischemia. The combination of these two techniques is a new therapeutic approach for the use of livers after extended or unclear periods in non-heart beating donors.

26

Effect of a Novel Potent Cytokine Suppressor on Toxic Liver Syndrome in the Pig Treated by Auxiliary Partial Orthotopic Liver Transplantation for Fatal Fulminant Hepatic Failure

S. Ishiguro, Y. Takada, K. Seino, H. Taniguchi, T. Kawamoto, K. Yuzawa, M. Otsuka, T. Todoroki, K. Fukao

Dept. of Surgery, Institute of Clinical Medicine, University of Tsukuba, Tsukuba City Ibaraki, Japan

Introduction: Auxiliary partial orthotopic liver transplantation (APOLT) for fulminant hepatic failure (FHF) has the outstanding advantages of permanently stopping immunosuppressive therapy with withdrawal of the auxiliary graft and allowing recovery of full native liver function. However, it is supposed that "toxic liver syndrome", in which devitalized liver tissue may have adverse effects on the graft, can lead to considerable morbidity and mortality in some clinical cases. The "cytokine storm" may be one of the causes of the toxic liver syndrome. ONO-SM-362 is a novel potent cytokine suppressor which strongly inhibits releasing tumor necrosis factor alpha (TNF-α) and interleukin-6 (IL-6). The purpose of this study was to evaluate the effect of ONO-SM-362 on the graft function of the pigs after APOLT procedure for fatal FHF.

Methods: Male pigs weighing 15 to 20 kg were used. To induce FHF, pigs were intraportally administered 0.1 mg/kg of α-amanitin (AMA), toxin extracted from the mushroom *amanita phalloides*, and 1 microgram/kg of lipopolysaccharide (LPS). Pigs were divided into four groups. In group 1, a control FHF group, pigs received no treatment after the induction of FHF. In groups 2, 3 and 4, pigs underwent left hemihepatectomy after administration of toxins and received APOLT procedure 8, 24 and 24 hours after induction of FHF, respectively. Just before starting APOLT procedure, pigs in group 4 were intraportally administered 0.3mg/kg ONO-SM-362.

Results: Group 1 pigs showed a number of clinically relevant features of FHF (including elevated liver enzymes, coagulopathy, metabolic disorder and encephalopathy) and all of them died within 5 days after the toxin injection. All of the pigs in group 2 survived more than two weeks after APOLT. On the other hand, all of the pigs in group 3 died within 5 days after the transplantation. By using ONO-SM-362, group 4 pigs showed 100% two weeks survival with sufficient graft function. Regeneration of the diseased native liver was histologically confirmed in group 2 and 4.

Discussion: The difference in outcome between groups 2 and 3 was associated with the timing of APOLT. Although pigs in group 2 were successfully treated with APOLT, group 3 pigs died of graft failure immediately after the transplantation which were performed at the more aggravated state of FHF. The better survival in group 4 suggests that suppression of the cytotoxic cytokines by ONO-SM-362 could improve the graft function.

Conclusion: A novel potent cytokine suppressor ONO-SM-362 improved the graft function after APOLT procedure against fatal FHF.

27

Can we Guarantee the Safety of Donor Operation in Living Donor Liver Transplantation? Analysis of 52 Donors

N. Ohkohchi, M. Shoji, K. Fujimori, N. Kawagishi, S. Tsukamoto, S. Satomi

Division of Advanced Surgical Science and Technology, Graduate School of Medicine, Tohoku University, Sendai, Japan

Introduction: In living donor liver transplantation, safety of the donor operation should be guaranteed. We retrospectively evaluated the safety of donor operation according to blood loss, blood transfusion, operation time, duration of hospitalization, and complications.

Subjects and Methods: Fifty-two of donors for living donor liver transplantation (LDLTx) received the liver resection in Tohoku University Hospital from July 1991 to December 2001. Age ranged from 17 to 64 year old and ratio of male/female was 25/27. Donor operations were classified into four groups as follows, I) lateral segment (LS) group: the graft was the lateral segment (n=24), II) left lobe (LL) group: the graft was the left lobe without the middle hepatic vein (n=17), III) left lobe with the middle hepatic vein (LLM) group: the graft was the left lobe with the middle hepatic vein (n=10), and IV) right lobe (RL) group: the graft was the right lobe without the middle hepatic vein (n=1). Examination items: blood loss, blood transfusion, operation time, liver function tests after operation, duration of hospitalization, and complications. All the donors stored the 400 ml of autologous blood before operation.

Results: Mean value of blood loss was 496 ml in LS group, 720 ml in LL group, 1266 ml in LLM group ($p<0.05$: vs LS and LL group) and 1005 ml in RL group. In all groups serum bilirubin increased up to 2-3 mg/dl a few days after the donation but no significant differences were recognized among the four groups and values decreased within a normal range in a few weeks. In LS Group mean operation time was 7.3 hours, which was 2-3 hours less than those of the other three groups ($p<0.05$: vs LL and LLM group). Requirement of autologous blood transfusion in LS group was also significantly less, compared with the other three groups. 21 of 52 donors donor did not receive blood transfusion. Only one donor needed the heterologous blood transfusion. Duration of total hospitalization was from 10 to 15 days in all groups except 5 donors who had complications. Even in RL group the donors were discharged on the 8th post operative day and liver function tests became within a normal range two weeks after the operation. Major complications following the donor operation were bile leakage in 5, abdominal abscess in 2, and prolongation of liver dysfunction in 1, but all these complication occurred within early period from the beginning of LDLTx. These complications were overcome within 3 months and all the donors were doing well without any abnormal laboratory data.

Conclusion: Safety of the donor operation is guaranteed when every lobe of the liver is used as the graft for LDLTx, but in meticulous management of the operation is required for prevention for complications.

Organ and Tissue Transplantation II

28

Sensitivity, Specificity and Prognostic Value of E-Cadherin During Preservation of the Porcine Pancreas with Histidine-Tryptophan-Ketoglutarate Solution or University of Wisconsin Solution

P. Demetter, R. Troisi, C. van den Broecke, C.A. Cuverlier, U.J. Hesse

Ghent University Hospital, Ghent, Belgium

Background: The adhesion molecule E-cadherin is important for the maintenance of normal epithelial integrity and inflammatory conditions. We have recently reported that porcine pancreas epithelial integrity after flushing segmental pancreatic grafts with either HTK (histidine-tryptophan-ketoglutarate) solution or UW (University of Wisconsin) solution can be correlated to cytoplasmic or epithelial expression of E-cadherin in exocrine tissue. It was the purpose of this study to detail and quantify these findings to define its sensitivity, specificity and the predictive value.

Methods: Segmental porcine pancreatic grafts were flushed with either HTK (n=9) or UW (n=4) solution. Grafts were autotransplanted after 24 (n=9) or 48 (n=3) hr of cold storage. Routine haematoxylin-eosin staining and immunohistochemical staining for E-cadherin (clone 36, Transduction Laboratories) were performed at time of pancreatectomy, before reperfusion, at time of reperfusion and 30 minutes after reperfusion. Daily glucose values (<100 mg/dl) and an intravenous glucose tolerance test were performed to evaluate metabolic control. The Student's T-test and a Fischer exact test were used ($p< 0.05$ significant) for statistical analysis. The stainings were evaluated by 2 independent pathologists and scored from 0 to 3+ at 100 to 400x magnification (Piaciucci at al Am. J. Pathol. 1998).

Results: E-cadherin was expressed in 4/9 (44%) on the membrane and 4/9 (44%) in cytoplasm in non-functioning grafts and in 5/5 (100%) on the membrane and 4/5 (80%) in cytoplasm of functioning grafts ($p=0.078$). Simultaneous membraneous and cytoplasmic expression was present in 0/9 (0%) of non-functioning and 4/5 (80%) of functioning grafts ($p=0.005$). PPV=1, NPV=0.2, Sensitivity 80%, Specificity 100%.

Conclusion: Simultaneous membraneous and cytoplasmic E-cadherin expression on the acinar tissue is present in functioning pancreatic grafts after perfusion and storage with HTK or UW with a sensitivity of 80% and a specificity of 100% and a positive predictive value of 1 indicating that loss of exocrine cell integrity is responsible for impaired graft function.

29

Functional and Immunogenic Changes of Human Fetal Pancreatic Islet Following Long-Term Cultivation

G. Farkas[1], J. Csanády[4], Y. Mándi[2], A. Pál[3]

Department of Surgery[1], Institute of Microbiology[2], Department of Gynecology and Obstetrics[3], University of Szeged, Faculty of Medicine, Szeged; and Department of Pathology[4], County Hospital, Kalocsa, Hungary

Introduction: Transplantation of human fetal pancreas is a viable alternative method for the cure of diabetes. Earlier studies have shown that our long-term culturing method is efficient in increasing the islet mass by producing pseudoislet. In the present study the effects of long-term culturing on the islet function and immunogenicity were examined.

Methods: Fetal pancreatic islets were isolated from 10 human embryos aged 18-22 weeks following spontaneous abortion by modified collagenase digestion technique and were cultured in Eagle's medium supplemented with 20% human AB serum and L-glutamine for 10 weeks at 37°C in 5% CO_2 in air. The hormone production of different islet cells was measured by glucagon, insulin and somatostatin RIA, and the morphometric changes were determined by immunocytochemistry. The islet MHC class II expression was examined by immunostaining of the islet with monoclonal antibody (Dianova, Hamburg, Germany).

Results: During the long-term culturing period the glucagon production decreased continuously (from 375±31 to 8.5±1.25 pg/ml), the somatostatin concentration increased slightly (from 47±5.1 to 62.5±6.5 pg/ml) and the insulin release was almost continuous (325±12 µU/ml). The different hormone productions correlated with the results of the immunocytochemical examinations on the islets: no glucagon positivity, an increased somatostatin positivity and constant insulin positivity of the cells were noted. Following the 10-week culturing, the effective elimination of intraislet class II MHC positive cells was proved by immunostaining of the islets.

Conclusion: These results indicate that long-term cultivation presents a useful method not only for increasing the islet mass, but also for changing the ratio of different cells i.e. reducing the immunogenicity, which can provide more possibility for the successful clinical islet transplantation. Supported by grants from ETT 5K090 A 1 30 2000 and Hungarian Széchenyi Research Grant.

30

Successful Islet Xenotransplantation Following Macrophage Blockade Induced by Repeated Gadolinium Chloride Injections in Rats

A. Paszt, G. Farkas, Z. Szász, G. Lázár Jr., J. Csanády, G. Lázár

Department of Surgery, University of Szeged, Faculty of Medicine, Szeged, Hungary

Introduction: The immunologic consequences of xenogenic islet transplantation remain unsolved. Gadolinium chloride ($GdCl_3$) depresses the reticuloendothelial activity, selectively blocking the function of the hepatic Kupffer cells. In this work, the effects of $GdCl_3$-induced long-term Kupffer cell blockade on the survival of human fetal islet xenografts were investigated.

Materials and Methods: Cultured fetal human islets (18 weeks old; 800 islets) were transplanted through the portal vein into the liver of male, inbred CFY rats with streptozotocin-induced diabetes. 24 hr before grafting and 2 and 4 weeks following islet transplantation, 8 diabetic rats were treated repeatedly with 1 mg/100 g body weight $GdCl_3$, while the control diabetic rats were untreated (n=6).

Results: In the control, $GdCl_3$-untreated transplanted rats, the decrease in blood glucose level was only transitory. In contrast, in the repeatedly $GdCl_3$-treated rats transplanted with human fetal islets, the normoglycemic condition remained for as long as 5 weeks during the observation period (blood glucose 5.98±1.78 mmol/l). Histologically, human fetal islets were seen in the liver of the rats treated with $GdCl_3$, without any inflammatory cell reaction. No human fetal islets were observed in the liver of the diabetic control rats not treated with $GdCl_3$.

Conclusion: These studies suggest that the Kupffer cells play significant roles in the recognition of xenoantigens and in the induction of xenograft rejection. The long-term Kupffer cell blockade promotes successful long-lasting islet xenotransplantation. Supported by grants from ETT 5K090 A 1 30 2000 and Hungarian Széchenyi Research Grant.

31

The Use of Octreotide in Pancreatic Transplants with Enteric Drainage: Results of a Prospective Randomised Single Centre Trial

H. van der Bracht, D. Meester, R. Troisi, B. Jacobs, B. de Hemptinne, N. Lameire, U.J. Hesse

Ghent University Hospital, Ghent, Belgium

Introduction: Pancreatic fistula from the capsule or an insufficiency of the anastomosis for pancreatic drainage either into the bladder or the intestine can have detrimental consequences for the outcome in pancreas transplantation. Octreotide has been recommended in the prophylaxis of fistula development in pancreatic transplantation, however the results are controversial. It was the purpose of this study to investigate the effect of octreotide in the perioperative course of pancreas transplants in terms of fistula formation, reflux-pancreatitis, hemorrhage and thrombosis.
Patients and methods: A total of 35 pancreas transplant recipients were prospectively randomised to either receive or not to receive octreotide 0.1 mg subcutaneously at the time of operation and 3x/day thereafter until day 7 postoperatively. The incidence of pancreatic leakage from the anastomosis or the content of peritoneal fluid drainage regarding amylase and lipase collected by abdominal drains were registered on day 0-10. Both groups were comparable for age, sex, onset of diabetes and surgical procedure.
Results: There were 33 simultaneous pancreatic-kidney transplants and 2 pancreas after kidney transplants. All had enteric drainage. 18 patients received octreotide and 17 did not. In 1 patient, receiving octreotide the pancreas had to be removed for septic complications due to an enteric fistula arising from the anastomosis (1/18 = 6%). The incidence on patients on octreotide versus non octreotide was 1 vs 0 for reflux-pancreatitis, 2 vs 3 for hemorrhage and 2 vs 1 for thrombosis resulting in a patient survival of 100 % in both groups and a pancreas survival of 89% vs 94 %. The amylase and lipase content into the peritoneum on day 0 to 10 post-operatively indicating pancreatic fistulisation was comparable in both groups except for day 6 (1076±591 U/l vs 333±235 U/l, $p=0.02$).
Conclusion: The use of octreotide following pancreas transplantation did not prevent pancreatic fistula formation from the anastomosis neither from the pancreatic capsule in pancreas transplantation. The adverse effect of octreotide for the occurrence of reflux pancreatitis and thrombosis has to be confirmed in a larger trial.

32

The Incidence of Rejection with Quadruple Immunosuppression, Including ATG or IL2 Antibodies and Mycophenolate Mofetil (MMF) Following Simultaneous Pancreas and Kidney (SPK) Transplantation

U.J. Hesse, B. Jacobs, R. Troisi, B. van Vlem, B. de Hemptinne, R. van Holder, F. Vermassen, J. de Roose, N. Lameire

Ghent University Hospital, Ghent, Belgium

Introduction: The multicenter EURO SPK I trial comparing TAC and CyA following simultaneous pancreas kidney transplantation reports a 40% rejection rate. This single center study analyses the frequency and clinical relevance of allograft rejection in SPK patients receiving ATG or the IL2 receptor antibody (Basiliximab) induction therapy, CyA, MMF and steroid based immunosuppression. Between 15/1994 and 01/01/2002, 47 consecutive patients received a pancreas transplant (SPK=44) (PAK=3) at our institution with a mean±SD age of 42±7.5 years, 32 males, 15 females. Out of these 33 patients were treated with ATG Fresenius (Rabbit) 3-5 mg/Kg for a mean±SD of 4±2 days, Cyclosporine Neoral (CyA) (trough levels 350-4000 ng/ml), MMF 3 g/day and low dose steroid therapy. 14 SPK patients were treated with Basiliximab (Simulect, Novartis 20 mg on day 0 and 4 days post-transplantation) instead of ATG. The patients had an average HLA mismatch of 3.9/6 and a negative cross match. All patients remained on triple drug therapy. Five patients were switched to FK instead of Neoral for CyA intolerance. The mean±SD cold ischemia time of the organs was for the pancreas 10.0±2.5 hours and for the kidney 9.7±3.3 hours.
Results: Biopsy proven rejection occurred in the kidney of 5 ATG-patients (15%) and responded to steroid bolus therapy. Two patients (15%) with Basiliximab induction developed renal allograft rejection which resolved after treatment. All patients except 2 patients (95%) were free from rejection in the pancreas as measured by urine amylase levels and glycemic control without the need of exogenous insulin with a mean HBA1C of 6.2±2.1% and a serum creatinine of 1.5±0.9 mg/dl in a mean follow-up period of 22±12 months (median 24, range 2-79).
Conclusion: Triple drug immunosuppression including Cyclosporine, MMF and low dose steroids with ATG or IL2 receptor antibodies induction therapy appears to be a very suitable immunosuppressive regimen for combined pancreas-kidney transplantation and PAK with a marked reduction in the incidence of rejection.

33

Acute Small Bowel Rejection and Mucosal Perfusion in CD4, CD40 and CD28 Knockout Mice

G. Dindelegan, H. Liden, G. Kurlberg, O. Nilsson, A. Aneman, N. Lycke, M. Olausson

Institute for Surgical Sciences, Department of Surgery, Göteborg University, Göteborg, Sweden

Introduction: The relative importance of CD4 T cells and CD40 and CD28 pathways in allograft rejection remains controversial. Experimental studies suggest that different T-cell subsets may have different roles in rejection, depending on the model used and the organ studied. The intestine is the most immunogeneic organ compared to all other solid organs. This unusually strong immune response may be related to different mechanisms of rejection. The aim of this study is to compare acute intestinal rejection in wild-type mice to rejection in CD4-/-, CD40-/- and CD28-/- mice. We have previously shown that acute small bowel rejection in the mouse is clearly defined by histology and by mucosal laser-Doppler flowmetry at 6 days postoperatively.
Methods: Intestinal allografts from Balb/c mice were heterotopically (paratopically) transplanted into C57BL/6 recipients using microsurgical technique. Recipient groups consisted of wild-type mice as well as CD4-/-, CD40-/- and CD28-/- mice. Mucosal perfusion was measured by laser-Doppler flowmetry at 6 days posttransplantation both in the native and in the grafted intestine. Histology specimens were obtained at the same time and graded for rejection.
Results: Acute rejection occurred in all groups. Significant difference in mucosal perfusion was noted between the graft and the native intestine inside each group. Graft perfusion was also significantly decreased in the CD28-/- group compared with graft perfusion in wild type group. On the other hand, no significant difference was noted in terms of graft perfusion between CD4-/-, CD40-/- and wild-type groups. Histology showed medium-grade rejection in wild-type, CD4-/- and CD40-/- groups but advanced rejection in CD28-/- group.
Conclusion: Our study demonstrates that the absence of CD4+ T cells, or the separate blockade of CD40 or CD28 pathways seem not to impair the acute rejection process in mice small bowel transplantation. Furthermore, blocking the CD28 pathway was subsequently followed by a stronger rejection compared with the wild-type or with CD4-/- and CD40-/- mice, probably by overreaction of other components involved in the acute intestinal rejection. This difference in rejection was demonstrated both by histology and by mucosal laser-Doppler flowmetry. The method of measuring mucosal blood flow by laser-Doppler proved to be a reliable indicator of acute rejection in small bowel transplantation.

34

Moderating of Oxidative Stress by Ischemic Preconditioning: Role of Cellular Signal Mechanisms in Small Bowel

A. Ferencz, B. Borsiczky, Z. Szántó, K. Kiss, J. Szeberényi, K. Kalmár-Nagy, Ö.P. Horváth, E. Rőth

Department of Experimental Surgery, Department of Surgery, Department of Medical Biology, Pécs University, Faculty of Medicine, Pécs, Hungary

Introduction: One cause of limitation of small bowel transplantation is that the intestine is extremely sensitive to ischemia-reperfusion injury. There are few data regarding the beneficial effect of preconditioning on ischemic tolerance of the bowel. We aimed to investigate, beside the protective effects of preconditioning the activation of cellular signal transduction mechanisms prior to autotransplantation.
Methods: In group I (GI) and group II (GII) total orthotopic intestinal autotransplantation was performed in 20 mongrel dogs. In GI grafts were perfused by mesenteric artery and stored in the cold University of Wisconsin solution. In GII before this procedure we preconditioned the intestine by 4 cycles of 5-min ischemia, 10-min reperfusion of the mesenteric artery was employed. In GI and GII after 3 hours of preservation, 1 hour of reperfusion was allowed to test graft viability. In group III (GIII) after laparotomy the intestines were preconditioned by 4 cycles without preservation. In GI and GII bowel samples were collected after laparotomy (control), and at the end of preservation and reperfusion periods. To monitor oxidative stress we determined malondialdehyde (MDA), reduced glutathione (GSH) concentrations and the activity of superoxide dismutase (SOD) in bowel tissue homogenates. In GIII we detected NF-κB activity after laparotomy (control); 15, 30 min and 1, 2, 3 hours followed by preconditioning in mucosal cells by gel electrophoretic mobility shift assay of mucosal cells.
Results: Our results showed that in non-preconditioned group the tissue GSH concentration increased slightly by the end of the reperfusion. The SOD activity decreased significantly during the same period (GI 266.3±16.2 control, to 110.2±37.7 IU/g $p<0.01$). In preconditioned group the GSH level elevated more markedly, indicating the activation of endogenous antioxidant system. We also observed better preservation of SOD activity (GII 192.4±14.3 IU/g). In GIII we detected the presence of NF-κB in control samples. However we observed gradual activation of NF-κB peaking by 1 to 2 hours, and falling 3 hours past preconditioning.
Discussion: One of the methods to reduce oxidative stress of small intestine is by way of ischemic preconditioning. Our findings confirm protection is afforded by preconditioning prior to small bowel preservation, moderating the severity of oxidative stress and activating endogenous cellular adaptation. This model demonstrates that activation of transcription factor NF-κB may play an important role at the field of these processes.
Conclusion: Ischemic preconditioning of the small bowel may open a new perspective for reducing ischemia-reperfusion injury, but further studies are needed to elucidate the mechanism of these changes.

35

Effects of Ischemic Preconditioning on the Graft Microcirculation During Small Bowel Transplantation

A. Wolfárd, J. Kaszaki, L. Szalay, S. Varga, Á. Balogh*, M. Boros*

Department of Surgery*, Institute of Surgical Research, University of Szeged, Szeged, Hungary

Introduction: In addition to immunologic reactions, ischemia-reperfusion injury of the intestine contributes to the high complication rate of small bowel transplantation (SBTX) and limit the widespread clinical application. Amelioration of reperfusion injury is an important experimental and clinical aim and ischemic preconditioning (IPC - short periods of ischemia and reperfusion before induction of longer ischemia) was found to be effective against reperfusion injury in several organs, including the small intestine. However, the exact macro-, and microcirculatory background and the underlying mechanisms are not yet fully understood. Therefore our study was designed to examine the most important macrohemodynamics and the microcirculatory parameters of the intestinal graft following small bowel autotransplantation with or without IPC.
Methods: Orthotopic SBTX was performed in two groups of mongrel dogs. In group 2 IPC was performed by clamping the superior mesenteric artery (3 times for 5 min) 60 min before ischemia induction. Superior mesenteric artery blood flow (SMAF) was continuously recorded, mucosal microcirculation and villus structure (thickness of the epithelial layer) was monitored with intravital videomicroscopy using orthogonal polarization spectral (OPS) imaging technique (Cytoscan A/R, Cytometrics, PA, U.S.A.). Functional capillary density (FCD) of the intestinal villi was calculated. Leukocyte-endothelial cell interactions (rolling and adherence) in the postcapillary venules of the mesentery were monitored with intravital fluorescent microscopy, leukocytes were stained with rhodamine 6G. Data evaluation was performed off-line, using a computer-software. For statistical analysis, non-parametric methods were used.
Results: SMAF decreased significantly during reperfusion as compared to pre-ischemic values. The fall in SMAF was significantly less in group 2 with IPC. The FCD of the villi decreased in group 1 during the reperfusion and IPC significantly attenuated this change. Significant epithelial shortening was detected in the I-R group and epithelial narrowing was less severe in the IPC group. Reperfusion was accompanied by an increase in leukocyte-endothelial cell interactions in the postcapillary venules and IPC significantly reduced both leukocyte rolling and adhesion.
Discussion: I-R induces a fall in SMAF, capillary hypoperfusion of the villi and leukocyte-endothelial cell interactions. IPC when applied 60 min before ischemia preserved SMAF, improved capillary perfusion, and attenuated leukocyte activation within the graft.
Conclusion: IPC significantly improves the intestinal microcirculation and reduces leukocyte-mediated tissue injury, thus it can be an effective tool to limit reperfusion injury during small bowel transplantation. Supported by Research Grant OTKA T035275

36

Protective Effects of Exogenous Fructose-1,6-biphosphate Added to University of Wisconsin Preservation Solution in Rat Intestinal Transplantation

A. Sola[1], J. de Oca[2], V. Alfaro[3], C. Xaus[1], G. Hotter[1]

Department of Medical Bioanalysis[1], IIBB-CSIC, IDIBAPS, Department of Surgery[2], C.S.U.B. Hospital "Princeps d´Espanya" University of Barcelona, Department of Physiology[3], Faculty of Biology, University of Barcelona, Barcelona, Spain

Introduction: F16BP is a high energy glycolytic intermediate therapeutically effective in ischemia and post-ischemic reperfusion. The aim of this study was to assess the protective effect of the addition of exogenous fructose-1,6-biphosphate (F16BP) to the preservation solution [University of Wisconsin storage solution (UW)] used during an experimental procedure of small bowel transplantation in rats.
Methods: We studied the levels of tissue nucleotides, the histological changes, and the associated deleterious processes such as bacterial translocation produced during cold ischemia, further transplantation and reperfusion period.
Results and Discussion: The groups of rats treated with F16BP showed the lower levels of hypoxanthine/xanthine and uric acid, the higher levels of adenosine, and the lower level of histological damage and lactate dehydrogenase (LDH) release to bloodstream. Consumption of intestinal hypoxanthine during reperfusion was lower in the groups treated with F16BP. Moreover, the incidence of bacterial translocation was lower in the groups treated with F16BP.
Conclusions: The addition of F16BP to UW solution provides protection to small intestinal tissue during experimental transplantation in rats, being this protection related to a reduced availability of substrates of xanthine oxidase (XO) for free radical generation during reperfusion.

37

Xanthine/Adenosine and NO Modifications During Rat Intestinal Cold Perservation Modulates the Apoptotic Response

M. Genesca, A. Sola, L Palacios, F. Pi, G. Hotter

Department of Medical Bioanalysis, IIBB-CSIC, IDIBAPS, Barcelona, Spain

Introduction: Tissue injury related to ischemic preservation can compromise the viability of the organ upon transplantation. The main factor determining graft survival in intestinal preservation is the duration of the ischemic process. During cold ischemia, mucosal damage has been attributed both necrosis and apoptosis. In this study, we have evaluated whether substances that are modified proportionally to the duration of the ischemic process (xanthine and adenosine) could determine cell demise (apoptosis/necrosis), and if adenosine effects could be mediated by NO.
Methods: A model of isolated perfused rat intestine was used. The following groups were done: Cold ischemic group (CI); CI+Xanthine, to assess the effect of xanthine; CI+Theophylline, to

evaluate the effect of adenosine by blocking its receptor; CI+Theophylline+Xanthine, to know the effect of xanthine by itself; and CI+Theophylline+NONOs to evaluate if the action of adenosine was mediated by NO. Measurement of xanthine and adenosine levels, caspase 3 activity, DNA fragmention and NO generation were done. Histological analysis were also assessed.
Results/Discussion: Xanthine treated rats showed increased levels of caspase-3 activity and DNA fragmentation. In contrast, in theophylline treated rats, decreased levels of these parameters were found. Administration of xanthine or NONOs to theophylline treated rats the observed effects were reverted. Histology evaluation agreed with the previous results.
Conclusions: Our study indicates that xanthine and adenosine induce the apoptotic response in cold ischemic preservation. The action of adenosine is mediated by NO.

Organ and Tissue Transplantation III

38

Different Pictures of Autogenous Infection and Rejection in Human Skin Allografts

W.L. Olszewski, M. Moscicka, D. Zolich

Dept. of Surgical Res. and Transplantation, Medical Research Center, Polish Academy of Sciences, Warsaw, Poland

Introduction: The human hand transplantation has revived the interest in the rejection process of grafted skin and its control with antirejection drugs. Clinical application of isolated skin grafts has so far been limited because of risk associated with high doses of immunosuppressive drugs required. The most important clinical conclusion from hand allografts was that large mass of allogeneic skin can be accepted and function as in a normal extremity. New problems have arisen from these observations. First, early diagnosis of skin rejection, the other, recognition of skin reaction against infection. The actual question is how to discriminate the alloreactive and inflammatory bacterial changes in the skin graft.
Aim: To study the biopsy pictures of rejecting and/or infected human skin.
Methods: Fragments of human skin from lower leg were transplanted to CB-17/SCID mice. After 14 days grafts were ready for further studies. Bacterial strains residing on skin surface were isolated and cultured. Human blood mononuclear cells allogeneic to the grafted skin were isolated. Group 1. 10^7 bacteria in 0.1 ml were injected intradermally. They were *E. coli*, *Staph. epidermidis*, *Aerococcus*, *Corynebacterium*, *Micrococcus*. Twenty-four and 72 h later skin fragments were harvested for histology. Group 2. 10^7 PBM were injected intradermally and biopsies taken 72 h and 144 h later for histology. Changes in graft epidermis and dermis as well as grafts bed were evaluated. For discrimination between mouse and human cell infiltrates, staining with mouse class I moAb was performed.
Results: Group 1. Advanced changes were seen after infection with *E. coli* and *Staph. epidermidis* but not other strains. The mid-portion of epidermal graft was affected. Subepidermal granulocyte infiltrates (+++) with focal necrosis of epidermis were seen. In dermis limited infiltrates (+) were observed. These infiltrates resolved after 72 h without treatment. Injected mouse skin bacterial strains did not produce any evident changes. Group 2. Intravenous injection of PBM caused major changes in dermis but not epidermis with necrosis and perivascular infiltrates. These were mostly mononuclear cells of human origin (mouse MHC I-negative). Seven days after administration of PBM the entire graft was necrotic. Intradermal injection of allogeneic PBM produced necrotic changes already on day 3, also affecting epidermis.
Conclusions: Autologous skin surface bacteria evoke subepidermal granulocyte infiltrates not affecting deeper layers of dermis. Allogeneic mononuclear cells injected i.v. produce major perivascular infiltrates, spread into entire dermis and cause its necrosis. These topographical and phenotypic differences may be helpful in evaluation of skin biopsies after limb transplantation.

39

The Mechanisms Involved in Initiation of Skin Allograft Rejection - Inhibition of Antigen Presentation by CsA and Prograf

J. Mijal, H. Galkowska, W.L. Olszewski

Dept. of Surgical Res. & Transplantation, Medical Research Center, Polish Academy of Sciences, Warsaw, Poland

Introduction: Skin allografts are acutely rejected even under high dosage of immunosuppressive drugs. The mechanism of this phenomenon remains unclear. It has been suggested that immunosuppressive chemicals are ineffective in downregulating the antigen presentation by skin veiled cells. Antigen presentation by skin veiled cells (VC) to lymphocytes (LY) proceeds through a direct contact of both cell types (cluster formation). Inhibition of clustering would presumably down regulate the alloantigen recognition in skin allografts. The question arises as to whether CsA or FK506 used *in vivo* or *in vitro* would inhibit VC-LY clustering.
Methods: Dog skin lymph served as a source of VC and LY. Dog blood served as a source mononuclear cells (MNC). Lymph was collected by cannulation of the hind limb lymphatics. In dogs with experimental lymphoedema it was obtained by direct percutaneous puncture of dilated lymphatics. In group 1, VC were cultured with allogeneic LY for 6 days. Then, clusters of VC with LY were disintegrated and put into 4 h cultures *de novo*. In group 2, CsA was injected into canine skin draining lymphatics, 3 times per week, to reach the lymph level of 0.43+0.32 mg/ml. On day 7, lymph collected, VC and LY isolated and cultured *in vitro* as in group 1. In group 3, VC and autologous LY were cultured *in vitro* as in group 1, but in the presence of normal lymph and lymph with CsA. In group 4, VC were cultured with autologous LY or allogeneic MNC, like in group 1. In group 5, VC were cultured with autologous LY or allogeneic MNC for 6 days in the presence FK506 at concentration of 0.4mg/ml. In group 6, VC were cultured with autologous LY or allogeneic MNC for 6 days in the presence normal lymph. In group 7, VC were cultured with LY or MNC in the presence FK506, in normal lymph.
Results: Group 1. There was 33.0+6.0 % of clusters formed after 4h incubation. Group 2. There were 30.2+6.0 % of clusters with VC-CsA treated cells and 34.3+7.4% in LY-CsA treated cultures (NS).

Group 3. There was no difference in cluster formation by autologous VC and LY in presence of normal lymph or lymph with CsA (39.3+18.1% and 43.3+5.8%, respectively). Group 4. There were 38% of clusters with autologous LY and 72% with allogeneic MNC. Group 5. There were 30% of clusters with autologous LY and 39.8% with allogeneic MNC, in the presence FK506 ($p<0.05$ compared with group 4). Group 6. There were 30% of cluster with LY and 66% with MNC. Group 7. There was a difference in cluster formation in comparison with group 5, with 12% of clusters with autologous LY and 48 % with allogeneic MNC, in the presence FK506 ($p<0.05$ compared with group 4).
Discussion and Conclusions: The *in vivo* treatment of VC or LY with CsA at concentrations used for routine allograft immunosuppression did not affect the cluster formation rate of cutaneous VC and allostimulated LY. CsA had no effect on autologous cell cluster formation *in vitro*. In contrast, FK506 was found a potent inhibitor of lymph cell clustering.

40

Damage of Graft by Ischemia and Rejection Results in Release of DNA and its Accumulation in Recipient Tissues

B. Interewicz, W.L. Olszewski, J. Stanislawska, E. Szyper, M. Maksymowicz

Dept. of Surgical Res. and Transplantation, Medical Research Center, Polish Academy of Sciences, Warsaw, Poland

Introduction: Warm and cold ischemia as well as immune rejection of transplanted organ or tissue bring about destructive changes in graft cells. Endothelial and parenchymal cells are affected. Fragments of disintegrated cellular organelles are phagocytized by recipient infiltrating macrophages and scavenger cells located in lymph nodes, spleen and liver. The question arises as to whether DNA from the damaged cells is enzymatically lyzed and eliminated or its fragments are retained in recipient phagocytic (macrophages, dendritic) cells. Beside the putative effect on immunity or tolerance the level of donor DNA in recipient blood and tissues may be a measure of the degree of damage of the transplanted organ.
Aim: To measure donor DNA in recipient tissues 7 days after transplantation of syngeneic and allogeneic organs and tissues.
Methods: Male BN (RT1An) and LEW (RT1Al) rats served as donors and female LEW (RT1Al) as recipients. Free skin flaps (SK), heart (H), bone marrow cells (BMC), bone marrow cell debris (BMCd) and naked DNA isolated from BMC were tx. Seven days later blood (B), bone marrow (BM), skin (SK), lymph node (LN), spleen (SPL), liver (L), and heart (H) were harvested. After isolation genomic DNA was amplified with rat Y sex determining region (Y-Sry) specific primers, PCR products were analysed by PAGE. The presence of donor DNA was expressed in OD units. Statistical analysis was done with 95 percent Tukey HSD.
Results: After grafting of syngeneic and allogeneic SK, H, BMC and BMCd donor DNA was detected in all analysed recipient tissues. Following i.v. injection of naked DNA, only its traces could be detected in recipient skin and lymph nodes. Comparing syngeneic and allogeneic grafts, there were no differences in donor DNA OD after H tx. In contrast, statistically significant differences in OD between syngeneic and allogeneic DNA, in favor of allogeneic, were found after SKtx in recipient skin 0.7 and 3.6, spleen 0.9 and 4.7 and heart 0.4 and 3.3, respectively. Following BMCtx the values for syngeneic and allogeneic DNA were in skin 0.3 and 5.8, and in spleen 2.1 and 6.3. In case of BMCd and naked DNAtx the levels of donor DNA were higher in recipient organs after syngeneic than allogeneic tx. Tx of BMCd brought about the DNA values in spleen 18.2 and 2.0, and in liver 17.4 and 1.8. Infusion of naked DNA was followed by its detection in spleen at levels of 1.33 and 0.15.
Conclusions: Donor DNA is present in recipient tissues at least 7 days after allo- and syngeneic grafting. Rejection of allografts is followed by higher levels of released donor DNA than following syngeneic tx. Syngeneic DNA may originate from ischemically damaged cells, whereas allogeneic DNA in addition from rejecting cells. Higher levels of syn- than allogeneic DNA after BMCd and naked DNA tx probably resulted from fast administration of material and various tempo of syn- and allo- DNA elimination.

41

Experimental Model of Heterotopic Uterus Transplantation in Rat

P.L. Jiga, C.M. Lupu, B.S. Zoica, M. Ionac

"Victor Babes" Univ. Med. Pharm., Timisoara, Romania

Introduction: Transplantation of genital organs is reserved today only to experimental work due to ethical and perceptual issues, since uterus is a life generating, rather than life sustaining organ. Although there might be indications for the transplantation of human genitalia, information regarding both the technique and the immunology in this field is still lacking.
Methods: Fifty adult female Sprague-Dawley rats with 200 g average weight were used as donors and recipients of the graft. Whole uterus and ovaries allograft based on aorta and both uterine vessels were transplanted heterotopically by standard microsurgical technique. The grafts were explanted at 24, 48, 72 hours. Standard hematoxilin-eosin and Masson coloration was used for microscopy. For the immunocytochemistry studies specific monoclonal antibody trays were used.
Results: Two animals died during the observation period and were excluded from the study. Postoperative survival was 100% at 24 hours. The anastomotic patency rate was 100% at 24 hours, 37% at 48 hours and 0% at 72 hours. The cellular appearance suggests an anaphylaxis phenomenon rather than the classical pattern of acute organ rejection.
Discussion: The rat is one of the standard animals used in studies regarding solid organ transplantation and transplant immunology. In the first report of transplantation of fallopian tube and ovary in rats Scheidel (1985) only half of the uterus and its ovary is used. Based on ovarian pedicle this model has the advantage of an easier harvesting technique. In contrast, this model presents the transplantation of the whole uterus and ovaries based on the uterine vessels. Although the harvesting technique is more difficult, it has the advantage of using the whole organ with both ovaries attached to it. The heterotopical placement of the graft (inguinal region) makes it more accessible for *in vivo* observation and biopsy.
Conclusion: Before clinical transplantation of the uterus it should be considered that there are important issues to be solved as toxic effects of immunosuppression on the embryo and other major psychological factors. The presented experimental model is proposed as a valid tool for further studies regarding this topic.

However, the mechanism for this reduction in bone stiffness remains unclear. To maintain bone quality in CTA, new treatment modalities that don't require irradiation or modern combination immunotherapy need to be evaluated.

42

Elastic Properties of Bone in Composite Tissue Allotransplantation

M. Vossen, G. Perez-Abadia, C. Maldonado, M.J. Voor, V.S. Gorantla, C. Francois, P.C.R. Brouha, L. Perez-Laurentin, J.H. Barker, M. Kon

Department of Plastic, Reconstructive and Hand Surgery at the University Medical Center in Utrecht, The Netherlands and the Division of Plastic and Reconstructive Surgery and the Department of Orthopedic Surgery at the University of Louisville, Louisville, USA

Introduction: Composite tissue allotransplantation (CTA) is a clinical reality that offers many advantages over conventional reconstruction. To prevent allograft rejection, conventional immunosuppression has been used clinically and tolerance induction using mixed allogeneic chimerism (MAC) has been tried experimentally. The long term effect that these treatment modalities have on the elastic properties of autologus and transplanted bones in CTA are not known. Immunosuppression with tacrolimus and mycophenolate mofetil (MMF) and irradiation used to induce MAC, have been reported to cause loss of bone mass and thus, reduce strength. The purpose of this study was to examine and compare the long-term effect that immunosuppression and irradiation for MAC induction have on the elastic properties of bone in a rat CTA model.
Methods: Tibiae from age-matched male Wistar Furth (WF) and ACI rats were used in the study. In Groups I (n=7) and II (n=7), tibiae were harvested from naive WF and ACI rats, respectively. In Groups III (n=7) and IV (n=7), WF rats received an ACI hind limb, and were immunosuppressed with tacrolimus (1 mg/kg/day i.p.) and mycophenolate mofetil (15 mg/kg/day p.o.). Group III tibiae were from the transplanted ACI limbs, and Group IV tibiae were from contralateral recipient WF limbs. In Groups V (n=7) and VI (n=7), WF rats were made into ACI $\rightarrow$ WF chimeras by being conditioned with 950 cGy and infused with 100×10^6 donor ACI bone marrow cells. ACI $\rightarrow$ WF chimeras received an irradiated (1050 cGy) ACI hind limb. Group V tibiae were from the transplanted ACI limbs and Group VI tibiae were from contralateral recipient WF limbs. All animals were sacrificed at 5 months post-transplant. Acoustic velocity (v) was measured using a longitudinal ultrasound transmission technique while density (rho) was measured using Archimedes principle. Longitudinal elastic coefficient was calculated (E= rho x v2), as indication of bone stiffness.
Results: (mean±SD) E was significantly reduced by both immunosuppressive therapy and irradiation for MAC induction. Group I (36.5±1.0) vs. Group IV (30.6±2.4) and Group VI (28.80±2.1) $p<0.001$, and Group II (35.3±1.7) vs. Group III (29.48±1.6) and Group V (29.08±0.2), $p<0.001$. There was no significant difference in the degree of reduction of E between all tibiae receiving immunosuppression or irradiation.
Results for v were similar to E, however, there were not differences of rho between all groups.
Conclusions: These findings indicate that long-term immunosuppressive therapy and irradiation for MAC induction reduced the acoustic velocity and the elastic coefficient of transplanted and autologus bone. The degree of reduction induced by either treatment modality was similar at 5 months in all groups. Other time points should be studied to determine the time course of these changes.

43

CK-MB/CK Serum Values after Heart Transplantation Do Not Correlate with Cardiac Damage

J.H. Fischer[1], S. Jeschkeit[1], F. Kuhn-Régnier[2], R. Switkowski[3]

Institute for Experimental Medicine[1], Department of Cardiothoracic Surgery[2], Department of Clinical Chemistry[3], University of Cologne, 50931 Cologne, Germany

Introduction: The creatine phosphokinase isoenzyme ratio CK-MB/CK is widely used for diagnosis of myocardial damage. In transplant experiments in pigs we found rather constant values of this parameter irrespective of the acute myocardial damage. Thus correlations of post-transplant CK-MB/CK serum values with values in various tissues were performed.
Methods: Hearts of 27 pigs (Duroc x German Landrace) of 28±3 kg body weight were grafted and stored for 14 hr in HTK-solution (Custodiol), UW-solution (ViaSpan), Euro-Flush-solution or modified HTK containing hyaluronidase combined with coronary oxygen persufflation (mHTK-COP). Control hearts were stored for 3 hr in HTK. Orthotopic transplantation was performed and after 2 hr attempts were made to wean from cardiopulmonary bypass. Functional measurements (left ventricular pressure development, dp/dt, heart rate, aortic and central venous pressure, cardiac output) were performed up to 3 hr posttransplant and any 30 min blood serum samples tested for total CK activities (CK-NAC monotest). CK isoenzymes were determined using agarose gel electrophoresis (Helena Lab., Beaumont, Texas). In addition tissue samples of various organs of the donor animal or recipients own heart (n=5) were collected for CK isoenzyme measurement of the normal tissue.
Results: After 14 hr preservation only the hearts which had been preserved by mHTK-COP were able to maintain the circulation of the recipient without any mechanical support, a functional recovery, which was similar to that of the short term preserved control hearts. In contrast to this functional outcome the CK-MB/CK serum ratios in all groups remained stable in the range of 2.0-3.0 an average, only in one group (14 hr HTK storage) higher values around 5.0-6.0 were found, but existed already before the transplantation. CK-MB/CK values in the tissues were 3.2±0.9 for the left ventricular myocardium (mean±SD), 6.2±1.1 for the liver, 16.7±1.0 for the lung, 41.9 ± 4.8 for the intestine and zero for the skeletal muscle.
Discussion: Good or bad function of hearts after 3 hr or 14 hr preservation and orthotopic transplantation can not be reflected in more or less elevation of CK-MB/CK serum values as the isoenzyme ratio in the healthy myocardium is only 3.2 on average. But this situation does not seem to be a speciality in pigs. An analysis of the papers presenting measurements on human tissues supports the hypothesis that healthy myocardium also in humans has low CK-MB levels and only predamage of hearts tends to elevate the CK-MB/CK ratio.
Conclusion: Intestinal or lung tissues are a much more likely origin of elevations of CK-MB/CK serum values than the heart in the post-

transplant situation. A reevaluation of CK-MB and CK values in human tissues thus should clarify the origin of increasing CK-MB/CK values after transplantations or in other clinical situations.

44

Preserved Endothelial Function of Large and Small Coronary Vessels After Prolonged Storage Including Coronary Oxygen Persufflation

M. Bosse, S. Dahnken, J.H. Fischer

Institute for Experimental Medicine, Cologne, Germany

Introduction: Previous studies performed have indicated that storage time of donor organs especially hearts can be notably extended by including gaseous coronary oxygen persufflation (COP) in the storage regime. Even after preceding normothermic ischemia (non heart beating donor) subsequent preservation is possible with life supporting recovery. The aim of this study was to ascertain the begin of endothelial damage caused by COP and to determine the maximum storage time possible without causing endothelial dysfunction.
Methods: Hearts were taken from 100-120 kg pigs at the abattoir, the right coronary artery was freed by blunt dissection, flushed with and then stored in Krebs-Henseleit solution (10°C) for transport. Different regimes were then followed: 3 h storage in modified HTK solution (mHTK = Custodiol + hyaluronidase) + COP and 18 h storage in mHTK + COP, each was followed by 75 minutes reperfusion with electrolyte solution. Rings of 5 mm length were taken from the arteries before (control) and after preservation as well as after the reperfusion period and tested for endothelial derived relaxation (EDR). Indomethacin was applied to eliminate endothelial prostacyclin activity. Then Substance P was used to trigger relaxation after precontraction with PGF2α EDR is expressed in % of the PGF2α contraction. In a second approach rabbit hearts were grafted under anaesthesia and then stored for 18 hours in mHTK + COP. Reperfusion was performed according to Langendorff. Endothelial function of the resistance vessels was tested during Substance P infusion by online flow measurements using a transit time flowmeter which were calculated in % of the initial flow. All values are expressed as mean values ±SD.
Results: EDR in the control group amounted to 81%±7 (n=13), 3h mHTK + COP resulted in 75%±4 (n=7) and 76%±4 (n=7) after reperfusion. After 18h mHTK + COP a significant reduction of EDR to 67% ± 8 was found, after reperfusion however EDR was restored to 78%±6 (n=4). The rabbit hearts stored for 18 h in mHTK + COP showed a coronary flow increase during Substance P infusion of 52%±16 (n=5), the increase in unpreserved control hearts was 30%±7 (n=3).
Discussion: Our experiments on rabbit and pig hearts demonstrate that up to 18 hours storage in mHTK + COP guarantees recovery of physiological function in large coronaries as well as small resistance vessels. Only immediately after 18 h preservation + COP without reperfusion a transient impairment of endothelial function was found.
Conclusion: An extension of heart preservation time to 18 hours using the COP technique seems to be possible without damaging the endothelium or impairing endothelial relaxation mechanisms.

Traumatology and Orthopedics

45

Long-Term Preservation with UW Solution Improves Revascularization and Viability of Transplanted Bone Versus LPD and EC at 4 °C

M.H. Kirschner, L. Suess, A. Wanders, G.O. Hofmann, K. Messmer

Trauma Center Murnau and Institute for Surgical Research, University of Munich, Germany

Introduction: Open fractures of the long bones and in the knee joint region are likely to become infected. In many cases there is no alternative to resecting large parts of the bone, sometimes the whole joint. Since Ilizarov-technique or arthroplasty could not be performed due to technical reasons, we introduced a new approach by allogenic grafting of vascularized human bones and knee joints under immunosuppression to keep a mobile lower extremity and to prevent amputation. Up to now the problem of bone and joint preservation has still been unsolved. To allow a quantitative analysis of revascularization and viability of bone transplants a model was designed in nude mice. Three standard preservation solutions used in transplant surgery were tested.
Material and Methods: Femora of adult outbred nude mice (CD1 nu/nu, female, age 8-10 weeks, 18-25 g) were cut in slices of 300±10 m and stored in University-of-Wisconsin-Solution (UW), Low Potassium Dextran (LPD) and Euro-Collins-Solution (EC) for 30 hours at 4 °C. Following bone preservation dorsal skin fold chambers were implanted in host animals and the bone was transplanted into the chamber. Oxytetracycline (100 mg/kg BW) was administered s.c. for later visualization of the bone borders on day 0. FITC Dextran was given i.v. prior to intravital microscopy (IVM). IVM was performed on days 3, 6, 8 and 10 post transplantation (pTx). Microcirculatory observations were recorded on video tapes and analyzed off-line with a computer-assisted analysis system. Functional vessel density in periosteal tissue around the bone (FVDp) and on bone tissue (FVDb) were determined as parameters of bone-induced angiogenesis and revascularization of transplanted bone. FVD was defined as the length of vessels stained with FITC dextran per area (1/mm). On day 14 pTx serial histological sections were taken and stained with H.E. in order to calculate living osteocytes (O*) and non viable cells (O-). Transplant viability (TxV) was defined as the ratio of O*/(O* + O-) given in percent. All data were analyzed using the Kruskal-Wallis Test and the Student-Newman-Keuls-Test. The data are presented as mean values ± standard error of the mean.
Results: Significantly higher values of FVD and TxV were found for UW (2.88±0.43/mm, 46.8±5.3%) vs. LPD (1.48±0.29/mm, 21.6±7.0%) and EC (0.51±0.15/mm, 14.0±4.5%), $p< 0.05$.
Conclusions: In long-time preservation at 4°C UW solution should be used to protect long bones and whole joints for vascularized allotransplantation.

46

MedEdit: Computer-Assisted Orthopedic-Trauma Surgery Planner System

K. Ollé[1], A. Kuba[1], E. Varga[2]

Department of Applied Informatics[1], Department of Traumatology[2] University Szeged, Hungary

Introduction: Surgery of the fractured bones often has complexity. The fixation of these bones has to be designed very carefully. This is the reason why trauma surgeons try to build a geometrical and mechanical model of the treated bone. Following simulation and analysis of the behavior of the bone, surgeons can test several virtual surgical methods on the virtual bone and they can define the optimal treatment for the patient. A new computer software has been developed by our team: it is called MedEdit.
Methods: The system has three main parts. The first part builds geometrical model of the treated bone. CT scans are used for this procedure. Then the segmentation of the bone parts is·followed. A 3D structure is constructed from the segmented model. Usually we get a very complex geometrical model so we use a kind of mesh simplification algorithm to eliminate the complexity of the surface. In the third part we created a medical planner where one can test several surgical methods. We implemented some 3D editing functions like implant insertion, boring or slicing.
Results: We show that our geometrical model generated from the patient CT scans and the medical planner user interface is easy to use by the surgeon.
Discussion and Conclusion: Minimal invasive technique means less interventions, percutaneous methods, as small implants as possible and as stable configuration as possible. The optimal surgery can be performed with the help of computers. The MedEdit software can be useful to design new minimal invasive surgical techniques. These procedures could be made safer both for the patients and the surgeons.

47

Trauma of Soft Tissues and Bones Evokes Local Inflammatory Reaction Expressed in the Lymphatic System

G. Szczesny, W.L. Olszewski, M. Zaleska

Dept. Surg. Res. and Transpl., Med. Res. Centre, Pol. Acad. Sci., 02106 Warsaw, Poland

Introduction: Trauma of human lower limbs with fracture of bone is often followed by prolonged edema of the extremity. The site of injury remains erythematous and hyperthermic for months or years. The lymphoscintigrammes reveal dilatation of lymphatics and enlargement of inguinal lymph nodes. This can be observed also in closed injuries without damage of skin. The described clinical observations point to the presence of a protracted local inflammatory reaction reflected in the regional lymphatic system. The question arises what kind of autologous antigenic reaction takes places in the nodes.
Aim: The aim of study was to evaluate the changes in phenotypes and responsiveness of cells from lymph nodes draining the injured tissues.
Materials and Methods: Experiments were performed on male (WAG) rats under ether anaesthesia. Group 1. A tibia mid-shaft closed fracture using three-points limb bending. Group 2. A direct contusion of sural muscles. Group 3. Whole mid-calf soft tissue trauma with single energy 3.7J/g . Group 4. Toeweb injections of syngeneic bone marrow cells (BMC)(10^6 in 0.1 ml of saline). Group 5. Toeweb injections of syngeneic venous blood (B) (0.1 ml). There were 8 experiments in each group. The contralateral limbs served as controls. After 7 days the popliteal and iliac lymph nodes (LNs), as well as tissue specimens from the site of injury were harvested. The LNs were weighed. Lymphocytes were isolated and cultured for measuring the autotransformation and responsiveness to increasing concentrations of PHA. The staining with mAbs W3/13 (leukocytes), W3/25 (CD4), OX8 (CD8), OX 12 (B cells), OX7 (stem cell marker), OX6 (class II) and ED1 (macrophages) was carried out. Statistical analysis was made using Student t-test.
Results: Lymph node mass: There was an increase in group 1 by a factor of 6 compared with the non-injured side ($p=0.0045$). The respective values in other groups were 1.5, 1.5, 1.46 and 1.58 (all $p<0.05$). The difference in LN mass increase between fractured bone and soft tissue injury and BM and B extravasation groups was significant ($p<0.05$). In all groups the autotransformation rate of LN cells was higher than in controls with a mean index of 2.4 in group 1 ($p=0.018$) in group 1 and 1.4 to 2.2 in other groups (all $p<0.05$). On histology, dilated marginal sinuses filled with W3/13 leukocytes, enlarged OX12 B-cell follicles, accumulation of ED1 and OX6 macrophages in the paracortical and medullary regions were seen. Most pronounced changes were observed in group 1.
Conclusions: Increased mass of lymph nodes, high level of node lymphocyte responsiveness and inflammatory changes in nodes on histology suggest an immune response to own antigens released from the injured tissues. Bone fracture evoked most advanced changes. The nature of the reaction including lack of immunization against autoantigens remains unclear and requires studies on the mechanism of cross-tolerance to own antigens during wound healing.

48

Intraarticular Leukocyte Activation During Acute Clinical Haemarthrosis

B. Borsiczky, B. Fodor, J. Lantos, G. Jancsó, E. Rőth, J. Nyárády**

Department of Experimental Surgery, University of Pécs, Pécs, Hungary

Introduction: In vitro investigations have proven that single or a limited number of intraarticular bleeding episodes result in cartilage damage, in which cytotoxic oxygen metabolites derived from the interaction between mononuclear cells and red blood cells are supposed to play a role. However, cellular activation and its place in the order of pathogenic events have not been investigated in clinical cases of acute haemarthrosis (HA). The study aims to assess the leukocyte activation in the joint fluid of patients with acute traumatic haemarthrosis.
Method: Paired samples of peripheral blood and articular effusions were obtained from 22 patients following 18.27±17.2 hours after the injury. Leukocytes were separated and stained with fluorescein isothiocyanate (FITC)-conjugated mouse anti-human CD11a, CD18 and CD97 monoclonal antibodies for flow cytometry.

Results: Distribution of leukocyte population in the synovial samples was similar to the venous blood, showing moderately increased ratio of polymorphonuclear granulocytes (PMN). Significant decrease of CD11a density on monocytes (venous blood: 224.20±54.23; effusion 188.37±56.83; $p=0.00167$), but markedly enhanced expression of CD97 (venous blood: 65.53±10.99; effusion 76.6±19.15; $p=0.00338$) and CD18 (venous blood: 285.41±52.45; effusion 345.98±53.34; $p=0.00945$) on PMN were found in the joint fluids as compared to the corresponding peripheral blood samples. Significantly increased proportion of CD97 positive lymphocytes was also detected in the same group of samples (venous blood: 22.69±16.34; effusion 38.88±20.5; $p=0.000149$).
Conclusion: Our results from the clinical investigations provide good evidence for leukocyte activation thus supporting the *in vitro* proven role of leukocytes in the pathomechanism of acute haemarthrosis. Since the timing of the activation precedes synovial inflammation, it is suggested that the leukocytes, especially PMN, play an important initiator role in the pathogenesis of acute haemarthrosis. Supported by Hungarian grant OTKA F-030630

49

DYNASTAB-T external stabilizer for open femoral and tibial shaft fractures

G. Szczesny[1,3], J. Deszczynski[2], J. Karpinski[2], A. Stolarczyk[2]

Dept. Orthop. and Traumatol.[1], Med. Acad., Warsaw, Poland, Dept. Orthop. and Rehabil.[2], Med. Acad., Warsaw, Poland, Dept. Surg. Res.[3], Med. Res. Centre, Pol. Acad. Sci., Warsaw, Poland

Introduction: External stabilization is a widely used nowadays technique for treatment of long bones fractures. The aim of study was to evaluate the usefulness of external stabilization using DYNASTAB-T (for long bone fractures) for treatment of open, comminuted fractures of tibial and femoral shaft fractures. The telescopic construction of unilateral DYNASTAB-T stabilizer allows controlled, with range from 1 to 5 mm, axial movements at the site of fracture. Three-dimensional, tent-like insertion of screws fixating frame of the stabilizer to the bone ensures the proper stiffness of the stabilization reducing rotational and angular dislocations.
Patients and Methods: 26 patients with open, comminuted fractures of the femoral and tibial shaft were treated using DYNASTAB-T stabilizer for 16-40 weeks (21±7 weeks).
Results: In all cases clinical as well as radiological signs of fracture union occurred without significant reduction of range of motion of joints of affected extremity. All patients tolerated the chosen type of stabilization very well. In none of the cases any common complication that occur in plaster cast immobilization, like joint stiffness, were observed. Some minor suppurative complications at the place of implant insertion were treated conservatively.
Conclusion: We conclude that external stabilization using DYNASTAB-T is sufficient for long bone fractures treatment. Moreover this type of stabilization gives the possibility to maintain the range of motion in joints of the affected extremity during fracture healing process.

50

External Stabilization for Articular Fractures of Knee, Ankle and Elbow Joints Using DYNASTAB Stabilizers

J. Deszczynski[1], J. Karpinski[1], G. Szczesny[2,3], M. Ziółkowski[1]

Dept. Orthop. & Rehabil.[1], Med. Acad., Warsaw, Poland Dept. Orthop. and Traumatol.[2], Med. Acad., Warsaw, Poland, Dept. Surg. Res.[3], Med. Res. Centre, Pol. Acad. Sci., Warsaw, Poland

The aim of study was to analyze the usefulness of the articulated external stabilization for treatment of multifragmental, articular fractures of the knee, ankle and elbow. An analysis was performed using the articulated DYNASTAB-K (for knee fractures), DYNASTAB-S (for ankle) and DYNASTAB-L (for elbow) stabilizers, which construction allows to achieve proper stabilization with possibility of joints movements due to articulated segment mimicking the physiological joint movements (flexion - extension for ankle and elbow, and flexion-extension combined with sliding for knee).
Patients and Methods: Observations were made in group of 39 patients with multifragmental fractures of the knee joint (six patients), ankle (27 patients), and distal humerus (six patients) treated with DYNASTAB stabilizers for 6-10 weeks. Early passive joint movements were started on the second postoperative day, then active movements were allowed in controlled range of motion.
Results: In all cases the sufficient fracture healing process occurred with satisfactory final range of motion in the affected joint.
Conclusion: Application of articulated external stabilization technique allows the proper stabilization sufficient for fracture healing together with application of motion in the joint preventing from its stiffness.

51

Intramedullary Nailing in Ankle Arthrodesis: Anterograde vs Retrograde

M. Goebel, M.H. Kirschner, M. Militz

Berufgenossenschaftliche Unfallklinik Murnau, Murnau, Germany

Introduction: Posttraumatic arthrosis and severe deformity are common after injuries of the upper and lower ankle joint. An effective pain reducing procedure is in many cases only arthrodesis. Aim of the presented prospective study is to introduce the anterograde and retrograde technique of tibiotalocalcaneal arthrodesis using intramedullary nails and compare its results.
Methods: 15 patients with retrograde combined arthrodesis of the upper and lower ankle joint and 17 patients with tibiotalocalcaneal arthrodesis using the anterograde approach were available for standardized follow up (mean follow up 18 months). The patients were examined in dependence to the SF-36 with special attention to approach, osseous consolidation and postoperative quality of life.
Results: Bony consolidation and freedom from pain can be achieved in 82-90% with both techniques. Advantage of the transcalcaneal approach is not involving the knee-joint and plantar freedom from pain in most of the cases.

Discussion: Early retrograde intramedullary nailing of the ankle joint was performed and published by G. Küntscher. Since then, intramedullary implants, ranging from Steinmann pins to dynamic interlocking nails, were used more or less succesfully in tibiotalocalcaneal arthrodesis. However, ankle arthrodesis using an intramedullary nail has gained popularity in recent years. Berend et al. published a study proving that intramedullary nailing with interlocking screws provided significantly stiffer fixation in all bending directions compared to lag screw fixation. It has also been suggested that increased rigidity of fixation enhances the outcome of combined ankle and subtalar arhtrodesis. It has been reported that intramedullary nailing decreased the rate of non-unions compared with other techniques. With the possibility of dynamic interlocking screw fixation and the interfragmentary compression by the axial insertion of a compression screw we achieved an 85-89% fusion rate in this study. In our opinion, advantage of the transcalcaneal approach is not involving the knee pretibial proximal, where some patients still suffered from the anterograde approach after mean follow up time. Also, in case of deep infection, the knee-joint will not be affected. In addition to that, though the plantar approach, there hasn't been an increased number of patients with heel pain in the retrograde group. Most of the patients of both groups could gain quality of life with better mobility and less pain than before surgery. But the use of an intramedullary nail is not free of complications. Failures occurred in this series and reported in the literature have been associated with displacement of the intramedullary rod, malunion, nonunion, implant failure, infection and results leading to amputation. Nevertheless, with proper patient selection, operative planning, anatomic dissection and the use of modern implants with dynamic interlocking option and axial compression possibility by an insertion screw, we see good results of tibiotalocalcaneal fusion and limited complications.
Conclusion: Intramedullary nailing in ankle arthrodesis using the antrograde or retrograde approach is an innovative and suitable technique with very good results.

52

Vascular Tunnel Concept in the Surgical Treatment of Brain Swelling

A. Csókay

National Institute of Traumatology, Budapest, Hungary

Purpose: Decompressive craniectomy with durotomy is a possible last resort therapy for severe brain swelling. Although the method successfully diminishes the ICP, partial or total vascular insufficiency occurs in the herniated part of the brain. The actual cause of the insufficiency is most likely due to the compression of the cortical veins and arteries, caused by shearing and pressure forces between the dural edge and brain tissue. Furthermore venous congestion may induce edema in the protruding parts of the brain, thus further compromising neuron viability.
Methods: The new surgical technique consists of a stellate type durotomy and the creation of a vascular tunnel, around the main cortical veins and arteries, with the aim that the vessels do not become compressed by the dural or bone edge*. The effect of the novel vascular tunnel technique was proven by measuring the blood flow of the protected and non protected veins with Doppler-US, intraoperatively. Further space winning surgical methods were applied by scarification and stretching the skin or let it open.
Results: In the last two years 28 patients were operated on with this method. All were in severe GCS 3 or GCS 4 status, with more than 30 mmHg ICP. In comparison with the traditional treatment, the mortality rate was reduced from 80% to 40% and, recovery (GOS 4,5) rate increased significantly in these severe cases.
Conclusions: With this technique the ICP was significantly reduced and further edema and vascular insufficiency were prevented. This was due to protection of the arterial circulation and venous drainage of the herniated part of the brain, by the formation of a vascular tunnel at the durotomy edges.* Ref: A. Csókay et al. Acta Neurochir. (Wien) 143:173-175, 2001.

53

Surgical Consequences of the Polytrauma Equivalent Syndrome (PES) to the Spleen Injuries Treatment

G. Ács, A. Furka, T. Lesznyák, Z. Záborszky**, I. Furka, I. Mikó*

Department of Operative Techniques and Surgical Research, 2nd Department of Surgery*, Department of Traumatology**, Medical and Health Science Center, University of Debrecen, Debrecen, Hungary

Introduction: The injuries are the leading causes of the death at childhood and at the most active adult age-group, preceding the cardiovascular cases and tumors. These facts give us the reason for examining the possibilities of reducing the severity and fatal outcome. How can we describe the severity of the injury and the probability of the outcome? Certain scoring-systems try to give the answer by using anatomical and physiological parameters. Is there any reason for the usage of combined scores which contains dynamic and static components too? In the chain of survival the nowadays useable definitions and scoring-systems has got only limited results.
Methods: After the examination of the polytraumatized patients in the period 1996-2000, the analysis of the severe injured patients' prehospital care in 1999, first in 2000 we proposed a new definition: Polytrauma Equivalent Syndrome (PES). We can rank in this group of patients with single or multiple injuries that can lead to multiple organ failure, the ISS score of them is more than 18 and strategy of the treatment is similar to the polytraumatized one. The PES index is the ratio of the increasing and decreasing factors of the severity. In fact of an injury, not only the injury itself determines the survival chance, but the alterations and conditions the patients' already have got at the time of the injury, and the reactions started by the injury's stress and tissue damage. The injuries of the abdominal organs can occur as a monotrauma, but they can be a part of multiple injuries.
Results: We processed data of the therapy of persons who severely injured in 1999. Here we have found 256 severe injured patients, and at 42 of them arise the possibility of abdominal injury. By the data of the hospitals between 1996-2000 97 spleen injured were treated, in 91 cases were splenectomy and in 71 cases splenic autotransplantation attached to it.
Discussion: If it is possible we have to save the spleen or at least a part of the spleen by using bioplasts or by the Furka type interlacing suture line. If we have not got any possibilities to do it, the Furka type "spleen apron" method seems to be an optimal solution, where we make 20x10x1 mm size spleen chips from the injured spleen and we put them between the two sheets of the greater omentum.

Conclusion: The spleen injury can be directly critical itself, the adequate prehospital and preoperative trauma management and using of new operative methods makes the possibility to choose the most optimal solution to exempt the patient from the consequences of the PES.
This study was supported by OTKA No. 034211 and The Ministry of Welfare Research Grant No. 6100/1/2000/ETT No. 24/0003/2001/ETT.

54

A New Pressure-Free Intramedullary Reamer for Reducing Fat Intravasation: An Experimental Study in Sheep

H.U. Spiegel, A. Kröpfl, H. Redl, U. Frerichmann, C. Ortmann, A. Joist

Surgical Research - Dept. of Trauma and Hand Surgery, Münster University Hospital, Münster, Germany

Objective: Use of intramedullary reamers (IR) is typically associated with pressure generation during the reaming process, which may result in the introduction of fat and marrow particles into the venous system. Thus, a new system was designed in order to avoid pressure generation and thus reduce the risk of embolic events. The new pressure-free intramedullary reamer (PF-IR) was developed at the TU Clausthal (Germany) and the Ludwig-Boltzmann Institute (Vienna).
Materials and Methods: *In vitro* testing was carried out using pig femura. Intramedullary pressure was measured during drilling with either the new PF-IR (n=10) or a standard AO-IR (n=10). For *in vivo* testing, nailing of the femur was performed in sheep using either the PF-IR (n=7) or the standard AO-IR (n=7). Fat intravasation was measured using echocardiography and the Gurd-Test. Hemodynamic and pulmonary parameters as well as intramedullary pressure were continuously recorded during the experiments. The animals were then sacrificed an tissue samples were taken from all regions of the lungs. The incidence of lung fat emboli in histological sections was scored in a blinded manner. A finite element analysis was carried out to assess performance of the PF-IR under load. Statistics: Mann-Whitney U-test ($p<0.001$).
Results: The *in-vitro* tests showed that the new PF-IR resulted in significantly less intramedullary pressure (15±12 mmHg) than the standard AO-IR (813±247 mmHg; $p<00001$). These results were confirmed *in vivo*. Moreover, the PF-IR group had significantly less fat intravasation (Gurd-test) and better hemodynamic and pulmonary values than the AO-IR group. The incidence of fat microemboli in the lungs was reduced by 90% in the PF-IR group. Finite element analysis showed that the new drilling system performed well under load.
Conclusion: The newly developed pressure-free IR clearly outperformed a standard AO-IR. Use of the new PF-IR was associated with a low intramedullary, significantly less fat intravasation, and a markedly lower incidence of fat emboli in the lung. This, in turn, may have been the reason for the better hemodynamic and pulmonary values in the PF-IR group.

Shock and Ischemia-Reperfusion I

55

Regulation of the Ischemia-Reperfusion-Syndrome in Liver Ischemia by Transcription Factors - A Clinical Trial

S. Kersting, T. Zimmermann, G. von Gagern, D. Ratayczak, S. Albrecht, D. Ockert, H.D. Saeger*

Dept. of Surgery, Dept. of Gynaecology*, Technical University Dresden, Dresden, Germany

Introduction: Transcription factors like NFκB regulate the release of numerous mediators (immediate early gene products) in ischemia and reperfusion during liver resections. Earlier findings suggest that disturbance of the intracellular redox equilibrium by reactive oxygen species, normally maintained by seleno-enzymes PH-Gpx and thioredoxin-reductase, lead to activation of NFκB with a simultaneous raise of the inactivating factor of NFκB, IκBα . Until today the detailed mechanism of regulation has not been fully understood.
Methods: In order to evaluate the factors of the redox equilibrium *in vivo*, the authors investigated these processes on a molecular level in 40 patients undergoing liver resections, comparing operations under ischemic conditions (by clamping of the hepatoduodenal ligament) and operations without interruption of the blood supply. Blood samples were taken pre-op, intra-op (ex portal vein and v. cava) and directly post-op, +6 h, +24 h, +48 h and +72 h.
Reactive oxygen species (ROS) were determined by means of chemiluminescence, the binding activity of the subunits of NFκB p50 and p65 by EMSA. Additionally, mRNA of TNFα, tissue factor, IκBα and MIF were traced by RT-PCR.
Results: Comparing both groups we find a significantly higher activation of NO in the clamping group, simultaneously with a relative overexpression of p50 over p65. The imbalance between p50 and p65 leads to a depression in the NFκB binding activity and to a consecutive lower exprimation of the immediate early gene products. The release of ROS and NO seems to be dependent on the liver tissue, not the MBCs since there is no proof for a iNOS activity in the examined samples.
Conclusion: A new aspect in the regulation of the ischemia-reperfusion syndrome is presented, which opens new approaches towards the reduction of the ischemia-reperfusion damage. Promising substances in the restoration of the redox balance, could be antioxidants, corticoids or NO releasing substances.

56

Role of Pyrrolidine Dithiocarbamate in the Induction of Ischemic Tolerance of the Liver: Heme Oxygenase 1 Induction and Sinusoidal Dilatation

K. Hata, Y. Yamamoto, K. Yonezawa, K. Taura, A. Nakajima, H. Uchinami, Y. Yamaoka

Department of Gastroenterological Surgery, Kyoto University Graduate School of Medicine, Kyoto, Japan

Introduction: Stress preconditioning provides the liver with ischemic tolerance and heme oxygenase-1 (HO-1) is thought to play a pivotal role in some situations. We have reported that pyrrolidine dithiocarbamate (PDTC) induces HO-1 in the liver tissue *in vivo*. Recently, some studies revealed that HO-1 induced hepatic sinusoidal dilatation. In this study, we examined whether HO-1 induction by PDTC could induce sinusoidal dilatation, resulting in ischemic tolerance.
Methods: Male Wistar rats were used. PDTC was injected intramuscularly (150 mg/kg b.w.), and HO-1 expression were assessed both in mRNA and in protein levels. To examine dose-effect relationship, doses from 0 to 200 mg/kg were also tested. The expression of HO-1 was evaluated immunohistochemically as well. Other rats were divided into 2 groups: the rats injected with PDTC (group P), and the rats with only vehicle (group C). Diameters of sinusoidal venules were measured using intravital microscopy (IVM) 24 hrs after injection. Rats in both groups were exposed to a 60-min partial hepatic ischemia and subsequent reperfusion (I/R) 36 hrs after PDTC injection. Serum transaminase levels and histological liver damage were evaluated 6 hrs after reperfusion. Survival rate was also examined in the model of 30-min total hepatic I/R.
Results: HO-1 protein was hardly detected in the control rat livers. HO-1 mRNA level peaked at 6 hrs after PDTC injection, and then gradually decreased. It disappeared by 24 hrs. Protein level of HO-1 reached to a maximum at 12~24 hrs after injection and its increase was in a dose-dependent manner. Immunohistochemical staining revealed that HO-1 was induced mainly in Kupffer cells, but it was also induced in the hepatocytes around central veins after high dose injection of PDTC. IVM study showed that sinusoidal venules in zone 1 were not so different between the groups (group C vs. group P: 7.99±0.13 vs. 8.36±0.15 micrometer in diameter, $p=0.099$), whereas those in zone 3 were remarkably dilated in group P (11.14±0.13 vs. 21.94±0.58, $p<0.0001$). In good agreement with this difference, serum transaminase level decreased significantly in group P (9343±1077 vs. 5570±703 IU, $p<0.05$). Survival rate was also dramatically improved in group P (2/10 vs. 10/10, $p<0.001$).
Conclusion: PDTC induced HO-1 protein in the liver with a remarkable sinusoidal dilatation, and thus contributed to an ischemic tolerance of the liver. Preconditioning of the liver using PDTC may be a useful, new strategy in place of other stress preconditioning.

57

Heat Shock Preconditioning Enhances JNK/AP-1 Cascade Following Hepatic Ischemia-Reperfusion

H. Uchinami, Y. Yamamoto, K. Hata, K. Taura, A. Nakajima, K. Yonezawa, Y. Yamaoka

Department of Gastroenterological Surgery, Kyoto University Graduate School of Medicine, Kyoto, Japan

Introduction: Heat shock preconditioning (HPC) protects the liver from ischemia-reperfusion (I/R) injury. AP-1 is a redox-sensitive transcription factor and activates itself during hepatic I/R. We have reported that HPC enhanced the activation of AP-1. In addition, c-jun N-terminal kinase (JNK), regulator of AP-1, was also rapidly activated during reperfusion phase. However, the consequence of JNK/AP-1 is still controversial. Some studies showed that JNK activation initiated apoptosis. Other studies revealed that AP-1 induced the expression of heme oxygenase-1 (HO-1), a cytoprotective molecule, to maintain a redox state in cells. This study was conducted to investigate the role of rapid activation of JNK/AP-1 upon hepatic I/R injury after HPC.
Methods: Male Wistar rats were divided into two groups: Rats were bathed in a warm bath at 37° (group C) or at 42° (group HS) for 15 min. After 48-hr recovery, rats were exposed to a 30-min hepatic ischemia using Pringle's maneuver and allowed to reperfuse. The liver samples were collected at specified time points after I/R. DNA binding activity of AP-1 was examined by gel shift assay. The expression of mRNA was evaluated using RT-PCR. JNK activity was examined by *in vitro* kinase assay. Phosphorylation of c-jun was evaluated using Western blot analysis. Apoptosis was assessed by TUNEL reaction and by DNA fragmentation ELISA system.
Results: JNK activation was observed at 1-2 hrs postreperfusion in group C, but its activation was advanced to 30 min postreperfusion in group HS. Consistent with the time shift of JNK activation, DNA binding activity of AP-1 in group HS was also advanced from 2 hrs postreperfusion in group C to 1 hr postreperfusion. Phosphorylation of c-jun was also delayed in group C compared with in group HS. The mRNA expression of HO-1 in the livers, which was not observed in the preischemic phase, increased 2 hrs postreperfusion in group HS and was stronger than in group C. The degree of apoptosis 6 hrs postreperfusion was reduced in group HS.
Conclusion: Rapid activation of JNK/AP-1 cascade during hepatic I/R by HPC resulted in the increasing HO-1 expression and suppressed apoptotic cell death. This result was very rational in the light of attenuated I/R injury after HPC. However, contrary to a popular opinion *in vitro*, apoptotic cell death was rather suppressed with the rapid activation of JNK/AP-1 in this *in vivo* model of I/R. We should be careful when we deduce the theory of molecular cascade reaction *in vitro* to *in vivo* phenomenon.

58

Involvement of ELR (-) CXC and CC Chemokines in Hepatic Ischemia/Reperfusion Injury in Mice

D. Takeuchi, H. Yoshidome, Y. Morita, H. Ito, F. Kimura, H. Shimizu, A. Togawa, Y. Shimizu, M. Ohtsuka, A. Kato, M. Miyazaki

Department of General Surgery, Chiba University Graduate School of Medicine, Chiba, Japan

Introduction: Hepatic injury induced by ischemia and reperfusion is an important clinical problem in hepatic resection or transplantation. We reported that the ELR (+) CXC chemokines are upregulated causing neutrophil accumulation and activation, and leading to both local and remote organ injury. However, whether other mediators are involved has been undefined. The objective of this study was to investigate the expression of ELR (-) CXC chemokine, interferon-gamma inducible protein-10 (IP-10) and CC chemomines, monocyte chemoattractant protein-1 (MCP-1) and macrophage inflammatory protein 1-α (MIP1-α). We also examined distribution of recruited leukocytes.
Methods: C57BL/6 mice were subjected to 90 minutes of partial hepatic ischemia followed by reperfusion. Hepatic MCP-1, MIP1- α and IP-10 mRNA expression were measured by quantitative RT-PCR (LightCycler). Serum levels of these chemokines were measured using ELISA. Hepatic leukocyte accumulation was examined by histology. Hepatic neutrophil accumulation was also assessed by myeloperoxidase (MPO) content. Hepatocyte injury was assessed by serum ALT levels and liver edema quantified by wet to dry weight ratio. Recruited lymphocytes in the liver were separated and analyzed by fluorescence activated cell sorter (FACS) using TCR-ß and NK1.1 antibodies.
Results: Hepatic MCP-1 and MIP1-α mRNA expression were increased at 4 hours of reperfusion and remained elevated until 24 hours. Serum MCP-1 levels were elevated at 4 hours of reperfusion (Sham: 25±1 pg/dl, 4 hr: 112±13 pg/dl. $p<0.0001$). IP-10 mRNA expression was increased from 4 to 8 hours after reperfusion. Hepatic MPO content was increased 3 hours after reperfusion and continued to be elevated up to 24 hours. In histological examination, neutrophils were recruited at 4 hours after reperfusion, and accumulated neutrophils in hepatic pericentral parenchyma (zone 3) causing hepatocyte damage were observed 8 hours after reperfusion. Lymphocytes were accumulated in the liver more than neutrophils at 4 hours of reperfusion. At 8 hours, however, the number of lymphocytes was not increased as compared with neutrophils. FACS analysis of the lymphocytes showed decrease in TCR-ß positive and NK1.1 positive fractions at 4 hours of reperfusion as compared with sham control.
Conclusion: These data suggest that ELR (-) CXC chemokines and CC chemomines are upregulated, and lymphocytes, as well as neutrophils are recruited in the liver after hepatic ischemia/reperfusion, which may be involved in the inflammatory cascade.

59

Role of Selective COX-2 Inhibition by Meloxicam in the Ischemia/Reperfusion Injury of the Liver

R.H. Tolba[1], K. Yonezawa[2], Y. Yamamoto[2], K. Taura[2], A. Nakajima[2], K. Hata[2], H. Uchinami[2], T. Minor[1], Y. Yamaoka[2]

Div. of Surgical Research[1], University of Bonn, Germany and Department of Gastroenterological Surgery[2], Kyoto University, Japan

Introduction: Ischemia-reperfusion injury (I/R) is one of the major clinical problems in liver and transplant surgery. Livers adjusted to warm ischemia *in vivo*, often show a severe dysfunction and the release of numerous inflammatory cytokines and arachidonic acid metabolites. COX-2, is the inducible isoform of an intracellular enzyme that converts arachidonic acids into prostaglandins. The aim of the study was to evaluate the effect of COX-2 inhibition and the role of Kupffer cells in the ischemia-reperfusion injury of the liver.
Methods: Male Wistar rats (250-280 g BW) were anesthetized with i.p. application of pentobarbital (50 mg/kg BW) and atropine (0.05 mg). All animals were subjected to a 30-min warm ischemia of the liver (Pringle's maneuver) and 60 min of reperfusion after median laparotomy. The control group achieved no additional treatment. In the COX-2 inhibitor group (COX-2I), the animals received 10 mg/kg/BW meloxicam prior to operation. The Gadolinium chloride ($GdCl_3$) (10 mg/kg/BW) was given 24h prior to operation in the $GdCl_3$ and $GdCl_3$+COX-2I groups for the selective depletion of Kupffer cells. The $GdCl_3$+COX-2I group received also 10 mg/kg/BW meloxicam prior to operation.
Results: After 30-min warm ischemia *in vivo*, a severe hepatocellular damage and an increase in serum creatinine was observed in the control group. These impairments could be significantly prevented by a selective COX-2 inhibition and the depletion of Kupffer cells.

	GPT (U/L)	LDH (U/L)
Control:	3240±1262	19075±5986
COX-2I:	973±649*	6765±4462*
$GdCl_3$:	1611±600*	12100±2870*
$GdCl_3$	1511±575*	11223±3694*

	Creatinine (mg/dl)	TNF-α (pg/ml; serum)
Control:	1.2±0.2	16.3±11.7
COX-2I:	0.65±0.15*	3.5±1.5*
$GdCl_3$:	0.94±0.15*	8.05±3.5
$GdCl_3$	0.82±0.09*	7.7±2.3*
+COX-2I:		

(n=6; mean±SD, Statistics: ANOVA and Dunnet-Test;*$p< 0.05$ vs Control)

Conclusion: It was suggested that COX-2 was mainly expressed in Kupffer cells in the liver and the inhibition of COX-2 suppressed the activation of Kupffer cells, resulting in the inhibition of TNF-alpha release as an initiator of inflammatory reaction in hepatic I/R. Selective COX-2 inhibition is a possible therapeutic approach against the warm ischemia-reperfusion injury.

60

The Influence of Phosphodiestherase-Inhibition on the Ischaemia-Reperfusion Injury of the Liver

A. Zaránd[1], R. Banafsche[2], M. Kume[4], H. Uchinami[4], M.M. Gebhard[3], T. Gondos[1], F. Perner[1], E. Klar[2]

Clinic of Surgery and Transplantation[1], Semmelweis University Budapest, Hungary, Dept. of General Surgery[2] and Dept. of Experimental Surgery[3], University of Heidelberg, Dept. of Gastroenterological Surgery[4], Kyoto University, Japan

Introduction: Milrinone, a phosphodiestherase-3 inhibitor, was examined using a hepatic warm ischaemia-reperfusion model (1 hr of ischaemia, 6 and 12 hrs of reperfusion), to determine the efficacy of this drug on an induction of tolerance against a warm ischaemia-reperfusion injury of rat livers.
Methods: Male Wistar rats were divided into two groups; group A: control group with Ringer infusion, group B: milrinone pre-treatment group. Quantification of the hepatic microcirculation was performed at 6 and 12 hours after reperfusion by intravital fluorescence microscopy. Microcirculation data were performed with analytical software. Blood samples were taken from the aorta after the observation of the microcirculation. Alanine aminotransferase (ALT) and lactate dehydrogenase (LDH) were determined by the UV spectrophotometric enzymatic assay. Wilcoxon test was used for the analysis for all the data.
Results: Hepatic microcirculation failure was quantified by four parameters. (a) Sinusoidal perfusion failure indicated no-reflow phenomenon after reperfusion. The percentage in group A was significantly higher (19%, 24% vs 12%, 20%). (b) The number of sticking leukocytes in the sinusoidal area indicated a pathological process of contact and reaction between leukocytes and endothelial cells at the reperfusion. According to the time after reperfusion leukocyte sticking kept on increasing in group A. There was no difference between the two groups after 6 hrs reperfusion but there was significant difference after 12 hrs reperfusion (28 vs 16). (c) The rolling leukocytes in post-sinusoidal venules indicated modification on the cell surface and subsequent interactions between reperfused leukocytes and endothelial cells in this area. The numbers of rollers in group B were significantly lower than that in group A (337,220 vs 580,565). (d) Treatment by milrinone also avoided severe leukostasis in post-sinusoidal venules. In the comparison between the two groups there was a significantly difference (591,234 vs 261,92). Hepatocellular viability and damage: reflecting the microcirculatory recovery after reperfusion, in group A ALT (259,258 vs 402,389) and LDH (638,766 vs 698,996) enzyme levels as parameters of liver damage were significantly lower after reperfusion.
Discussion: Milrinone pretreatment stimulates immediate accumulation of cAMP in the liver tissue. Through the activation of the cAMP dependent protein kinases, cAMP may be involved in nuclear transcriptional activities such as activation of cAMP response element binding protein and cAMP response element modulator, or negative regulation of nuclear factor-kB activation.
Conclusion: Milrinone induces ischemic tolerance which means an ameliorated hepatic microcirculation and a protected liver tissue injury.

Shock and Ischemia-Reperfusion II

61

Local Intravascular Coagulation and Inhibition of Fibrinolysis with Subsequent Fibrin Deposition due to Intestinal Ischemia and Reperfusion in Rats

E.H.P. Roossink, I.G. Schoots, P.B. Bijlsma, M. Levi, T.M. van Gulik

Department of Surgery (Surgical Laboratory) and Internal Medicine, Academic Medical Center, Amsterdam, The Netherlands

Introduction: Postischemic accumulation of fibrinogen has been demonstrated in the microvasculature of the intestines, early after the onset of reperfusion. This fibrinogen deposition, mainly occurring onto the endothelial cell surface, promotes platelet adhesion, which is likely to contribute to the "no reflow" phenomenon and intestinal ischemia and reperfusion (I/R) injury. The aim of this study was to assess post-ischemic intravascular coagulation and fibrinolysis, and subsequent intravascular fibrin deposition in the splanchnic circulation following mild and severe intestinal I/R in a rat model. These findings were related to structural and functional alterations of the mucosal epithelium.
Methods: After induction of intestinal ischemia by superior mesenteric artery occlusion (SMAO) for 0 (n=7), 20 (n=8) or 40 (n=9) min, a 3-hr luminal perfusion of an *in situ* closed intestinal loop was performed. The clearance of water (ClH_2O), glucose (Clglucose) and disodium fluorescein ($ClNa_2Fl$) from the intestinal loop was measured, reflecting the absorptive and barrier function, respectively. During reperfusion, portal blood was collected at 5, 60 and 180 min and systemic blood at 180 min, to analyse activation of coagulation and fibrinolysis.
Results: 20 min of SMAO showed only mild structural and functional intestinal changes after 3 hours reperfusion whereas 40 min of ischemia resulted in more pronounced intestinal injury (LDH; 417±42 and 656±140, resp., vs. 376±37 U/L (control), αGST; 37±10 and 77±23, resp., vs. 21±8 ng/L), morphological changes (Park-Chiu classification: range 0-1 and 1-4, resp., vs. 0) and functional defects (ClH_2O 10.3±4.8 and 13.1±2.6, resp., vs. 13.9±2.3 µl/min*g, Clglucose 81.6±26.8 and 41.6±10.7, resp., vs. 81.6±14.8 µl/min*g, $ClNa_2Fl$ 12.8±4.2 and 12.5±3.7, resp., vs. 9.4±4.5µl/min*g). Portal blood samples after 20 and 40 min ischemia showed a marked thrombin generation, as reflected by a 2.9- and 4.1-fold increase in thrombin-antithrombin complex levels (15.6±0.7 and 21.6±2.4 vs. 5.4±0.8 ng/ml, $p<0.05$) and a gradual decrease in antithrombin (80.2±3.3 and 84.0±3.1 vs. 98.7±0.9 IU/ml, $p<0.05$). Portal fibrinolysis was markedly suppressed due to a 3-4-fold increase in levels of plasminogen-activated inhibitor-1 (22.4±2.7 and 20.6±1.8 vs. 5.6±0.7 IU/ml, $p<0.05$), the principal inhibitor of fibrinolysis. Fibrin degradation product (D-dimer) levels showed that activation of coagulation and depression of fibrinolysis indeed resulted in portal fibrin formation, which was confirmed by detection of fibrin deposition at histological examination.
Conclusion: These results demonstrate that local activation of coagulation following intestinal I/R precedes epithelial dysfunction.

Marked thrombin generation and depression of fibrinolysis result in fibrin deposition that may further compromise the intestinal microvasculature and hence, contribute to irreversible intestinal injury.

62

Antithrombin III Substitution Inhibits Local Intravascular Coagulation and Fibrin Deposition after Intestinal Ischemia in Rats.

I.G. Schoots, E.H.P. Roossink, P.B. Bijlsma, M. Levi, T.M. van Gulik

Department of Surgery (Surgical Laboratory) and Internal Medicine, Academic Medical Center, Amsterdam, The Netherlands

Introduction: In a previous study, we demonstrated local intravascular coagulation and inhibition of fibrinolysis with subsequent fibrin deposition following intestinal ischemia and reperfusion in rats. These phenomena resulted in epithelial dysfunction of the intestine. The aim of this study was to investigate the salvaging effect of systemic heparin and antithrombin III (ATIII) administration upon local intravascular coagulation and thrombotic obstruction in the splanchnic microvasculature following intestinal ischemia.
Methods: Rats were divided into 3 groups: control (n=24), heparin (n=18) and ATIII (n=18). Intestinal ischemia was induced by superior mesenteric artery occlusion (SMAO) for 0, 20 or 40 min. Saline, heparin (375 IU/kg) or ATIII (250 IU/kg) were administered 15 min before reperfusion. During reperfusion, portal (local) and systemic blood samples were analysed for activation of coagulation and fibrinolysis.
Results: SMAO resulted in mild to moderate intestinal injury as assessed by histological analysis, biochemical markers, absorptive capacity and barrier function. 20 and 40 min of intestinal ischemia and 3 hours reperfusion resulted in local intestinal thrombin generation and fibrinogen to fibrin conversion, reflected by a 2.9- and 4.1-fold increase in thrombin-antithrombin (TAT) complex levels (15.6±0.7 and 21.6±2.4 vs. 5.4±0.8 ng/ml) and a 2.9- and 2.8-fold elevation of fibrin degradation products (D-dimer) (154.6±7.4 and 147.9±15.2 vs. 53.9±6.5 ng/ml), respectively. Administration of ATIII resulted in reversion of ischemia/reperfusion-induced activation of coagulation, as shown by a 1.9- and 2.1-fold reduction of portal TAT levels and in a 1.5- and 3.2-fold decrease of portal D-dimer levels, after 20 min and 40 min of ischemia, respectively. Heparin infusion did not result in significant changes of activation of coagulation. After a short-lasting, initial activation of local fibrinolysis in the control group, plasminogen activator activity was subsequently suppressed after 20 and 40 min ischemia, as a result of an almost 4-fold increase in portal plasma levels of plasminogen activator inhibitor-1 during reperfusion. Both, heparin and ATIII administration did not change fibrinolytic activity or its inhibition. In the control group, activation of coagulation and depression of fibrinolysis resulted in fibrin formation, as confirmed by intravascular fibrin deposits at histological examination. No such fibrin deposition could be detected in the antithrombin-treated rats. Intestinal structural characteristics and functional parameters were however not improved.
Conclusion: Systemic substitution of ATIII but not heparin inhibits local activation of coagulation and reduces fibrin deposition in a model of 20-40 min ischemia and reperfusion in the rat. Intestinal dysfunction was however not improved.

63

Antioxidants and Ischemia-Reperfusion of the Rat Intestine in the Absence of Leucocytes

I. García-Alonso, I. Goicoechea, J. Caramés, B. Otero, J. Bilbao

Lab. of Experimental Surgery, Univ. of The Basque Country, Leioa, Spain

Introduction: Antioxidant drugs (AO) have proved to be quite effective at decreasing both the mucosal damage to the intestine and the mortality rate following reperfusion of the ischemic gut in the rat. We have also proved that AO improve all the hemodynamic parameters following reperfusion. Leucocytes are said to be the main responsible for all the reperfusion damage. We are assessing the effect of AO in a model of intestinal reperfusion *in vitro* without blood cells.
Methods: Male Wag rats have been used. The superior mesenteric artery and the portal vein are cannulated and the whole small intestine is excised, perfused with heparinized Ringer solution, and placed into a warming chamber for 60 minutes. Using a solution previously presented to this Society (which includes glucose, insulin and oxygen), the intestine is perfused during 30 minutes (12 ml/min; 100/60 mm Hg) restoring the cellular metabolism in the absence of white blood cells. Twelve rats were allocated to the control group, while 18 received folinic acid (0.21 µl/ml), α-tocopherol (1.6 µl/ml) and SOD (0.58 µl/ml) in the perfusate. Samples from the perfusate and the portal drainage were collected at 0, 5, 15 and 30 minutes of reperfusion. Afterwards, three samples of terminal ileum were obtained and embedded in paraffin.
Results: No statistically significant differences could be found between control and AO-treated groups, regarding analysis of the effluent fluid. The initial hyperkaliemia was reduced to normal values 15 minutes after starting reperfusion. The initial acidosis was also reduced after 15 minutes, stabilising at 0.06 below the perfusate's pH. Though [Ca^{++}] was initially low, by the end of the experiment it was within the normal range. The oxygen pressure of the effluent increased from 90 mm Hg at the initial moment to over 130 mmHg for the last 15 minutes. Damage to the intestine is being assessed on histological sections and by biochemical analysis of the effluent (LDH, CK).
Conclusion: When reperfusing the ischemic intestine without white blood cells, antioxidant treatment showed no benefit, which reinforces the hypothesis of these cells being the main agents of reperfusion injury to the intestine.

64

Changes of the Red Blood Cells Deformability Caused by Mesenteric Ischemia-Reperfusion Injury. An Experimental Animal Study

E. Bráth, I. Furka, G. Szabó, K. Pető, G. Ács, N. Németh, T. Lesznyák, T. Cserni, J. Papp Szekeres**, I. Mikó*

Dept. of Operative Techniques and Surgical Research, Dept. of Pediatrics*, Univ. of Debrecen, Medical and Health Science Center, Debrecen, Dept. of General Surgery**, Bács-Kiskun County Teaching Hospital, Kecskemét, Hungary

Introduction: Gut injury due to ischemia and reperfusion plays an important role in many clinical conditions, such as small bowel transplantation, heart or aortic surgery, hypovolemic shock, mesenteric infarct, and necrotizing enterocolitis in neonates. The cytotoxic effects of ischemia-reperfusion injury damages the cell functions. The free radicals can damage the membrane lipid molecules of the red blood cells by injuring the double bonds and terminating the connection between the membrane and the cytoskeleton. The aim of our experiments was to study whether mesenteric ischemia-reperfusion injury caused changes of the red blood cells deformability in laboratory animals, and if so, what the duration of this process was like.
Methods: This experiment was performed in 10 mongrel dogs that were divided into 2 groups. In the 1st group (n=5) superior mesenteric artery was isolated and clamped for 30 minutes (IR), in the 2nd group (n=5) was the control (sham operated) group (C). The blood samples were taken before operation and in the 1st, 2nd, 4th, 6th postoperative hours and on the 1st, 2nd, 3rd, 4th, 5th, 7th, and 9th days. The deformability of red blood cells was measured by St George FT-1 Filtrometer (Carat Diagnostics). 5 mm porediameter policarbonate filters were used. Two parameters were determined: IRFR (Initial Relative Filtration Rate) and RCTT (Relative Cell Transit Time). The two groups were compared by the help of Mann-Whitney Rank Sum Test ($p<0.05$).
Results: Mesenteric ischemia-reperfusion injury caused changes of the red blood cells deformability. The critical period was the 72nd postoperative hours. There was significant difference in the IRFR and RCTT values between the two groups. (RCTT values at the 72nd hours: mesenteric IR group=14.5±3.6; C group=9.67±2.14). There was no significant difference neither IRFR nor RCTT values between the two groups in all other period. There was a strong correlation, but no significant difference between the IR and C group at the 24th postoperative hours (RCTT values at the 24th hours: IR group=7.69±1.7; C group=4.56±0.93).
Discussion: Our results show that the rigidity of the red blood cell membrane increased. This process has an important role to decrease the movement of the red blood cell through the capillaries inducing disturbance of microcirculation.
Conclusion: With the help of this method it is easy and quick to detect the consequences of mesenteric ischemia-reperfusion injury. Probably it could help to follow the patient at the critical period. This study was supported by The Ministry of Welfare Research Grant No. 6003/1/2001/ETT.

65

Ischemia / Reperfusion-Induced Leukocyte-Endothelium Interactions in the Colon: Importance of P-Selectin, Lymphocyte Function Antigen-1 and CXC Chemokines

A.A. Riaz

Malmö University Hospital, Malmö, Sweden

Introduction: Leukocyte recruitment is a key feature in (I/R)-induced tissue injury. We have developed and validated a novel method to study molecular mechanisms of leukocyte-endothelium interactions in the colonic microcirculation *in vivo* by use of inverted intravital fluorescence microscopy.
Methods: The superior mesenteric artery was occluded 30 min in male C57/BL6 mice and leukocyte rolling and adhesion were analyzed in colonic venules using IVM after 120 min of reperfusion. Administration of oxygen free radical scavengers (allopurinol and superoxide dismutase) were used to assess the role of OFR in our model. The role of selectin, and integrin family of adhesion molecules was assessed using monoclonal antibodies directed against P-, E-, L- and control antibodies and LFA -/- mice. Furthermore the role of CXC chemokines in I/R-induced tissue injury in the colon was assessed using anti-KC and anti-MIP-II injected again just prior to reperfusion.
Results: It was found that 30 min of ischemia and 120 min of reperfusion induced the strongest and most reproducible leukocyte response, i.e. leukocyte rolling and adhesion was 29±3 cells/min and 75±25 cells/mm, respectively. Administration of allopurinol and superoxide dismutase dose-dependently reduced the I/R-induced leukocyte responses, validating the pathophysiologic role of oxygen radical generation in this model. The mechanisms of leukocyte rolling by inhibiting was investigated using anti L-, E- and P-selectin antibodies. We found that pretreatment with P-selectin antibody significantly reduced leukocyte rolling and adhesion by 88% and 85%, respectively, whereas antibodies directed against L- and E-selectin had no effect. Moreover, I/R-induced leukocyte adhesion was reduced by 95% in LFA-1 deficient mice, whereas leukocyte rolling was intact. Next we evaluated the role of CXC chemokines and found that injection of antibodies directed against MIP-2 and KC markedly reduced both leukocyte rolling and adhesion. Furthermore RT-PCR and ELISA demonstrated a marked increase in mRNA and protein levels of MIP-2 and KC in the colonic tissue after I/R.
Discussion and Conclusion: This study presents a new method to study I/R-induced leukocyte responses in the colon and provide evidence demonstrating that leukocyte rolling is mediated by P-selectin and that firm adhesion is supported by LFA-1 in I/R-induced injury in the colon. Moreover we show an important role for CXC chemokines (MIP-2 and KC) in mediating the leukocyte response in the colon. Taken together, this data may provide important targets to control pathological inflammation in I/R-induced tissue injury in the colon.

66

In Vivo Neuronal Nitric Oxide Synthase Stimulation Protects Intestinal Ischemic Injury

A. Sola, M.A. Peinado[1], E. Martínez-Lara[1], A. Jiménez[1], E. Gelpí, G. Hotter

Dept. of Medical Bioanalysis, Instituto de Investigaciones Biomédicas de Barcelona, Barcelona, Dept. Biología Experimental[1], Universidad de Jaén, Jaén, Spain

Introduction: Intestinal ischemia-reperfusion (IR) can produce a profound endothelial dysfunction that could lead to the intestinal barrier failure with the consequent translocation of enteric bacteria, sepsis and death. In this work, we have assessed *in vivo* which isoform of NOS is stimulated in a protective biological event before the I/R injury where the protective implication of NO have been clearly established (e.g. preconditioning). To address these issues, we have investigated how, where, when and which NOS isoform is implicated and activated in this process.
Methods: Intestinal ischemia and preconditioning was induced in Wistar rats by clamping the superior mesenteric artery. We determined NO production, the isoforms of NO synthase (NOS) implicated in the protection by localization and quantification of NADPH diaphorase histochemistry reaction (an enzyme that colocalizes with NO-synthesis activity) and by immunohistochemistry and Western blot of the different NOS isoforms. We also tested the inmunohistochemical and Western blot detection of nitrotyrosine that could also confirm the actual or the past presence of NO formation.
Results/Discussion: NADPH diaphorase is clearly enhanced in preconditioned animals. That was coincident and colocalized with the enhanced immunoreactivity for nNOS and with the increased protein expression. eNOS and iNOS immunohistochemistry and protein expression did not differ between groups.
Conclusion: *In vivo* stimulation of nNOS in intestinal tissue by a simple surgical method as preconditioning is able to produce NO that mediates protection against a subsequent and sustained ischemia.

67

Hemodynamic Effect of Intestinal Nitrite under Normoxic and Hypoxic Conditions

L. Szalay[1,2], F. Umar[1], A. Kozlov[1,3], H. Redl[1], S. Bahrami[1]

Ludwig Boltzmann Inst. for Experimental and Clinical Traumatology[1], Vienna, Austria, Inst. of Surgical Research[2], Univ. of Szeged, Hungary, Inst. of Pharmacology and Toxicology[3], Univ. of Veterinary Medicine, Vienna, Austria

Introduction: Recently, we have shown a nitric oxide synthase (NOS) independent formation of nitric oxide (NO) in ischemic intestine. Moreover, *in vitro* experiments performed with intestinal homogenates revealed their capability to reduce nitrite to NO, even more pronounced in the absence of oxygen. The aim of the present study was to determine whether intestinal nitrite might be the source of NO, affecting hemodynamic parameters under physiologic (normoxic) or hypoxic conditions.
Methods: Anaesthetized rats were instrumented for hemodynamic measurements, including mean arterial pressure (MAP), heart rate (HR) cardiac index (CI), stroke volume (SV), and total peripheral resistance index (TPRI). In order to install nitrite ($NaNO_2$) intraluminally, the animals were subjected to a midline laparotomy. After a 15 min stabilization period, 1 ml of Ringer's solution containing $NaNO_2$ (0, 0.2, 2, or 20 mg/ml) was injected into the proximal part of jejunum followed by monitoring hemodynamic parameters up to 12 min. Animals were allowed breathing spontaneously either room-air (normoxic group) or a gas mixture of 15/85% oxygen/nitrogen (hypoxic group).
Results: Intraluminal installation of $NaNO_2$ significantly reduced MAP and TPRI in a dose dependent fashion without affecting the heart function. Hypoxia significantly enhanced the reduction in TPRI.
Conclusion: Our data demonstrate that nitrite, present in the intestinal lumen, may become the source of NO generation, resulting in vasodilatation and hemodynamic alterations. Hypoxic conditions may augment the reduction of nitrite to NO thereby enhancing vasodilatation.

68

Adenosine/Xanthine Level Modulates NO Generation and Tissue Injury in Renal Ischemia

J. López-Martí[1], A. Sola[1], F. Pi[1], V. Alfaro[2], G. Hotter[1]

Dept. of Medical Bioanalysis[1], Instituto de Investigaciones Biomédicas de Barcelona, Dept. of Physiology[2], Faculty of Biology, University of Barcelona, Barcelona, Spain

Introduction: This study assessed the time-dependent changes of the tissular adenosine/xanthine levels during renal ischemia, and the effect of these nucleotide changes on the modulation of nitric oxide (NO) and superoxide (O_2^-)generation and subsequent renal injury.
Methods: Kidney ischemia/reperfusion (I/R) was experimentally induced in rats at different times (10, 30 and 60 min). The effects of the duration of ischemia during renal I/R were evaluated from the analysis of renal nucleotide levels (ATP, ADP, AMP, adenosine, xanthine and hypoxanthine), and from the effect of nucleotide level modulation (by addition of exogenous xanthine, adenosine or theophylline) on NO/O_2^- production, tissular injury and renal function.
Results/Discussion: Tissular levels of adenosine decreased as time of ischemia was longer, whereas xanthine/hypoxanthine levels increased concomitant with renal dysfunction and severe histological damage. NO production increased during early ischemia time but remained constant in subsequent times of ischemia, whereas lipoperoxidation increased parallel to the increase in the time of ischemia. The administration of theophylline reversed the early increase in NO production and adenosine administration enhanced significantly the NO generation. A deleterious effect of exogenous xanthine and adenosine on both renal function (reflected as increased creatinine and BUN) and histology was found.
Conclusion: The present findings show that the time of ischemia during renal I/R modulates lipoperoxidation and NO generation in a different way. NO/O_2^- production and the subsequent tissue injury and renal dysfunction may be modified by changes in the adenosine and xanthine levels of the injured kidney.

69

Thromboxane Release in Ischemia and Reperfusion Injury Studied by Microdialysis

M. Ionac, D. Bordos

Surgical Clinic 2, "Victor Babes" University of Medicine and Pharmacy, Timisoara, Romania

Introduction: Ischemia and reperfusion (IR) in the free tissues transfer represents a significant form of injury. Several lines of evidence implicate enhanced eicosanoid, and in particular thromboxane A_2 (TXA_2) synthesis as one of the IR mediators. Microdialysis, a new bioanalytical sampling technique, enables the monitoring of substances in the extracellular space. The present study aims to investigate the use of the technique in the *in vivo* measurement of TXA_2 levels in a model of IR injury in a free flap model in the rat.

Methods: Experimental model. Twelve male adult SD rats (average weight 320 g) were used. Gracilis semitendinosus free flaps were harvested and randomized into three groups. Four flaps were subjected to 2 hours, four were subjected to 4 hours and the last four to 6 hours of warm (37°C) ischemia. After the ischemic period the flaps were revascularized to the contralateral femoral vessels. A Cuprophan probe with a cut-off of 20 kDa was inserted into the muscle and perfused with 5 ml/min Ringer lactate. The samples were collected at 20 min during the equilibration, the ischemia period and the first 2 hours of reperfusion. Biopsies were taken from all flaps and contralateral nontransplanted control muscles and examined histologically for necrosis, inflammation and edema. Quantification of TXB_2. The release of immunoreactive TXB_2 was quantified for each sample in duplicate by sensitive ELISA using a monoclonal antibody for TXB_2 (clone 4E-TBR1). Data analysis. Statistical significance was calculated by the Fischer f-test. A p value of less or equal to 0.05 indicates a statistically significant difference between two sets of data.

Results: The mean level of TXB_2 during the ischemic period was 1785.34 ± 124.81 pg/ml and was considered base level. The mean levels of TXB_2 during reperfusion have been correlated positively with the duration of the ischemia, raising significantly ($p< 0.05$) compared to base level with 151.65% in the 2 hours ischemia group, with 192.33% in 4 hours ischemia and 294.69% in 6 hours. These values were also correlated with histologic observations.

Discussion: The present study reports the development of a new method for recovering immunoreactive TXB_2 from the extracellular fluid of an experimental free flap by implanting a microdialysis probe into the ischemic and reperfused tissue. The results demonstrate that the microdialysis technique permits monitoring of dynamics of TXA_2 release in interstitial space of an ischemic and reperfused free skeletal muscle flap. Our results may suggest thromboxane as a mediator of tissue necrosis in IR syndrome, since its increasing release correlates with histological tissue damage.

Conclusion: Microdialysis combined with a sensitive ELISA techniques proves to be a useful method for *in vivo* identification and monitoring of the release of TXA_2 and possibly other mediators of inflammation in experimental muscle free flaps during IR syndrome.

70

Gender Differences in Neutrophil Priming and Oxidative Injury Following Trauma and Hemorrhagic Shock

B. Toth, J.F. Kuebler, M. Schwacha, J. Hamar, K.I. Bland, P. Wang, I.H. Chaudry

University of Alabama at Birmigham, Birmingham, Alabama, USA

Introduction: Gender has been shown to influence immune and organ functions following trauma and hemorrhagic shock (T/H). Although neutrophils (PMN) play an important role following low flow conditions such as ischemia/reperfusion and hemorrhagic shock, it remains unknown whether gender affects PMN priming and free radical levels under such conditions.

Methods: Female Sprague-Dawley rats (3 months old) on the proestrus day of their menstrual cycle and age-matched male rats were used. Animals were subjected to a 5 cm midline laparotomy (i. e., induction of soft tissue trauma) and non-heparinized rats were then bled to a mean arterial pressure of 35 mmHg for ~90 min followed by fluid resuscitation (4 times the shed blood volume in the form of Ringer's lactate). At 2 hr and 24 hr following resuscitation or sham operation (n=6-11/group), circulating PMNs were isolated and tissue samples were harvested. PMNs were assessed for superoxide (O_2^-) production and various tissue samples were analyzed for myeloperoxidase (MPO) activity (a marker of PMN accumulation), thiobarbituric acid reactive substances (TBARS, a marker of lipid peroxidation) and tyrosine nitration (an index of peroxynitrite generation). One-way ANOVA and Student-Newman-Keul test were used for statistical analysis.

Results: PMN's O_2^- production in response to PMA stimulation was not altered by T/H or influenced by gender. In contrast, fMLP-stimulated O_2^- production was increased in PMNs from T/H rats. Gender influenced the PMN responsiveness following T/H as the levels of fMLP-stimulated O_2^- production by cells from T/H male rats were significantly greater than that of females. While T/H induced significant PMN accumulation (MPO activity) and oxidative injury (TBARS and tyrosine nitration) in the lung, liver and intestine of both male and female rats, the MPO activity, TBARS and nitrotyrosine levels in these tissues were significantly higher in males.

Discussion and conclusion: Male rats displayed significantly greater levels of T/H-induced PMN priming, activation and tissue sequestration as well as subsequent oxidative injury as compared to proestrus females. These observations suggest that the decreased PMN priming and activation in proestrus females, as compared to males, following T/H and the decreased tissue oxidative injury may contribute to the decreased cellular injury (i.e., TBARS and nitrotyrosine), lesser organ damage and improved outcome under those conditions. The co-localization of PMN accumulation and lipid peroxidation and tyrosine nitration suggests that PMNs play a significant role in tissue oxidative injury, specifically in males. (Supported by NIH Grant R37 GM39519)

Sepsis and Inflammation

71

Lactobacillus Plantarum 299v Reduces Endotoxin-Induced Bacterial Translocation in Rats

P. Mangell, M. Wang, S. Ahrné, G. Molin, H. Thorlacius, B. Jeppsson

Dept. of Surgery, Malmö University Hospital, Lund University and Dept. of Food Technology, Lund University, Sweden

Introduction: Translocation of enteric bacteria to extraintestinal sites is prevented by an intact intestinal mucosa. Disturbance of the mucosa may facilitate translocation of pathological bacteria and ultimately cause sepsis and multiple organ failure. Endotoxin is known to provoke bacterial translocation. However, it is not known whether probiotic bacteria, such as lactobacilli, may attenuate endotoxin-provoked translocation. In this study, we hypothesized that oral pretreatment with a probiotic bacterium may inhibit pathological translocation in rats.

Methods: Male Sprague-Dawley rats were pretreated with free access to regular drinking water (group A and B); unfermented oatmeal (group C) or *L. plantarum 299v* (mean intake 1010 CFU/day) in oatmeal (group D). After one week, groups B-D were given an intraperitoneal injection of lipopolysaccaride (LPS) from *E. coli* serotype O111:B4. After 24 hours, rats were sacrificed and mesenteric lymph node (MLN), liver, spleen and distal ileum were taken for bacterial culture.

Results: We found no translocation to MLN or liver in the control group (A). In contrast, LPS (group B) caused significant translocation of enteric bacteria to liver (7/8) and spleen (5/8). Pretreatment with unfermented oat (group C) further increased the LPS-induced translocation to MLN (6/8), liver (8/8) and spleen (6/8). Notably, pretreatment with *L. plantarum 299v* (group D) completely abolished translocation to MLN (0/8) and significantly reduced translocation to the liver (1/8). However, *L. plantarum 299v* had no significant inhibitory effect on translocation to the spleen (4/8). Moreover, there was no significant difference in the number of lactobacilli in the distal ileum between the groups. Nonetheless, LPS increased the level of Gram negative aerobes in the intestine.

Discussion: This study demonstrates that free access to *L. plantarum 299v* effectively reduced endotoxin-induced bacterial translocation. This protective effect of *L. plantarum 299v* appears to be unrelated to an increase in the absolute numbers of lactobacilli in the distal ileum. It is possible that the inhibitory effect of *L. plantarum 299v* on translocation may be attributable to secreted factors, which, however, was not addressed in the present study. It is interesting to note that unfermented oatmeal, a prebiotic, increased bacterial translocation in endotoxin-treated animals. The mechanism behind this effect is not known, but it may be speculated that administration of probiotics alone may predominately promote growth of the pathological flora under situations of endotoxemic stress.

Conclusion: Administration of *L. plantarum* 299v prevents pathological translocation of enteric bacteria provoked by endotoxin.

72

The Effect of Epidermal Growth Factor, *Lactobacillus Plantarum 299v* and Oat Fiber on Dextran Sulfate Sodium-Induced Colitis Model

C. Trably[1], D. Adawi[1], R. Ehrnström[2], B. Veress[2], M. Eklund[3], B. Jeppsson[1]

Departments of Surgery[1] and Pathology[2], Malmö University Hospital, Department of Surgery[3], Lund University Hospital, Sweden

Introduction: Epidermal growth factor (EGF) has been shown to play an important role in response to injury by promoting wound healing. EGF is capable of protecting the gastrointestinal mucosa from damage and enhances growth and mucosal repair of the gastrointestinal mucosa. The pathogenic mechanism of inflammatory bowel diseases (IBD) is not fully understood. The effect of colonic inflammation on intestinal microflora specifically lactobacilli are not clear although bacteriotherapy with lactobacilli has been reported to be effective both in ulcerative and pseudomembranous colitis. The interaction between EGF and lactobacilli and the possible beneficial effects on colonic inflammation are not known. The present study was performed to investigate the role of growth factors, *Lactobacillus plantarum 299v* and oat fibre, in DSS-induced colitis and the associated histological, intestinal mucosal and microflora changes.

Methods: Sprague-Dawley rats were used and divided into five groups. Colitis was induced by DSS 5 % (w/v) dissolved in drinking water for 7 days. EGF was administered through an osmotic minipump inserted subcutaneously in the suprascapular region. Severity of colitis assessed daily using a Disease Activity Index (DAI). Samples were collected on the 7th day for myeloperoxidase, mucosal mass analysis, different macroscopic and microscopic histological scoring, bacterial microflora and bacterial translocation.

Results: The DAI decreased on day 4 in the combined group DSS+Lac+EGF compared to DSS and DSS+Lac groups. DAI on days 5, 6 and 7 in the DSS+Lac+EGF group decreased compared to DSS, DSS+Lac and DSS+EGF groups, on the other hand in the DSS group increased compared to DSS+Lac and DSS+EGF groups. Macroscopic morphological damage, total histological scoring, mucus cell depletion score and crypt damage score in the distal colon in the DSS+Lac+EGF group decreased significantly compared to DSS, DSS+Lac and DSS+EGF groups. Bacterial translocation decreased in all the treatment groups compared to DSS colitis group.

Conclusion: Administration of EGF, *Lactobacillus plantarum 299v* and the combination of both decreased the Disease Activity Index but the combined treatment is more significant than EGF, *Lb. plantarum* alone. It also decreased macroscopic morphological damage, total histological scoring, mucus cell depletion score and crypt damage. The administration of *Lb. plantarum* and/or EGF decreased bacterial translocation to the extraintestinal sites. It seems that the combination of EGF and *Lb. plantarum* has beneficial effect in the DSS-induced colitis model although the exact mechanisms are not clearly understood.

73

Regulation of the Inflammatory Response on the Molecular Level in Mononuclear Blood Cells in Patients with Sepsis

T. Zimmermann, G. von Gagern, S. Albrecht, S. Kersting, H.D. Saeger*

Dept. of Surgery, Dept. of Gynaecology*, Technical University Dresden, Dresden, Germany

Introduction: Mononuclear blood cells (MBC) are a part of the inflammatory response network in patients with sepsis. The aim of our investigation was to figure out the role of MBC in the molecular regulation of the inflammation (transcription -mRNA synthesis- protein synthesis).

Methods: The authors examined 24 patients with S.I.R.S./sepsis (Apache III-Score with more than 69 Pts.) during 28 days (day 1, 3, 7, 14, 21 and 28). Lab. monitoring: NFκB binding activity in MBC (EMSA); mRNA expression of I Ba, MIF, TNFα , iNOS in MBC (RT-PCR); protein synthesis of MIF and IκBa in MBC (western blot), protein concentration of the target genes in plasma (ELISA)

Results: We found a higher NFκB binding capacity in survived patients during the whole time. Nonsurvived patients showed an I Ba depression on the third day. This was opposite to the surviving patients and persisted to the last day of the remaining time. The mRNA expression of the target genes (TF, TNFα , MIF, IκBa and iNOS) are higher in the survived patients. There are no correlatid between the mRNA expression in the nonsurvive patients in MBC with the distinctly higher protein concentration of TNFα , MIF and TF in plasma. The protein synthesis of MIF in MBC is distinctly elevated on survived and nonsurviving patients. We found MIF also in the nucleolus. The protein of IκBa was not detectable or only in small amounts.

Conclusion: There was a work inflammatory response in MBC in survived patients in relating on NFκB target genes. We found a less expression of the target genes in nonsurviving patients. A dysregulation of the normal function of MBC seems to play a key role for the letality of patients with S.I.R.S./sepsis.

74

The Role of IκBa on Regulation of Inflammatory Response in Septic Patients

T. Zimmermann[1], G. v. Gagern[1], H. Schikore[2], I. Alldinger[1], S. Kersting[1], S. Albrecht[3], H.D. Saeger[1]

Dept. of Visceral-, Thoracic- and Vascular Surgery[1], Dept. of Trauma[2], Dept. of Gynaecology[3], Univ. Hosp. "Carl Gustav Carus", Tech. Univ. of Dresden, Dresden, Germany

Introduction: NFκB plays a crucial role in the regulation of inflammatory processes. The uncontrolled expression of mediators can be influenced only at molecular level. Therefore it is unavoidable to clear up the effects of transcription factors (NFκB, AP-1) as well as of inhibitors of activation (IκBa) using molecular biological methods.

Methods: Binding activity of NFκB, AP-1, NFκB subunits (p50, p65) and expression/protein synthesis of I Ba have been evaluated in 24 patients suffering from S.I.R.S./sepsis (APACHE III score above 69).

Results: Distinctly increased NFκB binding activity on the third postoperative day has been registered. In addition there was a significant positive correlation to IκBa mRNA- expression. In the group of nonsurvivors the IκBa-expression decreased below 40 per cent on the third day. It continued to be expressed on a low level until death. In mononuclear blood cells of nonsurvivors there seems to be a protein synthesis malfunction of IκBa. In the group of survivors the IκBa expression was reduced.

Conclusion: In mononuclear blood cells IκBa plays a major part as a controller of NFκB activation. It means first a supervision of excessive NFκB binding activity in the group of nonsurvivors and secondly a missing output ("*de novo*" synthesis) of IκBa as a sign of reduced activation of NFκB for survivors (C.A.R.S.- reaction-immunoparalysis).

75

With or Without? Role of FAS in Sepsis

U. Glatzel[1], R.H. Tolba[2], M. Tinelli[1], M. Lysson[2], A. Wentzensen[1], T. Minor[2]

Div. of Orthopedic Surgery BG-Unfallklinik[1] Ludwigshafen, Surgical Research Div.[2] University of Bonn, Germany

Introduction: Multiple organ dysfunction syndrome (MODS) in trauma and sepsis is associated with mortality rates from 60% up to 98% if organ dysfunction involves three or more organs for 7 or longer days. Infections, specifically those involving lipopolysaccharide (LPS or endotoxin) may trigger for initiation of systemic inflammatory disease (SIRS) and MODS. Our aim was to investigate the role of Fas-activation and apoptosis with respect to topic organ dysfunction in LPS induced sepsis in the rat.

Methods: Male Wistar rats (260-300 g bw) were randomised into 3 groups. Sepsis was induced in 8 rats by LPS injection (single dose 4 mg/kg bw i.v.). Control animals (n=8) received corresponding amount of saline. Another 8 rats received LPS and an experimental receptor-blocking Fas-antibody (administered twice at a dose of 50 µg/g bw i.v. once with the LPS and again 24 h thereafter). On Day 3 all animals were sacrificed, organ samples as well as aliquots of central venous blood were taken for later analysis.

Results: FAS-receptor expression was investigated by immunohistochemistry using monoclonal antibody. LPS injection resulted in a significant ($p<0.05$) upregulation of FAS expression on lung alveolar cells but nor on hepatocytes. The histological distribution of FAS was parallelled by a significant increase in apoptotic (i.e. TUNEL-positive) alveolar cells/ high power field in the lung (5.6±2.6* vs 5.5±1.0* vs 0.6±0.8 -LPS/LPS+AB/control; * $p<0.05$ or better vs control, ANOVA and post-hoc test), but no apparent TUNEL reactivity on hepatocytes. A moderate FAS independent elevation of TUNEL-reactivity after exposition to LPS was however found on sinusoidal lining cells. Conventional signs of liver tissue damage were slightly elevated upon LPS challenge (serum bilirubine: 0.23±0.05* vs 0.15±0.13 vs 0.11±0.07 mg/dl; ALT: 149±121 vs 76±9 vs 64±5 U/l - LPS/LPS+AB/control), but more pronounced were sepsis-induced histological alterations in the lungs of "acute injury pattern": edema, membrane thickening, cellular infiltration) which, remarkably, were even massively enhanced upon systemic FAS-blockade. In particular, FAS-blocking antibody was followed by an

overwhelming increase of myeloperoxidase reactivity in the lungs after LPS challenge ($p < 0.05$), thus indicating exaggerated inflammatory tissue infiltration by activated granulocytes. Accordingly, in our model sepsis was lethal in 2 out of 8 animals (75% survival) versus 100% survival in controls, but the blockade of FAS-receptor reduced survival of the septic animals to only 25%.
Conclusion: We conclude from these results, that FAS mediated apoptosis does not seem to be a prevailing mechanism for end organ dysfunction in LPS-induced sepsis. Systemic application of FAS blocking agents actually does not reduce end organ failure but seems to prevent FAS mediated down-regulation of circulating leukocytes, eventually leading to exaggerated tissue inflammation and dysfunction.

76

Antibiotic Prophylaxis in Clean Surgery. A Spanish Inquiry

M. Caínzos, F. Lozano, J.L. Balibrea, J. Culebras, D. Dávil, A.A. Gomez, I. Iturburo, S. Morales, B. Oller, J. Potel, L.M. Sánchez-Ortega, J.M. Tellado

Dept. of Surgery, Hospital Ciynico Universitario, Santiago de Compostela, Spain

Introduction: The objective of this inquiry was to define Spanish practice and the opinion of Spanish surgeons regarding the use of antibiotic prophylaxis in clean surgery.
Methods: One anonymous inquiry was sent to the members of the Spanish Association of Surgeons. This inquiry was open from 1st of September to 31st of December 2000.
Results: Of the inquiries sent, a total of 602 inquiries have been received valid for tabulation. Of these inquiries, only 8.6 per cent corresponded to residents and 87.7 per cent to staff surgeons. Some 76.2 per cent of the surgeons were working in public hospitals, 10.8 per cent in private hospitals and 9.6 per cent in public-private hospitals. The hospitals have a standard policy for surgical antibiotic prophylaxis in 76.1 per cent of cases. 11.5 per cent of the surgeons use antibiotic prophylaxis routinely in clean surgery, and 85 per cent use antibiotic prophylaxis in specific surgical procedures. Some 36 per cent use it in mastectomy, 26 per cent in hernia repair but 86 per cent in prosthetic hernia repair; 58 per cent in laparorraphy, 18 per cent in thyroid surgery and 16 per cent in parathyroid surgery; 64 per cent in non-traumatic splenectomy, 48 per cent in exploratory laparotomy and 13 per cent in varicotomy. Concerning the duration of antibiotic prophylaxis, 55.9 per cent of the surgeons use only one preoperative dose. The most used antibiotics are cepholosporins (63.9 per cent) and in particular the second-generation (32.7 per cent) cephalosporins, 26.6 per cent use ß-lactam antibiotics, and only 4.5 per cent use aminoglycosides. We compare these results with a similar inquiry realized in 1994 and we found statistical differences.
Conclusion: According to this inquiry in Spain, 11.5 per cent of surgeons were using antibiotic prophylaxis systematically in all types of clean surgery and 3.5 per cent never used it in this type of surgery. The remaining surgeons used it in specific types of clean surgery.

77

The Soluble Tumor Necrosis Factor Receptor I (STNFRI) is an Early Predictor of Local Infective Complications after Colorectal Surgery

R. Slotwinski[1,2], W.L. Olszewski[1], A. Chaber[2], M. Slodkowski[2], M. Zaleska[1], I.W. Krasnodebski[2]

Dept. of Surgical Research and Transplantology[1], Med. Res. Center, Polish Academy of Sciences, Dept. of General, Gastrointestinal Surgery and Nutrition[2], Med. Univ. of Warsaw, Warsaw, Poland

Introduction: The role of endogenous cytokine antagonists after surgery and in patients with postoperative infections is poorly understood. Naturally occurring cytokine inhibitors have been detected in increased concentrations after severe injury and in septic patients. The aim of the study was to measure the serum levels of pro- and anti-inflammatory cytokines in patients with colorectal cancer surgery and compare their level in groups of patients with and without postoperative complications at the site of anastomosis and in the abdominal wound.
Methods: Studies were carried out in 22 patients with colorectal carcinoma undergoing elective surgical tumor removal. Thirteen patients developed postoperative complications, as massive wound infections, intraabdominal abscess and anastomosis dehiscence. Serum IL-1β, IL-1ra, TNFα, SRNFRI, IL-6, IL-8, IL-10 concentrations were measured before surgery and on the days 1, 3, 7,1 0 and 14 thereafter, by ELISA.
Results: There was a significant increase in serum concentrations of IL-6, IL-1ra and STNFRI between day 1 and 14 following surgery. There were no statistically significant differences in IL-1β, TNFα, IL-8, IL-6, IL-1ra and IL-10 concentrations between the group with and without postoperative complications. Significantly higher serum median concentrations of STNFRI were observed in the group of patients with postoperative complications, compared with that without complications on day 1 ($p=0.01$), 3 ($p=0.04$) and 10 ($p=0.04$). The serum median STNFRI level reached following values: 2662, 2806, 2487, 2453 and 2050 pg/ml on day 1, 3, 7, 10 and 14, respectively.
Conclusion: Our results demonstrate that changes of STNFRI, IL-1ra and IL-6 serum concentration are sensitive indicators of the response to surgery, but only STNFRI is a sensitive early marker of local septic complications in patients with colorectal carcinoma.

Vascular and Cardiac Surgery

78

Correlation Between Plasma Homocysteine, Aortic Aneurysms and Vitamins

A.A. Warsi[1], D. Hullin[1], B. Davies[2], M.H. Lewis[1]

Royal Glamorgan Hospital[1] and University of Glamorgan[2], S. Wales, UK

Introduction: Elevated levels of homocysteine (>15 micromol/L) is a recognised independent risk factor in the genesis of vascular diseases. There is little data, which has examined the relationship between homocysteine and the development of abdominal aortic aneurysm (AAA), and the influence of vitamin B_{12} and folic acid blood levels. The aim of this study was to examine the possible relationship between plasma homocysteine, AAA and vitamins.
Methods: Ethical approval was obtained for this prospective, case control study with age matched groups. Fasting homocysteine blood levels were analysed using a fluorescence polarisation immunoassay technique. Serum was separated within one hour of blood collection from antecubital venous puncture into an EDTA primed tube, from 38 AAA and 36 case controls for analysis.
Results: 26 (68%) of the AAA patients had elevated levels of homocysteine compared to 2 (6%) in the case control group. The mean homocysteine level in the AAA group was 19.4 (SE 1.1) (95% CI 17.17 - 21.65) and in the control group was 10.9 (SE 0.47) (95% CI 9.95 - 11.88), ($p<0.001$). Mean Vitamin B_{12} in the AAA and control was 332.11 (SE 16.44) and 414.33 (SE 19.72) ($p<0.001$), respectively. Mean folic acid in the AAA was 8.02 (SE 0.71) and in control was 9.8 (SE 0.69) (ns). There was no correlation between the size of the AAA and the level of plasma homocysteine in the AAA group. There were no differences with regards to age and gender and the level of plasma homocysteine either in the AAA group or control group.
Discussion: Our data suggests that there is a significant correlation between plasma homocysteine and AAA. This supports data published previously, which are limited. Moreover, our data suggest that there is higher prevalence of hyperhomocysteinemia (68%) in AAA than previously reported (48%). The prevalence of hyperhomocysteinemia of 6% in our study is similar to 5-7% reported previously. However, unlike previous reports our data fail to show an association between the level of plasma homocysteine and the size of the AAA in the study. In addition, unlike previous studies we found no correlation between elevated homocysteine and age or gender either the AAA group or the control group. Vitamins are known to regulate the metabolism of homocysteine thus preventing hyperhomocysteinemia. Previous studies have demonstrated an inverse correlation between deficient serum vitamin B_{12}, folic acid, vitamin B_6 and plasma homocysteine. Boushey et al. have concluded in a meta-analysis that folic acid bears the strongest influence on the level of plasma homocysteine. However, our data suggests that vitamin B_{12} and not folic acid have a stronger influence on the plasma homocysteine.
Conclusion: This study confirms significantly higher levels of plasma homocysteine in AAA. Use of selected supplemental vitamins that lowers plasma homocysteine, may modify vascular disease progression and clinical trials in this direction are warranted.

79

Topical Wall Shear Stress and Intimal Hyperplasia at End-to-Side Anastomosis

H. Ishibashi, Y. Kiyota, H. Ikeda, M. Ojha

Cardiovascular Surgery, Aichi Medical University, Nagakute, Aichi, Japan

Introduction: It is well known that there is a close relationship between the localization of anastomotic intimal hyperplasia and wall shear stress. Our purpose in this study was to measure topical wall shear stress at end-to-side anastomosis and to investigate arterial wall remodeling after the surgery.
Methods: A) Rheological study. An end-to-side anastomosis was produced in rabbit common carotid arteries. A vascular cast of the anastomosis was made from the anastomosed artery by infusing a plastic casting compound into the vessel. An ultraviolet-transparent flow mold was made from this anastomosis. Shear stress was measured at various sites around the anastomosis using the photochromic tracer technique. B) Pathological study. Two weeks after producing the end-to-side anastomosis, BrdU was administered, the rabbits were sacrificed, and the anastomosis was harvested. Longitudinal sections of the anastomosis were prepared and then stained immunohistologically to measure the rate of cell division around the anastomosis.
Results: Intimal hyperplasia developed mainly on the toe, the blind pouch, and the distal floor opposite the toe of the anastomosis. Shear stress of the roof and proximal floor was low (0 to 1 dyne/cm^2) at mean flow rate. The top of the velocity profile shifted to the floor side and a stagnation point shifted distally at peak flow rate. Shear stress was -1 to -3 dyne/cm^2 on the proximal floor and 16 to 29 dyne/cm^2 on the distal floor. The rate of BrdU-positive-cell was 16% at the distal floor opposite the toe of the anastomosis. This value was higher than detected at other portions (4 to 10%). Shear stress on the distal floor opposite the toe oscillated from positive to negative with the cardiac cycle. The rate of cell division was high in this position.
Conclusion: Anastomotic intimal hyperplasia developed where shear stress was low. We suspect that shear-stress oscillation induced intimal hyperplasia at the floor.

80

Extracellular Matrix Substance Coating on Culture Dish Inhibits Vascular Wall Cell Growth for Tissue Engineering

T. Miyake, T. Shinoka, J. Kashiwagi, M. Watanabe, T. Konuma, N. Hibino, A. Murata, Y. Nation, K. Nakajima, H. Kurosawa

Dept. of Cardiovascular Surgery, The Heart Institute of Japan, Tokyo Women Medical University, Japan

Introduction: Currently used prosthetic or bioprosthetic materials lack growth potential and, therefore, subsequently require replacement in pediatric patients as they mature. Tissue engineering (TE) is a new discipline that offers the potential to create replacement structures from autologous cells and biodegradable polymer scaffolds. In May 2000 we started the clinical application of tissue engineered vascular grafts. Until December 2001, nine patients underwent TE graft implantation. An approximately 2-cm segment of peripheral veins were explanted and cells from its walls isolated. Cells were cultured and expanded. The biodegradable polymer conduit was designed to degrade within 8 weeks. Ten days after seeding, the graft transplantation was performed. Cell growth in culture dish is a key point to create tissue-engineering structure. In this study we examined the effect of dish coating with several matrix protein and of fetal bovine serum (FBS) on cell growth.

Methods: Under general anesthesia with the patient in a supine position, saphenous vein was harvested from cruris. The venous tissue was minced with scalpel on non-coated dish and cultured for two weeks in culture media supplemented with heparin, penicillin-streptomycin, fungizone, VEGF, HGF, and b-FGF. Baseline cell counting was performed by cell count instrument. After cells were rinsed by PBS and trypsinized by trypsin-EDTA solutions, cells were evenly distributed into twelve culture dishes ($10x10^3$ cells/ml). The bottom surface of culture dishes were coated with collagen type I (Group I), collagen type IV (Group IV), fibronectin (Group F), gelatin (Group G), poly-L-lysine (Group L) and nothing (Group N). Cells in each six dish were cultured by two different culture media (with FBS or without FBS) for two weeks and final cell counting were analyzed.

Results: All results were expressed as mean ± standard deviation of the mean and analyzed by a statistical analysis software package (Stat-View Ver. 4.5). Analysis of variance (ANOVA) and Bornferroni test were used to compare the difference among groups. A p-value less than 0.05 were considered statistically significant. Cell counts after two weeks culture were as below. (X 10^3) Group N (+FBS) 103±18 Group N (-FBS) 31±3 Group I (+FBS) 15±3 Group I (-FBS) 12±2 Group IV (+FBS) 67±2 Group IV (-FBS) 20±2 Group F (+FBS) 40±7 Group F (-FBS) 25±5 Group G (+FBS) 76±2 Group G (-FBS) 43±3 Group L (+FBS) 59±5 Group L (-FBS) 20±3 Cell counts of FBS-groups are significantly larger than the other group ($p<0.0001$). Group N showed the most cell count in all groups in Bonferroni/Dunn test ($p<0.0001$).

Conclusion: In this study, the surface coating of culture dishes with extracellular matrix protein did not improve vascular cell growth *in vitro* system. Cell-network formation might inhibit the cell growth in the presence of matrix protein in culture system. An addition of FBS into the culture media accelerated cell proliferation. At the present time supplement of FBS is necessary for cell growth in creating tissue-engineering structure.

81

Titanium Clips and Bioglue in Vascular Surgery

T. Kotsis, A. Pafiti, K. Katsenis, P. Dimakakos

Vascular Department, Aretaeion Hospital, Medical School, University of Athens, Greece

Introduction: Vascular reconstruction with conventional sutures results in immediate post-reconstruction bleeding through the penetrated vessel's wall, and late intima irregularities because of the injury and irritation provoked by the foreign material. In this comparative experimental study we used titanium clips and glue in angioplasties to reduce bleeding and to avoid penetration of the wall. Haemostasis and vessel histology was evaluated in comparison with conventional suturing.

Methods: Forty angioplasties in ten pigs (mean weight 27 kg), using a synthetic patch were carried out; isolated stitches were placed at the right carotid (10) and the infrarenal abdominal aorta (10), while titanium clips were used at the left carotid artery (10) and the abdominal aorta just above the bifurcation (10). Haemostasis following completion of angioplasty was achieved, in the first case by isolated stitches and in the second case by local use of haemostatic Bioglue. Blood samples for intra-operative histocombatibility were taken, while 4 weeks later the patency and durability of the angioplasties were evaluated by means of angiography and balloon dilatation; histological examination of the angioplasties was also carried out.

Results: Bleeding occurred even after using the clips-Bioglue combination but the blood loss was statistically significantly less than that of the classical suturing ($p<0.001$). The duration of the angioplasty as well as the total time of ischaemia of the tissues were also less ($p<0.001$) in the second case; similarly when angioplasties were performed with clips, the impermeability was higher, and one month later following angiography more vessels were patent, while the resistance of the repaired segments (durability) during balloon dilatation was similar in both methods. The endothelium of the reconstructed vessels in the angioplasties performed with clips was intact while the vessels repaired with sutures presented with microthrombi and inflammatory elements; the use of Bioglue resulted in no local or systemic response.

Discussion: Angioplasty with titanium clips and haemostatic Bioglue decreases the risk of intraoperative post-repair bleeding, the time of tissue ischaemia and by avoiding the penetration of the vessel's wall reduces the vessel's injury, while presents an at least equal functionality of the repaired segments permitting balloon dilatation without risk of rupture.

Conclusion: Cross-clamping time, haemostasis time and post-repair bleeding are important factors in vascular surgery; the combination of non-penetrating titanium clips and Bioglue seems that reduces the aforementioned factors, and as shown by our experiments represents an alternative method for vessel repair.

82

Long-Term Result of Crossover Bypass to the Lower Limb

Y. Hamada, A. Otaki, T. Ogata, Y. Morishita

Kitakanto Cardiovascular Hospital, Gunma University School of Medicine, Maebashi, Japan

Introduction: This study was designed to evaluate the long-term patency of crossover bypass grafting as the treatment for arteriosclerosis obliterans in the lower limb.

Methods: 31 cases including 28 men and 3 women (mean age: 67) were enrolled to this study. Patient data was collected from the medical record, mail inquiry or telephone interview. Primary patency rate and survival rate were evaluated.

Results: Preoperative symptoms were intermittent claudication in 30 patients and resting pain in one. Risk factors of arteriosclerosis obliterans were smoking in 28, hypertension in 20, hypercholesterolemia in 8 and diabetes mellitus in 2. The lesions were infrarenal abdominal aorta or bilateral iliac artery or the combination of both lesions in 6 and unilateral iliac artery in 25. External iliac artery or femoral artery were selected as the inflow artery. When bilateral iliac arteries or infrarenal aorta were obstructed, unilateral axillo-femoral bypass was constructed to secure the inflow artery (n=6). Five out of 6 cases had another obstruction in the superficial femoral artery; therefore, axillo-femoral bypass was extended to distal superficial femoral artery. The anastomosis between graft and the proximal femoral or deep femoral artery was made in a sequential fashion. In the unilateral iliac artery obstruction cases, 6 had another lesions in the superficial femoral artery and femoro-popliteal bypass was made concomitantly. Therefore, solitary crossover bypass cases were 19. Outflow artery was selected mainly at the contralateral femoral artery. Artificial grafts used were Gore-tex in 17, Gelsoft in 6, Technograft in 5 and others in 3. Postoperatively, one or two kinds of anti-platelet drug were given in all patients and warfarin was given in 10 cases. In all cases, survival rate was 90% in one year, 80% in 5 year, 80% in 10 year. Exclusive to crossover bypass without axillo-femoral bypass, primary patency rate was 96% in one year, 91% in 4 year, 82% in 8 year. In 6 cases that the inflow artery was secured with the use of axillo-femoral bypass, primary patency rate was 80% in one year, 60% in 4 year, 60 % in 8 year. There were no amputation cases.

Discussion: The long-term patency is good in the crossover bypass in the ilio-femoral region.

Conclusion: According to our result, crossover bypass is a recommendable method not only for high-risk patients, but also when sexual dysfunction is feared.

83

Ventricular Rate Control during Atrial Fibrillation with Stimulation of the AV-Nodal Parasympathetic Plexus

P. Soós, P. Horváth, P. Schauerte[1], E. Zima, A. Juhász-Nagy, B. Merkely

Semmelweis University, Budapest, Dept. of Cardiovascular Surgery; University of Aachen[1], Germany

Introduction: The drugs generally used for the atrial fibrillation (AF) therapy commonly have negative inotropic effect. The goal of our study was to clarify, whether stimulation of the parasympathetic plexus that innervates the AV-node can decrease the rapid ventricular rate during AF and to analyze hemodynamic changes during the parasympathetic plexus stimulation.

Methods: In 9 dogs the parasympathetic plexus was stimulated intracardially or epicardially. The electrophysiological examinations were performed using direct current in a voltage (U) range of 1 V-40 V, impulse duration (ID) range of 0.05 ms-2 ms, the frequency was changed between 1 Hz-100 Hz. Diagrams of dose-response relationship were created to show the ventricular rate changes and the appearing third degree AV-blocks at each stimulation U, ID and frequency.

Results: During the stimulation of the parasympathetic plexus the RR interval was continuously expandable until a maximum of 5.9 times of the control value (from 285 ms to 1690 ms). Increasing the parameters further caused third degree AV-block. At 10 to 50 Hz, 1-2 ms ID stimulation and changing the voltage between 20-40 V the RR intervals increased to 4.3±0.3-times of the control values (from 249.3±7.6 ms to 1018.4±68.8 ms). This was accompanied by a significant decrease of the left ventricular end diastolic pressure (from 18.0±1.2 mm Hg to 11.2±0.2 mmHg, $p<0.05$), but didn't cause any significant change in the arterial mean pressure and in the dP/dt. Intravenous administration of atropine (0.1 mg/kg, bolus) eliminated the negative dromotropic effect of the stimulation.

Conclusion: Our results show that during AF the parasympathetic plexus stimulation can decrease the associated rapid ventricular rate without any harmful hemodynamic effect.

Hepatobiliary and Pancreatic Surgery

84

The CD14+ Class II+ Blood Cells Reveal Predilection to Liver Adenocarcinoma Metastases

M. Stanczyk[1], W.L. Olszewski[2], A. Wesolowska[2], M. Maruszynski[1]

Central Clinical Hospital of Military Med. School[1], Dept. Surg. Res. and Transplantation[2], Med. Res. Ctr., Polish Academy of Sciences, Warsaw, Poland

Introduction: The local reaction of the host against tumor is expressed by tumor infiltrating lymphocytes (TIL). The knowledge, which populations of blood mononuclear cells reveal predilection to accumulate around and in the tumor tissue, may be important for two reasons: a) evaluation of their cytotoxic capacity, and b) isolation and culturing cells for transfection with cytokine genes or arming with antitumor chemicals for tumoricidal therapy.

Aim: To characterize the blood mononuclear cell populations with highest predilection to adhere to the tumor tissue.

Methods: Tumor. Liver tumors were induced by injection of 106 CC351 colon cancer cells in to the portal vein. Blood cells. Liver sinusoidal blood washout cells (LSWC) were obtained from normal rats and rats with liver CC531 metastases by liver perfusion. Peripheral blood mononuclear cells (PBM) were isolated from normal and metastatic rats. PBM and LSWC adherence test to tumor cryosections. To examine the binding of blood cells to the colon carcinoma metastases in the liver an *in situ* frozen section assay was used. The PBM or LSWC were applied in a concentration of 1.56 cells on liver with tumor frozen section and incubated under rotation for 30 min. Slides were fixed in 70% metanol. Adhering cells were distinguished under 200x magnification from cells located within the tissue by their different focal position. Quantitation of cells adhering to the normal and tumor tissue was performed using a calibrated ocular gird. Topography of cell binding was evaluated quantitatively using Olympus Microimage analysis software. To determine the expression of surface molecules of adherent PBM and LSWC staining with mAb against CD14, CD5, CD4, CD8, CD43, CD56, MHC II, CD11a, CD11b, CD18, CD54, and CD49d was performed.

Results: The mean number of PBM and LSWC from normal rats and rats with CC531 metastatic tumors adhering to the metastatic foci was significantly (2-4 times) higher than the number of cells adhering to the normal liver tissue ($p<0.05$). There were evidently more (2-4 times) PBM from normal rats and with CC531 metastases, adhering to the tumor and normal liver tissue in comparison to the LSWC isolated from the vasculature of normal and metastatic livers

($p< 0.05$). LSWC from metastatic livers showed 2 times higher numbers of adhering cells to the liver and tumor tissue than LSWC from normal livers ($p< 0.05$). The PBM from rats with CC531 revealed lower adherence properties than PBM of normal rats. The PBM and LSWC bound preferentially to the tumor stromal structures (40-55%) but not to tumor cells. Adhering cells of both PBM and LSWC populations showed high expression of CD14, MHC II, CD18, CD11a, and CD11b molecules.
Conclusion: The PBM and LSWC populations of CD14 MHC II phenotype showed the highest predilection to bind to the liver tumor foci. These cells are candidates for *in vitro* antitumor programming and administration to the tumor bearer.

85

Effect of Cyclophosphamide and Retinoic Acid on Hepatic Metastasis Following Liver Resection

J. Caramés, T. Palomares, A. Alonso, B. Castro, A. Pineda, I. García-Alonso

Lab. of Experimental Surgery, Univ. of The Basque Country, Leioa, Spain

Introduction: In the previous congress of this Society we presented our results showing an antiproliferative effect of all-trans retinoic acid (a drug that promotes cell differentiation) on liver metastases in a rat model. We have continued our studies to explore the possible additive effect between a classic chemotherapeutic agent as cyclophosphamide (Cy) and retinoic acid. The experimental model used, resembles the condition of a patient who, after removing the primary tumour, underwent metastasectomy in the liver.
Methods: Rabdomyosarcoma cells were inoculated into the spleen of male Wag rats in order to induce the formation of liver metastases; 5 minutes later, the spleen was removed to avoid the existence of a primary tumour. The left lateral lobe of the liver was removed 10 days later, to stimulate the growth of the tumour cells. At the end of the experiment, the animals were sacrificed, and a meticulous necropsy was performed: the number of macroscopic metastases was assessed, both in the liver and in the lung, and these organs were embedded in paraffin for histological study of microscopic foci. Cy was administered i.p. on days 10th and 15th. Retinoic acid was administered i.p. from day 7 to day 26. Each experimental group consisted of 5-7 animals, randomly allocated to the control or treated group.
Results: Those animals treated with two doses of cyclophosphamide (100 mg/kg) do not develop macroscopic metastases on day 21, but show a mortality rate over 40% and a clear weight loss. Cutting by half the doses (50 mg/kg) all of the animals survive, there is no weight loss (though the ponderal curve is flattened) and both liver and lung metastases are reduced on day 21st ($p< 0.05$). With a more prolonged follow up, the reduction in the number of liver metastases is still significant on the 50th day (while non-treated animals usually die before the 28th day), expressed as "No. of metastases/liver": Control group: day 21 (14.8); Cy group: day 21 (1), day 28 (0.14), day 35 (0), day 45 (8.6), day 50 (11.5). Cy-treated animals have also shown a reduction in the number of metastases to the lung, which on day 35 present a mean of 55 against more than 100 in the control group ($p< 0.05$). When Cy was associated to retinoic acid, animals sacrificed on day 50th showed a reduced number of liver metastases (2.5 vs. 13; $p< 0.05$). Regarding the lung, it was not possible to find any differences in the mean number of tumoral foci, as in both series the number was over 100; however, only in those animals not receiving retinoic acid, lung metastases were developed as "buttons" bigger than 3 mm.
Conclusion: Cy has proved to be a useful agent in this experimental model, and its cyto-reductive effect is enhanced when associated to retinoic acid.

86

The Survival Benefit of Surgical Treatment for Recurrence of The Remnant Liver and Lung after Hepatic Resection for Colorectal Metastases

H. Yoshidome, H. Ito, F. Kimura, H. Shimizu, A. Togawa, Y. Shimizu, M. Ohtsuka, F. Shimamura, D. Takeuchi, M. Miyazaki

Department of General Surgery, Chiba University Graduate School of Medicine, Chiba, Japan

Introduction: Hepatic resection is an effective treatment for colorectal metastases. Recurrence of the remnant liver and extrahepatic, especially lung, metastasis after hepatic resection for colorectal metastases is concerned as significant prognostic factors. We documented that regional adjuvant chemotherapy could reduce recurrence of the remnant liver. However, chemotherapy may not prolong survival in patients with recurrence of the remnant liver and lung. The objectives of this study were to investigate the significance of surgical treatment for the recurrence of local or extrahepatic metastasis.
Methods: We identified 207 patients undergoing hepatic resection for colorectal metastases. The records of these patients were reviewed for age, sex, location and stage of primary colorectal cancer, location and number of hepatic and pulmonary metastases, type of hepatic and pulmonary resection, preoperative carcinoembryonic antigen (CEA) levels, and pathology of primary tumor, hepatic metastases, and pulmonary metastases. Overall survival rates were evaluated by Kaplan-Meier method. The univariate analyses were estimated by log rank test. The multivariate analysis was verified by Cox proportional hazards models. Differences were considered significant when $p< 0.05$.
Results: Recurrence of the liver and lung metastases after hepatic resection is seen in 88 and 49 cases, respectively. Thirteen cases underwent repeated hepatic resection, and fourteen patients underwent pulmonary resection including 4 synchronous hepatic and pulmonary metastases. Five year survival was 30% in patients undergoing repeat hepatic resection, while 3 year survival was 7% in patients undergoing chemotherapy without surgical treatment. In metachronously pulmonary resected cases, 3 patients are alive and disease free survival is 34, 79, and 121 months after the second resection. In resected cases, overall 2 and 5 year survival is 60 and 19%, while in non-resected cases 4 and 0%. Univariate and multivariate analyses revealed that time of metastasis and number of metastases are significant prognostic factors.
Conclusion: Hepatic and pulmonary resection could result in long-term survival in selected patients with recurrence of the remnant liver or pulmonary metastases.

87

Pringle Maneuver Improves Lesion Size in Radiofrequency Application. Experimental Study in Porcine *In Vivo* Model

F. Burdío, A. Güemes, A.C. Navarro, R. Sousa, T. Castiella, I. Cruz, O. Burzaco, S. Strassmann, J. Torcal, R. Lozano

Department of Surgery, University Hospital Lozano Blesa, Zaragoza, Spain

Introduction: Radiofrequency (RF) is an effective method used in the treatment of malignancies - both primary and secondary - of the liver. To achieve 1 cm free margins and to avoid excessive damage to vascular or biliary structures have to be taken into account in such procedures, so lesion size and predictable necrosis is still a major concern. Saline injection, bipolar electrodes and more powerful RF devices have been developed in order to improve the results. Pringle maneuver avoids the cooling effect of the blood flow and has also been used in experimental studies. But today surgical resection (if possible) is still the procedure of choice to treat liver malignancies. New electrodes and new animal models of RF application have to be tested prior to elective application of RF in the clinics.
Aim: To confirm that the bipolar saline-enhanced electrodes produce *in vivo* (in a pig liver model) larger lesions than conventional methods previously described with or without Pringle maneuver (vascular inflow occlusion of the liver). And to evaluate the feasibility and safety of creating such a large ablative lesions in the liver.
Methods: RF (480 kHz) was applied to the liver of a total number of 16 healthy farm pigs with (group B, n=8) or without (group A, n=8) Pringle maneuver via laparotomy. We used a new bipolar electrode, saline enhanced at a flow of 100 ml/min. The pigs were followed and euthanized on the seventh day of the experiment. The livers were removed for histological assessment. Time of the procedure, impedance, current, power output, energy output, temperatures in the liver, central temperature of the pig (Tc) and volume of the lesion were determined and compared across the groups. Additionally a regularity ratio (RR) was determined by gross examination of the specimen and scored (0-3) taking into account regularity and predictability of the lesion with pathologist' assessment.
Results: With both methods ellipsoid shaped lesions were created between the two electrodes. In both groups, tissue impedance fell progressively (beta = -.47, $p< 0.01$ and beta = -.34, $p< 0.05$, in groups B and A respectively). The mean lesion size achieved with Pringle maneuver was the largest lesion described in the literature for any RFA method *in vivo* and was greater in group B than in group A ($p< 0.05$) (123.22 cm^3±49.62 and 52.40 cm^3±23.59, respectively). A better regularity and predictability evaluated by RR was observed in group B compared to group A (1.88±1.35 and .40±.55, respectively, $p< 0.05$). Five major complications (including four lesions to adjacent structures) were described and attributed, primarily, to failure in isolation from hyperthermic lesions.
Conclusion: Our new bipolar saline-enhanced electrode with Pringle maneuver achieves in *in vivo* pig liver large hepatic ablations. These large lesions are well tolerated by the pig when thermal injuries to adjacent structures are avoided.

88

Angiostatin Inhibits Experimental Liver Fibrosis

J.M. Vogten, T.A. Drixler, E.A. te Velde, M.F.B.G. Gebbink, E.E. Voest, I.H.M. Borel Rinkes

Departments of Surgery and Medical Oncology, Univ. Medical Center, Utrecht, The Netherlands

Introduction: Liver fibrosis (LF) is a common endpoint for chronic hepatic damage that limits application of surgical therapy. Angiogenesis, the formation of new blood vessels from pre-existing vasculature, is important in several hepatic processes including tumor growth and liver regeneration. However, its role in vascular and proliferative events in the fibrotic liver are currently unclear. Angiostatin (AS) is a potent angiogenesis inhibitor and has been shown to inhibit endothelial cell proliferation, migration and tube formation (Ji et al. FASEB J 12:1731-8, 1998). In addition, AS has been reported to act on other cell types, including smooth muscle cells (SMC). Finally, the primary effector of LF, the hepatic stellate cell (HSC), proliferates and develops SMC-like characteristics during LF. Therefore, we hypothesized that AS can reduce experimental LF, possibly by impairing proliferation or activation of HSCs.
Methods: LF was induced by IP injection of carbon tetrachloride (CCl_4; 0.2 ml 10% CCl_4 in olive oil 3 times a week). Control animals (group A, n=5) received 0.2 ml olive oil 3 times a week for 5 weeks. Group B (LF, n=5) animals were exposed to CCl_4 for 5 weeks, while treated animals (group C, n=5) received AS (100 mg/kg/d in PBS; continuous administration via SC osmotic pump) during weeks 4 and 5, in addition to CCl_4 exposure for 5 weeks. After 5 weeks, animals were terminated and liver tissue was analyzed for fibrotic surface area using Sirius Red histostaining and computer image analysis. Fibrotic surface area was expressed as percentage of total hepatic area. Immunohistochemistry for Ki-67 and von Willebrand factor (VWF) was performed to assess cell proliferation and microvessel density, respectively.
Results: In normal liver (group A), fibrotic surface area was limited (0.6%±0.3). After 5 weeks of CCl_4 exposure (LF, group B), fibrotic area had increased to 5.9%±1.3 compared to controls ($p< 0.01$). In AS treated animals (group C), fibrotic area was significantly reduced to 2.6%±0.2 compared to untreated LF mice ($p< 0.001$). Immunohistochemical staining for VWF revealed increased expression in fibrotic areas of group B mice. In AS treated mice, the total expression of VWF had decreased, while expression of VWF within fibrotic areas remained unchanged. Finally, AS treatment induced no differences in cell proliferation as measured by Ki-67 expression.
Conclusion: Angiostatin inhibits the development of CCl_4 induced liver fibrosis. This inhibition is not associated with changes in VWF expression. Whether this effect can be attributed to inhibition of HSC activation is currently under investigation. Use of various treatment modalities can increase surgical options for patients suffering from liver disease.

89

Receptor-Mediated Acceleration of Hepatocellular Transport System as Measured by Near-Infrared Spectroscopy

A. Tanaka[1], H. Shinohara[2], Y. Yamaoka[3]

Dept. of Emergency Medicine[1], Kyoto University Hospital, Dept. of Gastrointestinal Surgery[2], Osaka Medical College, Dept. of Gastrointestinal Surgery[3], Kyoto University, Japan

Introduction: Hepatocellular transport system, including uptake through hepatocyte membrane, intracellular transport, and excretion to bile canaliculi, play an important role of liver failure which manifests as cholestasis. However, evaluation method of hepatocyte transport system has not been clinically available. It is known that glucagon causes receptor-mediated increase in intracellular calcium and cyclic AMP, resulting in contraction of bile canaliculi via calcium-calmodulin system. Therefore, we have developed a novel evaluation method for integrity of signal transduction and transport system in the down stream, using glucagon-induced acceleration of indocyanine green (ICG) excretion.

Methods: Kinetics of hepatocellular concentration of ICG was analyzed by *in vivo* near-infrared (NIR) spectroscopy with multichannel photodetector system. Absorbance of ICG, oxy- and deoxy-hemoglobin, oxidized and reduced cytochrome c oxidase, water and hemoglobin free liver were calculated by multicomponent curve fitting analysis of the spectrum from 700 to 1000 nm. After intravenous injection of 0.5 mg/kg ICG to the rabbit, NIR spectrum was measured at 2 second interval for 10 minutes. Absorbance of ICG increased by uptake through hepatocellular membrane and then decreased by excretion to bile canaliculi. The kinetics was analyzed by two compartment model: $ICG(t)=-A\exp(-\alpha t)+B\exp(-\beta t)$, where α and β (min^{-1}) indicate time constant of uptake and excretion, respectively. During the excretion phase, 40 µg/kg glucagon was infused via the portal vein. Immediately after glucagon administration to control rabbit liver, excretion was accelerated approximately for 10 seconds, and then returned to the previous exponential decrease. Integrity of hepatocellular transport system in response to signal transduction was evaluated by the presence of temporary acceleration of the excretion. In order to perturb glucagon-induced acceleration of hepatocellular transport, colchicine (microtubular conjugation inhibitor), ouabaine (Na-K ATPase inhibitor), wortmannin (myosin light chain kinase inhibitor), forskolin (adenylate cyclase activator), and ischemia-reperfusion insult were employed.

Results: Colchicine, ouabaine and wortmannin abolished temporary acceleration of ICG excretion in response to glucagon. These three inhibitors did not change time constant α, but significantly decreased β from the control value of 0.090±0.008 to 0.042±0.010, 0.030±0.008 and 0.018±0.008 (n=3), respectively. These inhibitor studies indicate that integrity of transport system is required for the glucagon-induced acceleration of ICG excretion. Ischemia reperfusion insult did not cause glucagon-induced acceleration and decreased both α and β to 0.50±0.08 and 0.042±0.007, respectively.

Conclusion: The NIR spectrophotometric method has a potential for a novel liver function test of signal transduction and transport system in the liver surgery, since β in human liver cannot be clinically used due to one-order smaller value as compared with that in rabbit liver.

90

Estrogen has a Potential Role in the Development of Hepatopulmonary Syndrome in Rats

S. Yol, S. Toprak, A. Kartal, L. Tavli, M. Sahin

Selcuk Univ., Fac. of Med., Departments of Surgery and Pathology, Akyokus, Konya, Turkey

Introduction: Hepatopulmonary syndrome (HPS) is defined by the presence of hepatic dysfunction or portal hypertension, a widened alveolar-arterial oxygen gradient with or without hypoxemia and intrapulmonary vasodilation. The potential role of estrogen has not been studied in the development of HPS.

Methods: Forty female Sprague-Dawley rats weighing 200-250 g were divided into four groups. Group I: Sham-laparotomy n=10, Group II: Common bile duct ligation (CBDL) n=10, Group III: CBDL+Bilateral oophorectomy n=10, Group IV: CBDL+exogen estrogen administration, n=10. Ketamine hydrochloride anesthesia (2 ml/kg, 10 mg/ml, i.p.) was used in all groups. Animals were caged for 5 weeks to induce cirrhosis. Meanwhile, the rats in Group IV received estradiol propionate (5000 U/kg, i.m.) in every 5 days. At the end of 5 weeks, blood samples were taken for gas analysis, estrogen level and biochemistry, lung and liver tissues were taken for histopathologic investigation. Intrapulmonary vessel diameters were measured by oculometry. One way ANOVA and Tukey HSD tests were used for statistical analysis.

Results: Biochemical and histopathological findings of CBDL were detected in all but sham animals. Blood estrogen levels were 37.2±5.8 pg/ml in Group I, 169.9±14.8 pg/ml in Group II, 14.5±3.5 pg/ml in Group III and >2000 pg/ml in Group IV. pO_2 values were 81.2±3.5 mmHg in Group I, 69.1±3.1 mmHg in Group II, 73.9±2.7 mmHg in Group III and 60.4±2.8 mmHg in Group IV. Blood estrogen level increased as high as 4 times in Group II than Group I, whereas pO_2 in Group II decreased significantly when compared with Group I. Blood estrogen level in Group III was lesser than half of Group I, whereas pO_2 in Group III was slightly better than Group II. Exogen estrogen administration decreased pO_2 to the lowest level. Intrapulmonary vessel diameters showed significant increase as the estrogen level increased but it decreased significantly when oophorectomy performed.

Conclusion: Increased estrogen level deteriorated the pO_2 levels and intrapulmonary vessel diameters in cirrhotic rats. The results of the study directed us to consider that estrogen has a potential effect in the development of HPS.

91

The Effect of Tamoxifen and Oophorectomy in Preventing the Development of Hepatopulmonary Syndrome in Cirrhotic Rats

S. Yol, S. Toprak, C. Vatansev, L. Tavli, M. Belviranli, A. Kartal

Selcuk Univ., Fac. of Med., Departments of Surgery and Pathology, Akyokus, Konya, Turkey

Introduction: Studies have shown that as many as 40% of cirrhotic patients have detectable intrapulmonary vasodilation and that up to 8% to 15% will develop impaired oxygenation. No clearly effective medical therapy for hepatopulmonary syndrome (HPS) has been found. In our previous study, we had shown that estrogen has a potential role in the development of HPS in rats. In the present study, we aimed to investigate the role of anti-estrogen therapies in outcome of HPS in cirrhotic rats.
Methods: Forty female Sprague-Dawley rats weighing 230-290 g were divided into 4 groups. Under ketamine hydrochloride anesthesia (2 ml/kg, 10 mg/ml, i.p.), all animals received a midline laparotomy. Sham animals (Group I, n=10) underwent mobilization of the common bile duct without ligation. The remaining three groups received common bile duct ligation (CBDL). No additional treatment was applied to the rats in Group II (n=10). Tamoxifen was given to the Group III rats (n=10) by orogastric gavage in a dose of 0.8 mg/kg daily for 5 weeks. Oophorectomy was performed during CBDL in Group IV (n=10). At the end of 5 weeks, blood samples were taken for gas analysis and biochemistry (total bil., direct bil., alkaline phos., AST, and ALT), lung and liver tissues were taken for histopathologic investigation. Intrapulmonary vessel diameters were measured by oculometry. One way ANOVA and Tukey HSD tests were used for statistical analysis.
Results: Histopathological cirrhosis was detected in all but sham animals. pO_2 values were 78.8±3.9 mmHg in Group I, 67.6±2.2 mmHg in Group II, 71.2±2.0 mmHg in Group III and 71.9±2.4 mmHg in Group IV. pO_2 was significantly lower in Groups II, III and IV when compared with Group I ($p< 0.05$). However, pO_2 in Group IV showed significant increase when compared with Group II ($p< 0.05$). The diameters of intrapulmonary vessels were 20.1±1.8 micron in Group I, 240.6±4.5 micron in Group II, 165.6±10.4 micron in Group III and 160.1±3.8 micron in Group IV. Intrapulmonary vascular diameters were significantly higher in Groups II, III and IV when compared with Group I ($p< 0.001$). Estrogen depressed animals in Groups III and IV showed decreased vascular diameters when compared with Group II ($p< 0.01$).
Conclusion: Either medical or surgical blockage of estrogen reduces the severity of HPS (hypoxemia and intrapulmonary vascular dilatation) in cirrhotic rats.

92

Importance of Cytokines, NO and Apoptosis in the Pathological Process of Necrotising Pancreatitis in Rats

L. Leindler[1], G. Farkas[1], Á. Morschul[2], F. László Jr.[2], Y. Mándi[3], J. Fejős[1], T. Takács[4], K. Jármai[4]

Dept. of Surgery[1], Univ. of Szeged, KOKI/Inst. Exp. Med.[2], Budapest, Inst. of Clinical Microbiology[3], Dept. of Internal Medicine[4], Univ. of Szeged, Szeged, Hungary

Introduction: Ischemia-reperfusion injury can be involved in the pathophysiology of acute necrotizing pancreatitis. The aim of this study was to determine the production of cytokines (TNF and IL-6), NO and apoptosis during this pathological process.
Methods: Acute pancreatitis was produced in male Wistar rats by the injection of 200 ml of 6% taurocholic acid into the main pancreatic duct, in combination with the temporary (15-min) occlusion of the inferior splenic artery. The animals were sacrificed at 6 or 24 hr following ischemia, and the serum amylase, TNF, IL-6, iNOS levels, apoptotic activity and the wet pancreatic weight/body weight ratio were measured. Histological examinations were also performed.
Results: 24 hr following the induction of pancreatitis, the mortality rate was 63%. During this period, the serum TNF and IL-6 levels were permanently high (50±15 U/ml and 7083±1610 pg/ml, at 6-24 hr respectively), while the iNOS activity demonstrated an increasing tendency (4.2±0.6 and 4.97±0.4 pmol at 6-24 hr, respectively). Severe necrotizing pancreatitis was confirmed histologically. Apoptotic activity significantly increased (4-27/mm^2) in the pancreas. In opposite this activity represents an inverse changing in the lung (49-11/mm^2, at 6-24 hr respectively).
Conclusion: The results indicate that ischemia-reperfusion increases the mortality rate in acute necrotic pancreatitis significantly, as a consequence of activation of the cytokine cascade, the production of inducible NO, and the systemic inflammatory reaction. The NO production and apoptotic process show a close correlation. Supported by grant from OTKA 5K296A 130 T/130 T/12 F/9032.

93

Changes of Quality of Life and Nutritional State in Surgically Treated Patients with Chronic Pancreatitis

B. Tihanyi, I. Farkas, Z. Csapó, R. Schwab, Á. Pap, T. Tihanyi

1st Dept. of Surgery, Semmelweis University, Depts. of Gastroenterology and Surgery, MÁV Hospital, Budapest, Hungary

Introduction: In our previous study we proved the suitability of the EORTC-QLQ C30 and the PAN-26 - originally designed for pancreatic cancer - questionnaires, to measure the quality of life (QOL) of chronic pancreatitis (CP) patients. The importance of this kind of study is, that comparing the effectiveness of the different surgical procedures might become more precise. The aim of this study was to compare the effect of different surgical interventions for CP on the QOL and nutritional status (NS).

Methods: We used the EORTC-QLQ-C30 and PAN-26 questionnaires. 119 patients were evaluated in total. 79 patients were assessed after operation, 65 patients before operation and 25 of them were controlled also after surgery. NS was measured to calculate the surgical risk and in support of the reliability of the subjective answers to the QOL questionnaires. In the interest of more precise evaluation of our patients state laboratory tests, pancreatic function tests and MRCP were performed. Distal resection (DR), decompression- techniques (DT), pylorus-preserving pancreato-duodenectomy (PPPD) and Frey-procedure (FP) were compared.
Results: The 25 pre- and postoperatively measured patients has an average 7.3 months follow-up time. Neither in the NS-parameters, nor the QOL-parameters showed significant differences in the DT-group (n=7, follow-up time: 5.3 months). FP (n=11, follow-up: 9.6 months) has significantly ($p<0.05$) better scores in the main, for CP characteristic QOL questions, and we have the best increase in the work-ability and in the NS-parameters. The patients after PPPD (n=7, follow-up: 6.8 months) showed significant results in the general QOL& health-score: $p=0.006$; pain-score: $p=0.011$; fatigability: $p=0.022$ QOL parameters. Nutritional recovery was found to be about 2% worse in the PPPD group, than after FP.
Conclusion: NS and the QOL questionnaires are important tools to compare the effectiveness of the different surgical procedures. It seems, that these measurements are sensitive parameters to indicate the success of the procedure. Early results suggest that local head resection with extended pancreatic decompression are acceptable procedures in severe cases of CP.

Molecular Biology, Gene Therapy in Surgical Diseases

94

Effect of Cycloprodigiosin on the Induction of Inducible Nitric Oxide Synthase by Interleukin-1β in Primary Cultured Hepatocytes

S. Teshima, H. Nakanishi, M. Kaibori, H. Toyokawa, A.H. Kwon, Y. Kamiyama, T. Okumura

First Department of Surgery, and Department of Medical Chemistry, Kansai Medical University, Moriguchi, Japan

Introduction: Cycloprodigiosin hydrochloride (cPrG), which is a product of marine bacterium *Pseudoalteromonas denitrificans*, acts as an H^+/Cl^- symporter and induces apoptosis in various cell lines. cPrG inhibited the activation of NF-κB in TNFα-treated HeLa cells, resulting in the enhancement of apoptosis. NF-κB plays an important role in the transcriptional regulation of proinflammatory gene expression. Interleukin-1β (IL-1β) induces the gene expression of inducible nitric oxide synthase (iNOS) through NF-κB activation, followed by production of nitric oxide, in hepatocytes. In this report, we examined whether cPrG influences the production of nitric oxide by IL-1β. We found that cPrG unexpectedly increased levels of nitric oxide production via the enhancement of NF-κB activation.
Methods: Hepatocytes were isolated from male Wistar strain rats (200-250 g) by collagenase perfusion method and cultured. Cells were incubated with IL-1β (1 nM) in the presence or absence of cPrG. Levels of nitric oxide production (as nitrite), iNOS protein, iNOS mRNA and NF-κB activation were measured. Activation of MAPK (ERK/JNK/p38) pathways was detected by immunoblotting with phospho-MAPK antibodies.
Results: cPrG (2 μM) increased levels of iNOS protein and mRNA in addition to the production of nitric oxide (2 to 3-fold), when hepatocytes were incubated with IL-1β. cPrG did not change the degradation of an inhibitory protein, IκB, of NF-κB, but delayed the recovery of IκB in the cytosol. Electrophoretic mobility shift assay demonstrated that cPrG significantly enhanced the levels of NF-κB activation, which was confirmed by the increase of p65, one of NF-κB component, in the nucleus. We reported that IL-1β activated MAPK pathways including ERK, JNK and p38. cPrG activated ERK, but neither of JNK nor p38, resulting in the increase of ERK activation in IL-1β-treated cells. PD-98059 (100 μM), a specific inhibitor of MEK (ERK kinase), completely inhibited the activation of ERK, but partially blocked the effect of cPrG on nitric oxide production.
Conclusion: These results indicate that cPrG enhances iNOS induction at a step of NF-κB activation at least in part via ERK pathway. Since nitric oxide plays cytoprotective or cytotoxic role in liver injury caused by endotoxemia, ischemia-reperfusion and surgical resection, manipulation of iNOS induction with clinical agent may contribute to a recovery of liver damage during inflammation.

95

Effect of Pirfenidone on the Induction of Inducible Nitric Oxide Synthase by Inflammatory Cytokine in Hepatocytes

H. Nakanishi, M. Kaibori, S. Teshima, H. Tsuchiya, A.H. Kwon, Y. Kamiyama, T. Okumura

First Department of Surgery, and Department of Medical Chemistry, Kansai Medical University, Moriguchi, Japan

Introduction: We recently have found that pirfenidone (PFD, 5-methyl-1-phenyl-2-(1H)-pyridone), which is evaluated clinically as an anti-fibrotic agent, prevented the endotoxin-induced liver injury following partial hepatectomy in a rat model of endotoxemia. In this report, we investigated whether PFD directly influences the induction of inducible nitric oxide synthase (iNOS) gene expression, which catalyzes the production of nitric oxide from L-arginine, in the liver of rats.
Methods: Hepatocytes were isolated from male Wistar strain rats (200-250 g) by collagenase perfusion method and cultured. Cells were treated with interleukin-1β (IL-1β, 1 nM) in the presence or absence of PFD. Levels of nitric oxide production (as nitrite), iNOS protein, iNOS mRNA and NF-κB activation were measured. iNOS promoter assay was done by transfection of iNOS promoter-luciferase construct (pRiNOS-Luc).
Results: PFD markedly inhibited the production of nitric oxide induced by IL-1β with the maximal effect at 1 mg/ml (5 mM). PFD also inhibited level of iNOS protein and its mRNA, indicating that the inhibition is at a step of transcription. Electrophoretic mobility shift assay demonstrated that PFD reduced the DNA binding of NF-B in the nucleus. Furthermore, co-transfection experiment with pRiNOS-Luc and NF-κB (p50/p65) revealed that PFD decreased the

transactivation activity of NF-κB. However, PFD could not prevent either degradation of an inhibitory protein, I B, of NF-κB or translocation of p65 (one of NF-κB component) to the nucleus.
Conclusion: These results indicate that PFD inhibits the induction of iNOS gene expression at a step of NF-κB binding to DNA, but not of NF-κB translocation to the nucleus, resulting in the inhibition of iNOS synthesis and nitric oxide production. Since NF-κB plays a critical role in the transcriptional regulation of proinflammatory gene expression in addition to iNOS, the inhibition of NF-κB activation by PFD may contribute to a protection against liver injury during inflammation.

96

Stromal Interaction Upregulates Gelatinase Activity in Pancreatic Tumours *In Vitro*

S.T. Ivanova, P.F. Ridgway, P. Ziprin, D.H. Peck, A.W. Darzi

Dept. of Surgical Oncology and Technology, Imperial College Faculty of Medicine, St. Mary's Hospital, London, UK

Introduction: Matrix proteolysis is a critical step in local invasion and metastasis. Despite its import, the antecedent mechanisms of proteolytic enzyme induction remain poorly understood. The authors hypothesize that bi-directional interaction between stroma and pancreatic tumour cell induce gelatinase expression.
Methods: Human pancreatic adenocarcinoma (PSN-1) monolayers were cultured in isolation or co-cultured (Direct) with human fibroblasts (MRC-5). A subgroup was co-cultured separated by an 0.4 mm filter (Indirect). Further characterisation was carried out using Fibroblast conditioned media applied to PSN monolayers for a period of 24 hours. Gelatinase A and B (MMP 2 and 9) activity was assessed using substrate zymography. Densitometric analysis was performed using Scion Image. Data was analysed using analysis of variance.
Results: A net upregulation of gelatinase B activity was observed in indirect co-culture (*p=0.016*). There was a trend toward augmented activity between direct co-culture group and controls implying an insoluble inhibitory factor. This did not reach statistical significance (*p=0.18*). No statistically significant differences were observed in MMP 2 activity. Application of conditioned media in various concentrations caused an upregulation of MMP 9 secretion in the tumour line, further implicating a soluble potentiator.
Conclusion: These findings support our hypothesis that bi-directional signalling exists between pancreatic cancer cells and stroma with respect to MMP 9 activity. Soluble factor mediated signalling suggests a putative mechanism for increased gelatinases activity *in vivo*.

97

Cepharanthine Conquers P-Glycoprotein-Associated Drug Resistance in Hepatocellular Carcinoma Cells

A. Nakajima, Y. Yamamoto, K. Hata, K. Taura, H. Uchinami, K. Yonezawa, Y. Yamaoka

Department of Gastroenterological Surgery, Kyoto University, Graduate School of Medicine, Kyoto, Japan

Introduction: The prognoses of patients with advanced hepatocellular carcinoma (HCC) are still unsatisfactory in spite of marked improvement of surgical skill. A major obstacle for treatment is its refractoriness to anticancer agents. P-glycoprotein (human MDR1 gene product), which is a 170 kDa ATP-dependent plasma membrane transporter, plays a key role in doxorubicine (DOX) resistance. Cepharanthine, a biscoslaurine alkaloid extracted from *Stephania cepharantha Hayata,* has been reported to inhibit the P-glycoprotein function. In the present study, we examined if CEP could conquer DOX resistance in human HCC cell lines overexpressing MDR1.
Methods: 1) We investigated P-glycoprotein expression of surgically resected HCC in our department (51 cases) by immunohistochemical staining. 2) Human HCC cell lines PLC/PRF/5, Hep3B and their DOX-resistant sublines PLC/DOR, 3B/DOR were used in the *in vitro* study. We examined the expression of MDR1 mRNA by RT-PCR, DOX sensitivity and the effect of co-administration of CEP by MTT assay, and intracellular DOX concentration by flow cytometry. Each assay was performed at least in triplicate.
Results: 1) Immunohistochemical staining of clinical samples showed that tumors of 42 cases (82%) had positive staining of P-glycoprotein. Among them, 8 tumors (16%) expressed higher levels of P-glycoprotein compared with non-cancerous lesion in the same cases. 2) DOX-resistant HCC cells expressed higher levels of MDR1 mRNA and showed significantly higher IC50 (average±SD μg/ml) of DOX than the parental cells (7.62±2.96 vs. 0.61±0.58 in PLC/PRF/5 and PLC/DOR, 3.53±1.33 vs. 0.20±0.06 in Hep3B and 3B/DOR). CEP itself showed cytotoxity to the HCC cells at higher concentrations than 2 μg/ml in regardless to MDR1 expression level. Co-administration of 2 μg/ml of CEP significantly augmented the sensitivity to DOX only in DOX-resistant cells (IC50 were 1.01±0.27 vs. 0.64 PLC/PRF/5 and PLC/DOR, 0.48±0.34 vs. 0.17±0.05 in Hep3B and 3B/DOR). CEP increased the intracellular concentration of DOX and inhibited the efflux of DOX in the resistant cells. This phenomenon was less remarkable in the parental cells.
Conclusion: The *in vitro* study indicated that CEP has a strong potential of conquering P-glycoprotein-mediated DOX resistance in HCC cells through both modulating P-glycoprotein efflux function and its direct cytotoxity. Considering the result of immunohistochemical staining, CEP seems to be a promising candidate for modulating P-glycoprotein-associated drug-resistance in clinical cases of HCC.

98

The Prognostic Significance of Proliferating Cell Nuclear Antigen in Colorectal Cancer. A Prospective Study with Clinical Correlation

R. Harisi[1], J. Dudás[2], G. Bodoky[3], T. Winternitz[1], L. Flautner[1], J. Weltner[1]

1st Department of Surgery[1], Semmelweis University, Budapest, Hungary, Dept. of Gastroenterology and Endocrinology[2], Georg August University, Göttingen, Germany, Dept. of Oncology[3], Teaching Hospital St. László, Budapest, Hungary

Introduction: The prognostic significance of proliferating cell nuclear antigen (PCNA) in colorectal cancer has not yet been settled, the relationship between PCNA expression and clinical outcome is unclear. The aim of our present study was to investigate the relationship between PCNA expression in colorectal cancer and tumor progression and prognosis.
Methods: Tumor tissues were obtained from 66 colorectal cancer patients who underwent curative resection. Their follow-up periods ranged from 13.2 to 49.7 months. The distribution of the patients according to modified Dukes classification was 22.72% stage B, 22.72% stage C, and 54.56% stage D. The expression of PCNA was determined by immunoblot analysis of tumor tissue and adjacent normal mucosa from 40 resected specimens of primary colorectal carcinomas and 26 liver metastases. The prognostic significance of PCNA expression was evaluated by univariate as well as multivariate analysis.
Results: PCNA expression was detected in tumor tissue or in the surrounding histologically tumor-free mucosa, as well as in normal liver tissue. Nevertheless, the expression level in tumor tissue is higher than in the surrounding mucosa. PCNA expression in tumor tissue from Dukes' D patients was higher than in stage B and C patients, this difference was even more enhanced in case of peritumoral tissue. We did not find correlation between the high expression of PCNA in tumor or surrounding tissue and subsequent local recurrence, metastasis and survival. The difference in PCNA expression of tumor and tumor-free surrounding tissue indicated tumorous progression, and the more this difference was enhanced the more tumorous invasion, recidiva and hepatic metastasis, or in advanced stage, metastasis progression was frequent. PCNA protein expression did not correlate with histological grade of tumors or DNA ploidy. PCNA expression was higher in colon tumors than in rectum located tumors.
Conclusion: By comparison of tumor and surrounding tissue PCNA expression we tried to get a glance into tumor growth. Analysis of tumors from individual patients, has shown that those whose tumor tissue possessed more times increased PCNA expression compared to surrounding tissue, were threatened with quick tumor progression. This finding has its particular significance in case of several Dukes' B and C patients, for whom more frequent control examinations are required, as well as adjuvant therapy is recommended for longer and event-free survival.

99

Identification and Validation of Candidate Genes in Pancreatic Cancer

R. Grützmann[1], I. Alldinger[1], M. Foerder[1], M. Peiper[3], R. Jesenofsky[4], D. Ockert[1], A. Rosenthal[2], C. Pilarsky[2], H.D. Saeger[1]

Dept. of Visceral, Thoracic and Vascular Surgery[1], Univ. Hosp. Carl Gustav Carus, Technical Univ. Dresden, Germany, MetaGen Pharmaceuticals[2], Berlin, Germany, Dept. of Surgery[3], Department of Internal Medicine[4], Univ. Hamburg, Germany

Introduction: Patients with pancreatic cancer (PaCa) still have a very poor prognosis. Despite of increasing knowledge about the molecular basis of PaCa no specific marker for earlier diagnosis nor a target protein for a new therapeutic approach have been identified so far.
Methods: 1. Using electronic northern (counting and statistical analysis of expressed sequence tags (EST) in EST pools from normal and tumor tissues) we could isolate 251 differentially expressed genes in PaCa out of assembled EST-libraries using newly developed software tools. 2. Using DNA microarray technology (GeneChip, Affymetrix) we investigated mRNA expression pattern of 9 PaCa cell lines (commercially available and cell lines from tumor of resected patients). Expression levels were compared to those of normal pancreatic duct cells. Second, mRNA expression profiling using DNA microarrays of 8 patients with PaCa was done.
Results: Differentially expressed genes, isolated by above mentioned methods, are presented, among them genes known to be involved in tumorigenesis and new candidate genes of yet unknown function.
Conclusion: Electronic northern and DNA microarray technology are useful tools for mRNA expression profiling. Genes of potentially significance for the development of PaCa have been selected for further investigation.

100

Detection of Occult Tumour Cells in Bone Marrow by Reverse Transcriptase-Polymerase Chain Reaction (RT-PCR) in Breast Cancer Patients

S. Dubecz[1], O. Csuka[2], K. Tóth[2], I. Köves[1], G. Péley[1], I. Láng[3]

Dept. of Surgery[1], Dept. of Pathogenetic[2], Dept. of Chemotherapy[3], National Institute of Oncology, Budapest, Hungary

Introduction: The presence of occult breast cancer cells in bone marrow (BM) has been reported to correlate with relapse-free survival and its adjuvant chemotherapy could improve the outcome of breast cancer patients. We have used RT-PCR to measure keratin 19 mRNA for detection of breast cancer cells in bone marrow.
Aim of study: correlation between BM micrometastasis and other prognostic factors: hormone receptors, node status, prognostic factors of primary tumours.
Methods: In a consecutive series of 87 primary breast cancer patients (of 42 histologically positive axillary node: 48.28%, of 45 negative:

51.72%, of 53 oestrogen receptor positive: 61%, of 34 receptor negative: 39%). BM aspirates - with no evidence of BM metastasis proved by scintigrapy - was investigated. Prognostic factors of the tumour (such as tumour size, histological grade, oestrogen receptors, erbB2, p53, nM23, c-met, axillar lymph node involvement) were compared to the RT-PCR examinations.
Results: Detecting the micrometastasis in BM correlated with the prognostic factors, such as a negative oestrogen receptor, metastasis in the axillary lymph node (18 of 42 lymph node positive: 42.9%, and 11 of 45 lymph node negative: 24.4%), primary tumour size, erbB2 and p53 expression. We could observe c-met overexpression and decreasing of nM23 also.
Conclusion: 1. Frequency of BM micrometastasis was 33.3%, by RT-PCR. 2. Positive correlation between oestrogen receptor negativity and BM micrometastasis, 3. High frequency of BM micrometastasis in node positive cases. 4. Correlation between BM micrometastasis and prognostic factors of primary tumours: high frequency of BM micrometastasis in HER2 and p53 tumours, low nm23 levels accompanied with BM micrometastasis, BM micrometastasis correlates with high level of c-met. Detecting micrometastasis in BM may have a role selecting a patient who would benefit from earlier adjuvant chemotherapy, and who would otherwise have been regarded free of bone metastasis.

101

Differential Gene Expression Profile in Monocytes (M) from Multiple Injured Patients

P. Biberthaler, B. Bach, V. Mayer, T. Mussack, W. Mutschler, M. Jochum

Chirurgische Klinik Innenstadt und Abteilung für Klinische Chemie und Biochemie, der Chirurgischen Klinik Innenstadt, Ludwig-Maximilians-Universität, München, Germany

Introduction: Development of the posttraumatic systemic inflammatory response syndrome (SIRS) is characterized by innate immune system alterations. In particular, monocytes (M) seem to play a pivotal role within this pathological process, although initial M mRNA expression as an early mediator of immunological alterations has not been evaluated so far. Therefore, the aim of this pilot study was to perform a serial differential mRNA expression analysis of isolated M from multiple injured patients using the microarray technique.
Methods: Patients (n=6) were enrolled presenting with blunt multiple injuries (Injury Severity Score: 22-57 points). Blood samples were drawn on admission and 6, 12, 24, and 48 hours after trauma. Differential gene expression profile was established by microarrays (Atlas human stress 1.2) performed on M isolated with anti-CD14 coated magnetic beads. For semi-quantitative analysis the mRNA expression pattern of the initial sample was set as the individual baseline and changes in the following samples were calculated as expression ratios compared to the baseline level. A ratio of 2 was accepted as significant alteration between initial and follow up samples.
Results: Out of the total spotted 1176 genes on the array a mean of 45±8 were expressed at least once within the observation period, and only 10 genes were permanently expressed in all patients during the whole 48 hour posttraumatic observation period.
Conclusion: We demonstrate for the first time a serial differential gene expression analysis on isolated M of multiple injured patients using microarrays. Probably due to the semiquantitative nature of the array data no significant trauma sensitive gene could be identified so far. Hence, we are presently performing quantitative RT-PCR for the clearly altered genes, which may allow a more detailed evaluation of trauma specific gene expression.

102

Liver Regeneration-Biochemistry-Insulin Uptake-PCNA Marking

T. Kotsis, A. Fotopoulos, I. Chondroudaki, A. Pafiti, M. Frangou, S. Kotsovolou, F. Nikolopoulou, K. Chondros, D. Rizos, B. Smyrniotis, J. Papadimitriou

Aretaeion Hospital, Medical School, University of Athens, Athens, Greece

Introduction: The regenerating liver is a valuable study-model of cellular proliferation. This experimental study aimed in detailing the rat's liver regeneration after 70% hepatectomy, along with DNA replication. Moreover, the application of the isolated perfused rat liver (IPRL) on postoperative day (POD) 1, 2, 3, 5, 7, 14 was used to assess the extraction of insulin from the regenerating liver.
Methods: Ninety rats were studied (BW 200-300 g), under general anaesthesia with ketamine and midazolam. A group of rats studied on POD 1 underwent a sham operation; control rats had no operation. In phase A the animals were subjected to 70% hepatectomy. In phase B, on POD 1, 3, 2, 5, 7, 14 the IPRL was applied. The regenerating liver was perfused with insulin (450 mU/ml) with portal flow 1.4 ml/g liver/min for 20 min. The perfusate was oxygenated (O_2 95%/CO_2 5%) with constant temperature at 37°C.
Results: Animal's weight, liver's weight, glucose, lactate, SGOT, SGPT, ALP, total bilirubin, albumin, urea, creatinine, PT, APTT, INR and insulin were evaluated during the 14 days. Additionally, the insulin clearance by the liver was estimated. The DNA replication was assessed via proliferating cell nuclear antigen (PCNA) immunohistochemistry, which demonstrated the remarkable regenerating activity of the liver on the 1st POD ($p<0.005$). We observed remarkable reduction of the liver's biochemical activities resulting in an increase of SGOT (684%), SGPT (532%), PT (27.7%), INR (72%), bilirubin (82.8%) on 1st POD, while a normalization of the essential liver's functions occurs on 5th POD. Insulin's extraction by the liver was reduced on 1st POD in the hepatectomized versus the control group (71+9.9 vs 165.88+12.3 μU/gr/min respectively, $p=0.0005$).
Discussion: The decreased insulin extraction by the regenerating liver is a phenomenon of the regeneration per se, probably due to the reduced posthepatectomy ability of the liver for glyconeogenesis, perhaps due to alteration of hepatocytes receptors for insulin. Further studies on this topic are recommended.
Conclusion: Liver regeneration after major hepatectomy is a synchronized growth process with the double role of saving the liver and the organism. Insulin and a constellation of other factors are involved. The unveiling of the mystery of regeneration will help solving other closely related mechanisms, like neoplasia.

New Surgical Techniques

103

A Systematic Approach to the Surgical Treatment of Gynaecomastia

B. Fruhstorfer, C.M. Malata

Department of Plastic and Reconstructive Surgery, Addenbrooke's Hospital, Cambridge, UK

Introduction: Numerous surgical techniques have been described for the correction of gynaecomastia and today the surgeon is faced with a wide range of excisional and liposuction procedures. There is, however, a paucity of literature on an integrated approach to the surgical management of this condition in general and the roles of the different treatment modalities in particular.
Methods: A review of all gynaecomastia patients operated on by a single surgeon over a two-year period was therefore undertaken. Forty eight breasts in 29 patients were treated; 31 breasts by liposuction alone (conventional=19, ultrasonic=12), 8 breasts by liposuction and open excision and 9 breasts by liposuction, open excision and skin reduction. Patient satisfaction was assessed using a linear analogue scale with a maximum score of 10.
Results: There were no early postoperative complications as haematoma, seroma and infection and 90% of patients were very satisfied (score 8-10) with their cosmetic outcome. The most frequently encountered complication was a residual subareolar lump in 5 breasts, which were all treated by conventional liposuction alone.
Discussion: In order to avoid the common complication of an uncomfortable residual subareolar nodule the threshold for open excision in patients undergoing conventional liposuction should be low. Ultrasonic liposuction extends the role of liposuction in gynaecomastia patients. Although skin excess remains a challenge, it can be satisfactorily managed without excessive scarring.
Conclusion: Based on our experience a practical approach to the surgical management of gynaecomastia, which takes into account breast size, consistency, skin excess and skin quality is proposed.

104

An Experimental Model for Alternative Blood Supply of the Kidney in the Aspect of Renal Function

T. Lesznyák, N. Németh, G. Ács, I. Mikó, I. Furka

Department of Operative Techniques and Surgical Research, Medical and Health Science Center, Univ. of Debrecen, Debrecen, Hungary

Introduction: Severe diseases can involve the renal artery and the vascular system of the renal parenchyma imperiling the renal blood supply and function. In these cases we have to ensure the blood supply by alternative ways to save the renal function. Since the 1930s omentonephropexy is a useable experimental method, which uses the great omentum for the neovascularisation of organs.
Methods: Mongrel dogs (n=8) were used in the experimental series, which consists of three operations. First we make median laparotomy, expose and decapsulate the left kidney. After it we spread the kidney surface with omental angiogenic factor (OAF) and cover with a part of the great omentum fixed with one-one stitches (1st operation). The OAF is a lipid type material extracted from the great omentum. Four weeks later we expose the left kidney again, mount and ligate the renal artery and cut it between the two ligatures (2nd operation). Recent four weeks later we remove the right kidney (3rd operation). In our experiments beside the basic hematological parameters, serum urea and creatinin levels we measured the red blood cell (RBC) deformability, urine N-acetil-β-D-glucosaminidase (NAG-ase) activity and we made SPECT examinations.
Results: We have only 3 survivor dogs from 8. The SPECT examination shows that their remaining kidney without renal artery is functioning. Significant differences were observed in serum creatinine (SeCrea) and urea values during the experimental series among the three operation periods (outstandingly in SeCrea: 28th postoperative day after 1st operation vs 1st postop. day after 2nd operation: $p=0.00109$; and in urea: 28th postop. day after 2nd operation vs 1st postop. day after 3rd operation: $p=0.000155$) and between the survival and the perished animal subgroups (the survivor dogs had lower level of creatinine values). Hematological parameters changed similarly after operation by operation and showed a moderate tendency towards anaemia. There were not significant differences in NAG-ase activity and RBC deformability values.
Discussion: Unfortunately the survival rate is low. The effectivity of the neovascularisation stimulated by OAF shows deviance in the different animals. Changes in the renal function could be observed during the experimental period showing interesting differences between survivor and perished animals. The background of these results could be found in individual sensitivity of the dogs, or previous renal status, or in the effect of other unknown factors.
Conclusion: In certain experimental circumstances omentonephropexy can be an alternative way to support the arterial blood supply of the kidney to save the renal function.
This study was supported by OTKA Nr. T 034211 and The Ministry of Welfare Research Grant Nr. 6100/1/2000/ETT. and Nr. 6003/1/2001/ETT.

105

A Combination of Endoscopic Laser Surgery and Segment Resection for the Treatment of Cricotracheal Stenoses

Z. Bella[1], L. Rovó[1], M. Brzózka[2], L. Tiszlavicz[3], J. Czigner[1]

Department of Otorhinolaryngology, Head and Neck Surgery[1], Dept. Anesthesiology and Intensive Therapy[2], Dept. of Pathology[3], Univ. of Szeged, Szeged, Hungary

Introduction: The treatment of cricotracheal stenoses pose one of the most difficult challenges in head and neck surgery. They develop as a result of long-term intubation or technical problems during tracheotomy in most cases. The patients are almost always (re)-tracheotomized, and definitive solution follows later, often in several stages. This study reports on a new two-step surgical concept for the treatment, which offers a fast solution to stenoses without tracheotomy.

Methods: Study design: prospective study of 12 consecutive patients (ages 20-65) who were diagnosed with stenosis in the cricotracheal region. In the first stage acute suffocation was solved without tracheotomy, by endoscopic CO_2 laser scar excision in Jet ventillation in 11 cases; in 1 case with endoscopic Nd-YAG laser excision. In the second stage - as a final solution - before the onset of restenosis (within 6-8 weeks of the laser excision) trachea resection is performed in a combined intratracheal and translaryngeal jet ventillation narcosis. The length of the resected trachea segment is 3 to 6 rings (3 in average). End-to-end anastomosis: tracheo-tracheopexy in 5, tracheo-cricopexy in 6 and tracheo-crico-thyreopexy in 1 case. The removed segments were histologically examined to detect the pathological changes caused by laser.
Results: Complete stenosis elimination was achieved in 10 cases. 30% and 50% restenosis developed in 2 cases where the stenosis spread nearly up to the glottic region. In the latter case retracheotomy was needed during a heart attack. Histology revealed a more or less severe thermal damage causing the structural weakening of the cartilage.
Conclusion: The above numbers indicate that our concept for cricotracheal stenosis treatment provide excellent results, even in cases of stenoses spreading to the subglottic region. (Re)-tracheotomy can be avoided with endoscopic laser vaporisation, and thus segment resection can be performed in the best possible circumstances, and on the shortest tracheal segment.

106

Laryngeal Reinnervation in Animal Experiments

A. Tóth[1], A. Szűcs[1], K. Matesz[2], C. Harasztosi[3], I. Furka[4], I. Mikó[4], I. Sziklai[1]

Departments of Otorhinolaryngology[1], Anatomy[2], Physiology[3], Operative Techniques and Surgical Research[4], Univ. of Debrecen, Medical and Health Science Center, Debrecen, Hungary

Introduction: The paralysis/immobility of the larynx can be unilateral or bilateral. In most of the cases medialisation can't support suitable voice quality, moreover laterofixation makes the voice quality worse. After the failure of the previously mentioned two surgical methods reinnervation could become the best solution. There are several techniques and outcomes of laryngeal reinnervation. Methods include direct anastomosis, nerve grafting with nerves such as the phrenic nerve or ansa cervicalis and laryngeal nerve-muscle pedicle. So far there is no technique that has wide clinical application. In this study we adopted the nerve-muscle pedicle.
Methods: Five mongrel dogs (2 males, 3 females, 12-23 kg) were used. After midline incision the strap muscles were retracted laterally and the sternohyoid muscle with the ansa cervicalis was identified on the affected side. The left recurrent nerve was dissected and resected, so we paralysed the left vocal fold. We prepared the ansa cervicalis-sternohyoid muscle pedicle and sutured to the left posterior cricoarytenoid muscle (PCA) with three interrupted stiches of 6-0 Prolene, then the wound was closed. One year later in average, the dogs were returned for a second surgery, at which videolaryngoscopy, electromyography data were collected. The nerve pedicle and its attached muscular fragments were harvested for histological examination.
Results: The video records demonstrate the return of motion of the denervated PCA muscle by using the muscle-nerve pedicle. EMG data from the four animals showed evidence of reinnervation of the PCA muscle with polyphasic potentials. With the immune-histochemical reaction we could demonstrate neurofilaments and the motor end plates in both sides.
Conclusion: By using an ansa cervicalis-sternohyoid muscle pedicle for selective reinnervation of the PCA muscle a remobilization obtained of the previously denervated vocal cord after one year as it was documented by videolaryngoscopy, EMG recording and histological examination.

107

A New, Minimally Invasive Treatment Concept for the Bilateral Vocal Cord Paralysis - A Prospective Study

L. Rovó[1], J. Jóri[1], M. Brzózka[2], J. Czigner[1]

Departments of Otorhinolaryngology, Head and Neck Surgery[1] and Anesthesiology and Intensive Therapy[2], Medical Faculty of University of Szeged, Szeged, Hungary

Introduction: Bilateral vocal cord immobility (BVCI) is often transient or temporary consequence of a nonlaryngeal malignancy, thyroid surgery, or a presumed viral insult etc., thus vocal cord recovery can be expected within the first 6-12 months. Hence, most of the patients must be tracheotomized because of the bilateral paramedian vocal cord position in this early period, because the common vocal cord lateralization techniques seriously damage the patients' voice. This study reports on a newly developed minimally invasive way of the treatment instead of tracheotomy, which provides an immediate adequate airway without the definitive loss of laryngeal function.
Methods: Study design: a prospective study of 36 consecutive patients (ages 25 to 81 years) who were diagnosed with a BVCI within 6 months of onset of paralysis. The surgical procedure is performed endoscopically with a modification of Lichtenberge's endo-extralaryngeal suture lateralisation technique. The abducted vocal cord position is achieved by inserting a non-resorbable thread around the vocal process tied on the prelaryngeal muscles. The laterofixation suture was removed under local anaesthesia from an external approach in the case of vocal cord recovery detected at least on one side. Regular spirometric measurements and radiological aspiration tests were conducted on the patients.
Results: Adequate postoperative airway was achieved in 35 patients. Significant spontaneous vocal cord medialization was observed in four cases within a year and in three patients in the second and the third year. Partial or complete vocal cord recovery was observed in 18 cases. Further voice improvement followed in 10 patients when the threads were removed, due to vocal cord medialization or recovery. The mild postoperative aspirations ceased in the first postoperative days in 35 patients, and tracheotomy was required only at two elderly patients.
Conclusion: The concept of "early" laterofixation satisfies the important criteria: it can provide an immediate and long lasting adequate airway, and it can be considered potentially reversible from the view of laryngeal functions. Thus it is a reliable primary treatment for bilateral BVCI.

108

The Experimental Examination of the Healing Process of Telescopic Anastomosis

G. Szűcs[1], I. Tóth[1], T. Barna[2], E. Bráth[3], K. Gyáni[1], I. Mikó[3]

Semmelweis Teaching Hospital, Dept. of General and Thoracic Surgery[1], Dept. of Pathology[2], Miskolc, University of Debrecen, M.H.S.C., Faculty of Medicine, Dept. of Operative Techniques and Surgical Research[3], Debrecen, Hungary

Introduction: The telescopic anastomosis technique is known in the literature since the turn of the 19th-20th century. This type of anastomosis with some significant improvement has been adopted and used in performing esophago-gastrostomas and ileo-colostomas successfully in our clinical practice for ten years. A 15-20 mm long part of the esophagus is invaginated into the lumen of the stomach and the procedure is the same with ileum after division of vessels invaginated it into the lumen of the large bowel. In both cases single layer interrupted suture is used. The reason for doing our examination was that data about the healing process of telescopic anastomosis had not been found in literature.

Methods: During our experiments 12 telescopic esophago-gastrostomas, 9 telescopic ileo-colostomas, 3 end to side ileo-colostomas were performed on mongrel dogs. Making groups the length of the invaginated part in case of esophagus was 10, 20 and 30 mm and in case of ileum 0 (end to side), 10 and 20 mm. The esophageal mucosa was fixed using interrupted suture to prevent its retraction. The survival time was 0, 7 and 21 days. Macroscopic morphological and histological examinations were made and the bursting pressure was measured.

Results: The invaginated esophageal and ileal part did not suffer from ischaemic or any other damage. The gastric and the colonic mucosa and the prolabing mucosal layer of the ileum covered the free surface of the invaginated esophagus and ileum. The bursting pressure of the telescopic anastomosis did not depend on the length of the invaginated part and the average bursting pressure increased significantly during the healing process. The bursting pressure values of esophago-gastrostomas were on 0 day: 48±4 mmHg, 7th day: 115±5 mmHg, 21st day, 10 mm: 184±2, 20 mm: 201±16, 30 mm: 188±10 mmHg. The bursting pressure values of ileo-colostomas were on 0 day, 0 mm: 26±2 mmHg, 0 day, 20 mm: 56±6 mmHg, 7th day: 154±49 mmHg, 21st day, 10 mm: 249±20, 20 mm: 298±2 mmHg.

Discussion: The mucosal, submucosal layer sliding forward onto the external surface of the invaginated esophagus and ileum isolating and protecting the suture line of the anastomosis. It is the reason why the generally detected inflammation during the healing process of anastomosis was not close to the suture line. This process is possible because of the loose submucosal layer of the stomach and the colon.

Conclusion: The telescopic technique is a simple, cheap and safe method for performing esophago-gastrostomas and ileo-colostomas.

Immunology

109

Chimerism and Tolerance through Vascularized Bone Marrow Transplantation: Fact or Fiction?

M. Vossen, V.S. Gorantla, G. Perez-Abadia, C.G. Francois, P.C.R. Brouha, L.A. Laurentin-Perez, D. Pidwell, C. Maldonado, M. Kon, J.H. Barker

Department of Plastic, Reconstructive and Hand Surgery, University Medical Center Utrecht, The Netherlands, Division of Plastic and Reconstructive Surgery, University of Louisville, and Transplant Center at Jewish Hospital, Louisville, KY, USA

Introduction: Current methods used for inducing tolerance through mixed allogeneic chimerism (MAC) require ablative host conditioning with irradiation or radiomimetic drugs to make "space" for the donor bone marrow (BM) cells to engraft. In contrast to BM cell transplantation, a vascularized bone marrow transplant (VBMT) provides its own "space" along with its own microenvironment (stromal cells, hematopoietic cytokines), such that ablative conditioning of the host is not required. Syngeneic VBMTs have been demonstrated to be a better source for BM reconstitution than transplantation of BM cells alone. The purpose of this study was to determine if an allogeneic VBMT could induce chimerism in the absence of ablative conditioning, while using tacrolimus and mycophenolate mofetil (MMF) to prevent limb rejection. We used levels of chimerism to quantify the allogeneic cell contribution that VBMTs provided to recipients in our rat hind limb transplant model.

Methods: Thirteen Wistar Furth (WF) rats were divided into three groups. In Groups I and II, MAC was induced by infusion of $100x10^6$ ACI rat BM cells (ab and gd T cell-depleted) into WF rats irradiated with 950 cGy. After chimerism was established, mixed allogeneic chimeras in Group I (n=4) received ACI limbs and those in Group II (n=3) received WF limbs. In Group III (n=6), naive WF rats received ACI limbs, and were treated with tacrolimus (1 mg/kg i.p. for 14 days, and twice a week thereafter) and MMF (15 mg/kg/day p.o.). Flow cytometry was performed before sacrifice to determine the percentage of peripheral blood lymphocytes bearing ACI or WF MHC class I antigens. Animals were assessed daily for signs of rejection or graft versus host disease (GvHD) and sacrificed at five months (end study), or earlier if signs of GvHD occurred.

Results: The levels of chimerism increased 8.0±0.7 % in Group I (pre-transplant: 90.3±0.8% vs. post-transplant: 98.3±0.3%*) and 7.3±4.6% in Group III (pre-transplant: 0 vs. post-transplant 7.3±4.6%*). The levels of chimerism decreased 86.0±3.8% in Group II (pre-transplant: 91.0±0.6% vs. post-transplant: 5.0±4.3%*). *=$p< 0.05$. All animals in Group I showed signs of lethal GvHD and survived for 20.5±2.1 days. Animals in Group II survived for the duration of study (5 months) with no sign of rejection or GvHD but a significant reduction in levels of chimerism was observed. In Group III, four animals experienced at least one episode of rejection, whereas two animals in this group were free of any rejection episode with the described immunosuppressive regimen. The mean level of chimerism of the animals that underwent rejection episodes was

8.6±5.8%, whereas the levels of chimerism of the animals that were free from any rejection episode were 0.5% and 1.7%.

Conclusions: The significant decrease of ACI donor lymphocytes in chimeric hosts in Group II provides evidence of the effectiveness of the VBMT in contributing donor-reactive WF cells that in this case decreased levels of chimerism. In Groups I and III, the contribution of cells by the VBMT was also apparent but in this case resulted in increased levels of chimerism indicating that ACI cells transplanted with the donor limb proliferated and contributed to increased chimerism. All together, we conclude that fully mismatched allogeneic limb transplants acting as VBMTs can induce peripheral blood chimerism without the need for ablative conditioning of the host. This study found no correlation between the level of chimerism and the occurrence of rejection. The continuous administration of immunosuppressive drugs may have interfered with the development of transplantation tolerance. It remains to be elucidated whether the continuous source of donor cells within the transplanted limb can maintain stable chimerism and eventually induce a tolerant state. Further studies are in progress to pursue these questions.

110

Mast Cell-Dependent Neutrophil Recruitment in the Skin is Importantly Mediated by KC and LFA-1: Inhibitory Mechanisms of Action of Dexamethasone

R. Schramm[1], T. Schaefer[2], M.D. Menger[2], H. Thorlacius[1]

Department of Surgery[1], Malmö University Hospital, SE-20502 Malmö, Sweden and Institute for Clinical and Experimental Surgery[2], University of Saarland, D-66421 Homburg/Saar, Germany

Introduction: Mast cells play a critical role in inflammatory leukocyte recruitment. The study was conducted to I) characterize signaling pathways and molecular mechanisms behind leukocyte recruitment and II) to define the mechanisms of the anti-inflammatory action of dexamethasone in mast cell-dependent skin inflammation.

Methods: The mast cell secretagogue compound 48/80 (CMP48/80) was used to degranulate mast cells in murine air pouches and exudates were harvested at different time points after challenge. Dorsal skinfold chambers and intravital fluorescence microscopy were used to characterize leukocyte-endothelium adhesive interactions.

Results: Mast cell activation triggered a dose- and time-dependent influx of leukocytes into the subcutaneous cavities. Maximum amounts of predominately polymorphonuclear leukocytes (PMNs) were found after 4 hours. As assessed by ELISA analysis of pouch exudates, KC production increased time-dependently and reached peak levels at one hour after mast cell activation, whereas MIP-2 and TNF-α were not detected at any time point. Local administration of a monoclonal antibody (mAb) against KC, but not against MIP-2 or TNF-α, significantly attenuated neutrophil recruitment by 44% upon mast cell activation. Intravenous injection of a mAb against P-selectin, but not against E- or L-selectin markedly reduced leukocyte rolling and firm adhesion by 53 and 58%, respectively. Moreover, CMP48/80-induced leukocyte firm adhesion and recruitment were greatly attenuated by 48 and 49%, respectively, whereas the amount of rolling leukocytes was not changed in LFA-1-deficient animals. Dexamethasone pretreatment caused a significant reduction of dermal neutrophil accumulation (40%) and leukocyte firm adhesion (70%) in response to mast cell activation, but did not interfere with leukocyte rolling. Interestingly, dexamethasone significantly reduced the levels of secreted KC in pouch exudates by 51% upon mast cell activation. However, KC-induced subcutaneous neutrophil infiltration was not sensitive to dexamethasone treatment.

Conclusions: We provide evidence demonstrating that leukocyte rolling and firm adhesion in mast cell-dependent skin inflammation is mediated by P-selectin and LFA-1, respectively. Moreover, KC, but not MIP-2, is a key CXC chemokine in signaling mast cell-dependent neutrophil recruitment. Furthermore, dexamethasone attenuates leukocyte adhesion and neutrophil recruitment in mast cell-dependent skin inflammation through downregulation of KC synthesis, whereas KC function is not sensitive to this corticoid. Taken together, this study elucidates important interactions between chemokines and adhesion molecules in mast cell-dependent tissue infiltration of neutrophils and provides new insights in the complex anti-inflammatory mechanisms of action of dexamethasone in dermal inflammation.

111

Conditioning of Donor Graft with Recipient Bone Marrow Cells Predisposes for Acute Rejection

M. Maksymowicz[1], E. Cybulska[1], W.L. Olszewski[1,2]

Dept. of Surgical Research and Transplantation[1], Medical Research Center, Polish Academy of Sciences, 5, Pawinski Str., 02106 Warsaw, Poland and Norwegian Radium Hospital[2], Oslo, Norway

Introduction: Replacement of donor allograft dendritic cells (DC) and endothelial cells (EC) by recipient phenotype cells from bone marrow precursors prior to transplantation (tx) could theoretically prevent acute rejection. Lethal irradiation of donor and transplantation with vascularized bone marrow (hind limb tx) from prospective recipient of repopulated heart graft should result in replacement of donor organs with recipient DC and EC. We followed the repopulation process of DC and EC in the prospective donor heart (H) by transplanted vascularized bone marrow from the prospective recipient, over a period of 14 days, and the survival time of tx repopulated H.

Material and Methods: All BN rat H donors were irradiated 8Gy. No $OX6^+$, $OX27^+$ (specific for BN) DC were found in H. In group 1, H were harvested on day 3 and tx to LEW. In group 2, LEW hind-limb was transplanted to BN on day 3 for a 14 days repopulation with LEW bone marrow derived DC. H DC were found of LEW origin $OX6^+OX27^-$. In group 3, in addition CyA i.m. 3 mg/kg and in group 4, FK506 i.m., 0.5 mg/kg were given for 14 days. On day 15, DC-repopulated BN H was harvested and tx to LEW. The level of MLR of LEW recipient lymphocytes against BN cells was measured.

Results: Group 1. BN H were rejected by LEW within 7±2 d. Group 2. BN H were fully repopulated with LEW DC before tx to LEW. Interestingly, on histology a +++ intravascular inflammatory reaction was found in harvested H. Repopulated H were rejected by LEW recipient within 5±2 days. Group 3. CyA inhibited H repopulation with recipient DC. H survival time was 7±2 days. Group 4. FK506 totally inhibited repopulation as in group 3. The MST was 10 days. No replacement of donor EC by recipient EC was observed 14 days after recipient VBMtx.

Conclusions: Neither depletion of H allografts prior to tx of own DC nor repopulation by recipient DC prolong H graft survival. Repopulation in non-treated rats leads to GVH-like reaction in the prospective donor heart. Lack of repopulation of H by DC during CyA and FK506 administration indicates these drugs inhibit migration of DC bone marrow precursors.

112

Studies on the Role of T Cells and T Cell Subclasses in Graft Rejection

T. Jánossy[1], G.A. Ceepil[1], C. Vizler[1], I. Ocsovszki[2], R. Benner[3], P. Végh[1]

Institute of Surgical Research[1] and Department of Biochemistry[2], University of Szeged, Szeged, Hungary, Department of Immunology[3], Erasmus University, Rotterdam, The Netherlands

Introduction: Permanent tolerance to A (H-2^a) skin allografts induced in newborn CBA (H-2^k) mice was abolished and grafts were rejected following the i.p. injection of spleen cells of normal CBA mice or CBA mice sensitized to A antigens. In this *in vivo* model, we analysed the graft rejecting activity of T cells and T cell subclasses as well as the effect of anti-T cell antibodies.
Methods: Tolerance was induced in newborn CBA mice by the i.v. injection of $2x10^7$ (CBAxA)F_1 spleen cells. Mice carrying an intact A skin graft for more than 120 days were considered as permanently tolerant. CBA mice were sensitized with A skin grafts and their spleens were removed 16 days after transplantation. $CD4^+$ helper (T_H) and $CD8^+$ cytotoxic T (T_C) cells were purified from the spleen cell suspensions by affinity columns. For coating with antibodies, spleen cells were incubated (4 °C, 60 min) in anti-T cell rat mAbs or in rabbit anti-mouse antithymocyte serum (ATS). The purity of the separated cells and the binding of antibodies to lymphocytes were checked by flow cytometry. Different groups of permanently tolerant mice were injected i.p. with untreated or treated sensitized and normal spleen cells, respectively.
Results: 10^8 normal and $2x10^7$ sensitized spleen cells caused graft rejection in the tolerant recipients with similar efficiency. $4x10^6$ sensitized $CD4^+$ T_H cells induced delayed graft rejection in 68.9% of the recipients, while 2 x 10^6 $CD8^+$ T_C cells did so only in 33.3% of them. If the separated $CD4^+$ and $CD8^+$ T cells were mixed, they were as efficient as the unseparated spleen cells. *In vitro* coating of the sensitized spleen cells with anti-CD3 mAb reacting with all T cells considerably inhibited their tolerance abrogating activity. Anti-CD4 mAb was more effective than anti-CD8 mAb. The graft rejecting effect of both normal and sensitized spleen cells was significantly reduced if they were incubated in polyclonal ATS *in vitro*. ATS treatment reduced the binding of anti-CD45, anti-CD90, anti-CD8, and, in the case of sensitized spleen cells, anti-CD4 mAbs, while that of anti-CD3 mAb was not diminished.
Discussion: $CD3^+$ T cells play a decisive role in the abrogation of transplantation tolerance. To induce normal graft rejection, the cooperation of $CD4^+$ T_H and $CD8^+$ T_C cells is needed. ATS contains antibodies to CD45, CD90, CD4 and CD8 cell surface molecules which are involved in the activation of T cells. These antibodies might play a role in the graft protective effect of ATS.
Conclusion: The results indicate that the abrogation of neonatal transplantation tolerance by cell transfer is an appropriate *in vivo* model for analysing the role of lymphoid cell (sub)populations in graft rejection as well as the mechanism of immunosuppression caused by antibodies.
This work was supported by the grants from OTKA (No. T26014), Ministry of Health (No. 480 05/2000), Hungary and NWO (No. 047-003040), The Netherlands.

113

Studies on the Prevention of Graft-versus-Host Disease (GVHD) by *in vitro* Pretreatment of Donor Cells with Anti-T Cell Antibodies

L. Szalai[1], M. Laurinyecz[1], G.A. Ceepil[1], C. Vizler[1], I. Ocsovszki[2], R. Benner[3], T. Jánossy[1]

Institute of Surgical Research[1] and Department of Biochemistry[2], University of Szeged, Szeged, Hungary, Department of Immunology[3], Erasmus University, Rotterdam, The Netherlands

Introduction: Earlier we found that, in adult CBA mice made neonatally tolerant to the histocompatibility antigens of the A mouse strain, the i.v. injection of A spleen cells induced an acute lethal GVHD. GVHD did not develop if A spleen cell donors were pretreated with rabbit anti-mouse antithymocyte serum (ATS) which inhibits T-cell-mediated immune responses. In this study, we investigated whether GVHD can be prevented by *in vitro* treatment of donor spleen cells with ATS or anti-T cell monoclonal antibodies (mAb).
Methods: Tolerance was induced in newborn CBA (H-2^k) mice to A (H-2^a) antigens by the i.v. injection of $2x10^7$ (CBAxA)F_1 semiallogeneic spleen cells. 95% of the tolerized CBA mice became permanently tolerant: they carried their A test skin allografts lifelong without any sign of rejection. GVHD was induced in 12-month-old tolerant CBA mice by the i.v. injection of $5x10^7$ untreated or antibody-treated A spleen cells. For coating with antibodies, spleen cells were incubated (4°C, 60 min) in rabbit anti-mouse ATS or in different mAbs. The binding of antibodies to leukocytes was checked by flow cytometry.
Results: Untreated A spleen cells induced acute GVHD with >30% weight loss and >80% mortality. *In vitro* coating of spleen cells with antibodies of ATS prevented the development of the symptoms and the mortality of GVHD. The treatment did not change the composition of the spleen cell suspension, but it decreased the expression of CD90, CD8 and CD45 cell surface molecules participating in the activation of T cells, while it did not modify that of others (CD3, CD4). The induction of GVHD was also prevented by an anti-CD90 mAb reacting with all mature T cells. It was significantly inhibited by an anti-CD4 mAb binding to helper T (T_H) cells as well as by an anti-CD8 mAb specific to cytotoxic T (T_C) cells. However, GVHD was not influenced by an anti-CD24 mAb reacting with all leukocytes except mature T cells and macrophages.
Discussion: The induction of GVHD was inhibited by *in vitro* coating of donor lymphocytes with anti-T cell antibodies. Inhibition of T cell activation and/or elimination of antibody-coated T cells in the recipient can be responsible for this effect. The decreased expression of CD8, CD45 and CD90 molecules on ATS-treated cells suggests that ATS might contain antibodies specific to these markers which can play a role in the immunosuppressive activity of ATS. The inhibitory effect of anti-CD4 and anti-CD8 treatment indicates that both T_H and T_C donor cells participate in the induction of GVHD.

Conclusions: GVHD can be prevented by *in vitro* coating of donor lymphocytes with anti-T cell antibodies. Both T_H and T_C donor cells participate in the pathomechanism of GVHD in this model.

This work was supported by the grants from OTKA (No. T26014), Ministry of Health (No. 480 05/2000), Hungary and NWO (No. 047-003040), The Netherlands.

114

Physiological Roles of Kupffer Cells in Liver Injury

G. Lázár[1], E. Husztik[1], E. Duda[2], G. Lázár Jr.[3]

Institute of Pathophysiology[1], Biological Research Center[2], Department of Surgery[3], University of Szeged, Hungary

Introduction: Kupffer cells, the resident hepatic macrophages, have diverse functions, including phagocytosis, endocytosis, immunomodulation, synthesis and secretion of biologically active products. Gadolinium chloride ($GdCl_3$) depress or destroy large Kupffer cells and has been used *in vivo* to investigate their role in a variety of hepatotoxic processes. In these experiments we studied the effect of Kupffer cell blockade on endotoxin sensitivity, endotoxin induced cytokine production and hepatocellular injury in rats with obstructive jaundice.

Methods: Surgery: Obstructive jaundice was induced by bile duct ligation (BDL). Kupffer cell blockade: The animals were given $GdCl_3$ in a dose of 1 mg/100 g body weight i.v. 24 h before testing.

Results: Obstructive jaundice greatly sensitized the animals to bacterial lipopolysaccharide (LPS) and LPS-induced tumor necrosis factor-α (TNF-α) production, and LPS-induced hepatic injury. Kupffer cell blockade significantly increased the resistance of animals with jaundice against bacterial endotoxin, reduced LPS-induced TNF-α production. $GdCl_3$ also significantly reduced the serum levels of GOT and GPT compared to controls 4 hours after the endotoxin challenge.

Discussion: Bacterial endotoxin and the release of cytokines are primarly responsible for the increased number of complications in patients with jaundice.

Conclusion: The results underline the importance of Kupffer cell function and the activation of inflammatory cytokines in the increased morbidity in obstructive jaundice.

115

Changes in Immune Defence and Heat-Shock Protein 70 Level in the Various Stages of Tuberculosis

J. Furák[1], I. Troján[1], T. Szőke[1], L. Tiszlavicz[2], Á. Balogh[1]

Departments of Surgery[1] and Pathology[2], University of Szeged, Szeged, Hungary

Introduction: An account will be given of the occurrence of $CD4^+$ T-helper, $CD8^+$ T-cytotoxic and $CD20^+$ B-lymphocytes and of heat-shock protein 70 (HSP70) in pulmonary tuberculosis before and after antituberculotic treatment. An assessment will be presented of the significance of the presence of HSP70 in the cells comprising the tuberculoma and in the adjacent lung tissue.

Method: A total of 40 patients operated on for pulmonary tuberculosis (TB) were divided into two equal groups, depending on whether they received antituberculotic treatment (group I) or not (group II) preoperatively. Immunohistochemical tests were performed on paraffin sections of TB samples from the two groups in order to determine the presence or not of $CD4^+$, $CD8^+$, and $CD20^+$ lymphocytes and HSP70. The strengths of the immunohistochemical reactions were graded on a scale of 0 to 4, and mean values were calculated for purposes of comparison. The Mann-Whitney test was applied for calculation of the significance level ($p<0.05$).

Results and Discussion: There was no significant difference in the incidence of $CD4^+$ ($p=0.516$), $CD8^+$ ($p=0.679$) and $CD20^+$ ($p=0.784$) lymphocytes in groups I. and II: mean 2.6 vs. 2.8, 2.05 vs. 1.9, and 0.8 vs. 0.6, respectively. The mean incidence of HSP70 in normal lung was significantly lower ($p=0.015$) in group I (1.5 vs. 2.2) than in group II, and it was almost the same level in the tuberculoma (1.6 vs. 2.5) in groups I and II. In the tuberculoma, the mean levels of HSP70 in the Ziehl-Neelsen-positive cases (2.1 vs. 2.5) were not significantly different in groups I and II ($p=0.137$), but higher than the values for acid-fast-negative cases (1.3 vs. 2.3, significant; $p=0.001$) in groups I and II. As concerns the cells constituting the tuberculoma, the occurrence of HSP70 in groups I and II was as follows: 2 vs. 2.68 in the Langhans cells (no significance; $p=0.27$), 1.6 vs. 2.5 in the lymphocytes (significant; $p=0.008$), 1.6 vs. 2.4 in the epitheloid cells (significant; $p=0.023$).

Conclusions: Independently of the stage of the infection, and independently of the performance of antituberculotic treatment, the occurrence of T-lymphocytes (participating to a much greater extent) and of B-lymphocytes (taking part to only a minor extent) is constant in the immune defence against TB. In contrast, the HSP70 levels, which are elevated in the early, untreated group II, are indicative of active infection. On the basis of the higher HSP70 levels in the Ziehl-Neelsen-positive cases, the presence of active mycobacteria may be concluded in the Langhans cells and the epitheloid cells.

116

Methotrexate as an Immunosuppressive Agent in a Life-Supporting hDAF Pig-to-Primate Xenotransplantation Model

R. Cadrobbi, A. Dedja, N. Baldan, F. Calabrese, M. Boldrin, F. Fante, M. Castagnaro, P. Carraro, F.M. Cancellotti, P. Rigotti, E. Cozzi, E. Ancona

Department of Medical and Surgical Sciences, Institute of Pathology, Veterinary Institute, University of Padua; Padua General Hospital; Institute of Health Animal Prophylaxis; C.O.R.I.T., Padua, Italy

Introduction: Methotrexate (MTX) is an antimetabolite drug which in combination with T-cell directed immunosuppressants, has been used successfully to achieve long-term survival in concordant xenotransplantation in rodents. Only limited data with MTX are available in the discordant pig-to-primate xenotransplantation model, as cyclophosphamide (CyP) is commonly used as an immunosuppressant in this pig-to-primate xenotransplantation model, and has led to the best results published to date. In an attempt to identify new immunosuppressive regimens using antimetabolite drugs for this model, we used MTX to replace CyP.

Materials and Methods: Ten bilaterally nephrectomised cynomolgus monkeys received a life-supporting kidney from hDAF transgenic pigs (Imutran/Novartis). MTX was administered according to three different regimens: group A (n=5) received 5 daily peri-operative MTX doses at 0.1-0.5 mg/kg; group B (n=3) received 4 preoperative MTX doses at 0.15 mg/kg; and group C (n=2) received 4 preoperative MTX doses at 0.15 mg/kg and 0.075-0.15 mg/kg twice weekly thereafter. Cyclosporine A (Neoral, Novartis) and tapering steroids were always part of the maintenance therapy in all the groups. In addition, mycophenolate sodium (ERL080, Novartis) was administered postoperatively in groups A and B. Close monitoring for levels of hemolytic anti-pig antibodies, serum biochemistry and blood counts was performed in all primates.
Results: There were no cases of hyperacute rejection in any of the groups. One animal died of anesthesiological complications. The remaining animals showed graft function with a nadir of creatinine levels between 61 µmol/L and 245 µmol/L by day 7. The animals' survival was: 6, 9, 9, 10, 39 days in group A; 16 and 34 days in group B; 0, 16 and 41 days in group C. Two animals from group A and 1 animal from group B were sacrificed between day 6 and 16 as a consequence of severe enteritis. The remaining animals were sacrificed between days 9 and 41 due to kidney failure associated with grade II-III acute humoral rejection in all cases. Acute cellular rejection was also observed in 3 animals in group A.
Conclusions: At the doses used in this study, MTX appears to be a compound with a very narrow therapeutic window in this recipient species. Moreover, a maintenance immunosuppression with MTX does not appear to confer any advantage over a maintenance therapy with previously tested immunosuppressants. Three animals nonetheless survived for more than one month. Irrespective of the capacity of immunosuppressive regimens with MTX to extend the survival of pig organs transplanted into cynomolgus monkeys, the high toxicity of this compound limits its potential application in this xenotransplantation model.

Thoracic and Esophageal Surgery

117

Telescopic Esophageal Anastomosis: Clinical Results and Data of Animal Experiments

G. Szűcs[1], I. Tóth[1], T. Barna[2], E. Bráth[3], K. Gyáni[1], I. Mikó[3]

Dept. of General and Thoracic Surgery[1], Semmelweis Teaching Hospital, Dept. of Pathology[2], Miskolc, Dept. of Operative Techniques and Surgical Research[3], University of Debrecen, Debrecen, Hungary

Introduction: There are two potential ways of decreasing the insufficiency and stricture rate of the esophageal anastomosis: to protect and restore the blood supply of the anastomosing organs, or to improve the anastomosis performing methods. Herein we report significant improvement with the latter method using the telescopic anastomosis which was first published at the turn of 19-20th century (Maylard, Sonnenburg).
Methods: The esophageal mucosa is fixed to its muscular wall using circularly inserted stitches in order to prevent the mucosal retraction. A 15-20 mm long part of esophageal stump prepared the above way is invaginated into the lumen of the other organ using single layer interrupted suture. The wall of the distally anastomosed organ is inverted by these stitches into the lumen adjoining the esophagus. It is important that the stitches do not include the mucosal layer. This way the wall of the other anastomised organ belts 3-4 mm width around the muscular wall of the esophagus. The stitches do not drain the lumen. We have performed telescopic technique for ten years for resection of esophagus because of 126 esophageal tumors, 5 esophageal strictures and because of for 75 cases of stomach/cardia tumor. We performed 108 collar anastomosis (106 esophago-gastrostoma and 2 oesophago-ileocolostoma), 41 intrathoracic and 57 intraabdominal. Altogether 206 telescopic esophageal anastomoses were performed in our clinical practice. The healing process of telescopic esophago-gastrostomas were examined on 12 mongrel dogs during our animal experiments.
Results: With regard to the collar anastomosis, anastomotic leakage of the esophago-gastrostoma occurred in 12 cases out of the total of 106 (11,3%). There were no reoperation or death due to insufficiency. The intrathoracic anastomosis and intraabdominal esophago-jejunostomas healed without complications. Stricture occurred in 12 cases always in collar position: in 9 cases after leakage and in 3 cases after "undisturbed" healing. Anastomosis-plasty had to be performed in 4 cases. In the animal experiments, no damage occurred in the examined esophageal part and it became covered with gastric mucosa due to the healing process. As evidenced by bursting pressure measurements, pressure tolerance of the anastomosis increased during the course of the healing process (0 day 48±4 mmHg, 7 day 115±5 mmHg, 21 day 201±16 mmHg).
Conclusion: The telescopic anastomosis technique improved by us is simple and cheap and therefore safe esophago-gastric and esophago-intestinal anastomosis can be performed using this technique.

118

Effect of Thoracic Epidural Anaesthesia During Experimental Gastric Tube Formation

G. Lázár[1], J. Kaszaki[2], S. Ábrahám[2], G. Horváth[1], K. Szentpáli[1], A. Wolfárd[1], A. Paszt[1], Á. Balogh[1], M. Boros[2]

Department of Surgery[1], Institute of Surgical Research[2], Szent-Györgyi Albert Medical Center, University of Szeged, Szeged, Hungary

Introduction: Gastric tube formation is a widely used surgical technique to re-establish the continuity of the gastrointestinal tract after esophagectomy. The inadequate vascularization of the gastric tube may result in serious post-operative complications including anastomotic leakage or stricture formation in the long run. Recent experimental and clinical studies demonstrated that thoracic epidural anaesthesia (TEA) prevents the decrease in gastric intramucosal pH (pHi), increases intestinal mucosal blood flow and beneficially affects the bowel function during abdominal surgery. On this basis we set out to study the consequences of TEA on hemodynamic parameters, gastrointestinal motility and tissue perfusion of the gastric tube.

Methods: The experiments were performed on 12 dogs under sodium pentobarbital anesthesia (30 mg/kg i.v.). The stomach was prepared for replacement according to the method of Akiyama. TEA was induced by Bupivacain (1mg/kg)) at the L3/L4 level. Mean arterial pressure (MAP), right gastroepiploic and superior mesenteric artery blood flow (Transonic Systems Inc.) were monitored, the small bowel motility was measured with strain gauge technique. All data were collected and analyzed with a computerized data acquisition system. Tissue perfusion changes of the stomach were investigated by determination of gastric intramucosal pH (pHi) and orthogonal polarization spectral imaging (OPS) technique.
Results: MAP was significantly reduced by 30% after epidural anesthesia and concomitantly the blood flow in the superior mesenteric artery and right gastroepiploic artery was significantly increased. After gastric tube formation the pHi in the proximal part of the tube diminished from 7.42±0.02 baseline to 7.15±0.1 values, red blood cell velocity (RBCV) in terminal arterioles of the upper part of the gastric tube decreased from 540±5 μm/s to 370±55 μm/s in the mucosa and 430±42 μm/s to 230±30 μm/s in the serosal side. After TEA the pHi significantly improved, the RBCV returned to the baseline level and the small bowel motility index significant increased from 4.8±1.2 to 9.4±2.2.
Discussion: These data show that TEA improves the intestinal motility and tissue perfusion of the distal portion of the gastric tube. We suggest that TEA is favorable and should be recommended during reconstructive esophageal surgery.

119

Usefulness of Phreno-Mediastinal Approach in Thoracoscopic Radical Esophagectomy

T. Kawano, K. Nagai, T. Nishikage, K. Ami, Y. Nakajima, K. Kawada, T. Iwai

Department of Surgery, Tokyo Medical and Dental University, Tokyo, Japan

Introduction: Video-assisted thoracoscopic surgery was recently introduced in thoracic esophagectomy. Although the thoracoscopic approach is less invasive and feasible for mediastinal lymph node dissection, it is less reliable for systematic lymphadenectomy. Moreover, thoracoscopic esophagectomy needs a specially trained surgeon(s), longer operative time, and involves higher costs. We devised a new technique for thoracoscopic radical esophagectomy using a new supportive approach called hand-assisted thoracoscopic surgery using an anterior phreno-mediastinal approach (HATS / APMA esophagectomy).
Patients and Methods: Between 2000 and 2001, fifteen patients with thoracic esophageal cancer were operated on by this new procedure. We could insert a left hand and / or therapeutic instruments through the anterior phreno-mediastinal route to the right thoracic cavity from the small upper abdominal incision and performed hand-assisted thoracoscopic surgery.
Results: All procedures in each patient were performed safely and the post-operative course was uneventful except one case with post-operative recurrent laryngeal nerve palsy and needed long hospitalization.
Conclusion: These procedures reduce stress on the surgeons, the number of thoracic ports, and costs as compared to simple thoracoscopic thoracic esophagectomy, and also reduce the operating time because the use of the hand yields a tactile sense and direct support.

120

The Role of the VATS in the Treatment of Hydrothorax

K. Kovács, G. Boross, M. Svébis, C. Oláh

Dept. of Surgery, Bács-Kiskun County Teaching Hospital, Kecskemét, Hungary

Introduction: Hydrothorax can be an accompanying symptom of many diseases. In most of the cases, proper treatment of the basic disease also abrogates hydrothorax formation, but when the primary cause of the disease is incurable, the complaints and symptoms of the patient can remarkably be reduced by terminating hydrothorax.
Methods: When thorax puncture is proved to be unsuccessful, different methods of video-assisted thoracic surgery (VATS, such as pleurodesis and pleurectomy) can be used not only to treat the hydrothorax of various origin, but also to lend support to the completion of diagnosis.
Results: During the last six years, 78 patients were treated with hydrothorax in our department; 47 men, and 31 women, the average age was 54/57 years. In all of the cases, the basic disease could clearly be identified before the thoracic surgical intervention. Thoracic punctures were examined cytologically and bacteriologically to confirm the correct diagnosis. After the traditional treatment had been proven to be ineffective, VATS interventions were performed in patients that could be operated in anaesthesia whereas isolated intubation in general anaesthesia was used. VATS interventions were performed in six diseases of different aetiology. Nine patients were treated in the proliferative phase of empyema thoracis. Thirty seven patients were treated with pleuritis carcinomatosa. In one patient, pericardial tamponade and right-side hydrothorax developed as a result of rheumatoid arthritis. Eight patients were operated with hydrothorax resulting from cirrhosis hepatis. Chronic pancreatitis was often accompanied by hydrothorax. In case of sixteen patients, VATS intervention was performed after medication and punctures could be proven to be unsuccessful. Six patients were operated for hydrothorax resulting from chronic heart disease. During VATS, pleura abrasion was performed on the parietal pleura with a diathermic knife, then talcum was sprinkled in the thorax. Partial pleurectomy was also performed in some patients.
Discussion: The authors state that pleurodesis with VATS and talcum suspension is effective in patients of recurrent hydrothorax with well defined symptoms. The average duration of the healing process was fifteen days. The method was successful in 83% of the cases with no major complications and without any mortality.
Conclusion: Based on our clinical experience derived from treatment of patients with hydrothorax, physical and chemical pleurodesis assisted with VATS is a suitable method for the treatment of hydrothorax when patients are in appropriate condition and the basic disease is treated satisfactorily.

121

Isolated Lung Perfusion with Gemcitabine in the Rat: Pharmacokinetics and Survival

B. van Putte, J. Hendriks, S. Romijn, B. Pauwels, G. Friedel, G. Guetens, P. van Schil

University of Antwerp, Edegem (Antwerp), Belgium; Catholic University of Leuven, Leuven, Belgium and Klinik Schillerhoehe, Gerlingen, Germany

Introduction: Currently, the only treatment to achieve long-term survival for isolated pulmonary metastases is complete resection, while systemic chemotherapy has no major benefit. Isolated lung perfusion (ILuP) is a promising technique to achieve high levels without systemic exposure. Toxicity and pharmacokinetics of gemcitabine (GCB) were evaluated in a rat model of IluP and compared to intravenous (iv) infusion.

Methods: CC531S adenocarcinoma cells were incubated *in vitro* for 24 hours with GCB. Cell survival was determined 4 days after GCB treatment with the sulforhodamine B test. Controls were incubated with a balanced salt solution. In a first *in vivo* experiment, Wag/Rij rats underwent left ILuP with 20 mg/kg (n=3), 40 mg/kg (n=6), 80 mg/kg (n=6), 160 mg/kg (n=6) and 320 mg/kg (n=6) of GCB. Animals were followed for 3 weeks postoperatively before a right pneumonectomy was performed to evaluate the effect of GCB perfusion on left lung function. In addition, survival was determined for rats treated with iv infusion of 40 mg/kg (n=10), 80 mg/kg (n=10), 160 mg/kg (n=10) and 320 mg/kg (n=6). Both ILuP and iv treated groups were observed for 90 days. In a second experiment lung and serum GCB levels were determined by chromatography for rats treated with iv infusion (160 mg/kg, n=6) and rats which had IluP (160 mg/kg, n=6; 320 mg/kg, n=6). A Student's t-test was applied for comparison of all data.

Results: Incubation of the CC531S adenocarcinoma cells with GCB led to a 50% decrease ($p<0.05$) in the number of cells at 24 hours compared to controls at a dose of 21.9 nM. The mortality for rats treated with 320 mg/kg iv GCB was 100% compared to 17% after ILuP for the same dose. ILuP with 160 mg/kg and 320 mg/kg resulted in significantly higher lung levels of GCB compared to iv therapy without any systemic leakage.

Conclusion: GCB ILuP is well tolerated to a maximum dose of 320 mg/kg and results in significantly higher GCB lung levels with undetectable serum levels compared to intravenous treatment. These results warrant further ILuP experiments with *in vivo* tumor rat models.

122

Variations in Flow, Duration and Concentration Do Not Change the Final Lung Concentrations of Melphalan after Isolated Lung Perfusion in The Rat

S. Romijn, J. Hendriks, B. van Putte, E. de Bruijn, P. van Schil

University Hospital Antwerp, Edegem, Belgium

Objective: Isolated lung perfusion (ILuP) with melphalan (MN) is superior to intravenous infusion in an experimental rat model for the treatment of lung metastases. We studied the influence of perfusion time, flow and concentration on MN lung levels in a rat model of ILuP.

Methods: To determine the level at which the lung is saturated by MN, ILuP was performed in WAG/Rij rats during 30 minutes by a single-pass system with 0.5 mg (n=5), 0.05 mg (n=5), 0.01 mg (n=5) and 0.005 mg (n=5) of MN. In a second experiment, the influence of perfusion time, dose and concentration was analyzed using the dose of 0.05 mg of MN. The lung perfusion was performed during 30 minutes with a flow of 0.5 mL/min (n=4) (group 1), during 60 minutes with a flow of 0.5 mL/min (n=4) (group 2) and during 30 minutes with a flow of 1.0 mL/min (n=4) (group 3). For comparison of MN lung levels the unpaired Student's t-test was applied. Statistical significance was reached at $p<0.05$.

Results: Melphalan lung levels of rats perfused with 0.5 mg (89.7± 47 µg/g) and 0.05 mg (25± 0.3 µg/g) were significantly higher compared to the lower doses (0.01mg: 0.6±0.3 µg/g; 0.005mg: 1.4± 0.2 µg/g). Perfusions performed with 0.5 mg were at a saturated level. Therefore 0.05 mg was chosen as the dose for the second experiment. No significant differences were seen in lung levels of MN between the groups with variation in perfusion time (2.0±1.1 µg/g), flow (2.9 µg/g) and concentration (1.3 µg/g).

Conclusion: Since no influence of perfusion time, concentration and flow was observed with a dose of 0.05 mg of MN, the only determinant of final MN lung levels is the dose administered.

Surgical Pathophysiology

123

How Do Redox-Sensitive Transcription Factors Influence the Inflammatory Reaction in Sepsis and Polytrauma?

G. v. Gagern, T. Zimmermann, S. Albrecht, S. Kersting, H. Schikore, H. Zwipp, H.D. Saeger*

Dept. of Surgery, Dept. of Gynaecology*, Technical University Dresden, Dresden, Germany

Introduction: The redox-sensitive transcription factor NFκB seems to be the central regulator of the inflammatory reaction in patients suffering from S.I.R.S. and sepsis. There is a strong correlation

(Zimmermann et al.) between changes in the activity of NFκB and mortality. The role of the transcription factor AP-1 with regard to sepsis still has remained uncertain. The initiating factor for activation of the AP-1 subunits c-jun and c-fos is the activation by oxidative and reductive processes. Aim of our study was to discover the role of these two transcription factors in septic and polytraumatised patients.
Methods: 50 polytraumatised patients and 15 patients with S.I.R.S./sepsis were included. Lab methods: 1) NFκB and AP-1 binding activity in mononuclear cells (EMSA), 2) AP-1 subunits (c-jun, c-fos) in mononuclear blood cells, 3) IL-6, 4) TNFα, 5) NO in the plasma. The Apache II and the MOF-Score (Goris) were recorded in course. Patients were divided into deceased and surviving patients.
Results: Deceased polytraumatised patients showed a significant increment of the NFκB binding activity on the 2nd and 3rd day ($p<0.005$). AP-1 showed a similar trend. Deceased septic patients also showed a significant and substantially stronger NFκB binding activity than surviving patients. TNFα and IL-6 were significantly different in the two groups (surviving/deceased). The subunits c-jun and c-fos of AP-1 were extremely elevated in the deceased patients.
Conclusion: The influencing of the activation of the transcription factors AP-1 and NFκB could be a therapeutical starting-point for antiinflammatory therapy. It should be investigated in further studies, how far a regulation of the redox status (antioxidative substances) or the administration of protease inhibitors (prevention of proteolysis and translocation of NFκB into the nucleus of a cell) can prevent further damage.

124

Evaluation of Phagocytic Function of Spleen after Splenic Artery Ligation in Secondary Hypersplenism

C. Vatansev, S. Tekin, M. Sahin, M. Avunduk, M. Serdengecti

SUTF General Surgery, Pathology and Nuclear Medicine, Konya, Turkey

Introduction: The aim of this study was to investigate the effects of splenic artery ligation on the phagocytic functions and morphology of the spleen in rabbits which were induced secondary hypersplenism by splenic vein ligation (SVL). Selective artery embolization and splenic artery ligation (SAL) are used by some centers in the treatment of secondary hypersplenism, though not very widely. However, effects of these procedures on the functions of the spleen are not exactly known.
Methods: 30 rabbits of New Zealand type were included in this study. The rabbits were separated into 3 groups, 10 subjects in each. The first group was applied laparotomy, and the second and third groups were applied laparotomy + splenic vein ligation. At the end of the fourth week, the first and second groups had laparotomy while the third group had laparotomy + splenic artery ligation. At the end of the eighth week, 1 cc blood was taken from all rabbits for hematological parameters. The rabbits were administered 0.1 mCi/kg Tc-99m sulfur colloid, and retention rates in the liver and spleen were determined. Spleens of the rabbits were removed and examined histopathologically.
Results: Liver/spleen retention rates were found to be 27.0±4.5 in the sham group, 28.3±3.8 in the SVL group and 57.4±8.1 in the SVL+SAL group. Retention rate in the spleen was significantly lower in the SVL+SAL group ($p=0.0001$). Leukocyte levels were similar among the groups while erythrocyte and thrombocyte levels were significantly lower in the SVL group than in the other two groups ($p=0.0001$). Histopathologically, wide congestion was observed in the SVL group while extended fibrosis and necrosis were observed in the spleen in SVL+SAL group.
Conclusion: Although application of SAL in secondary hypersplenism cases improves hypersplenism, it fails to improve phagocytic function of the spleen.

125

Endothelin-1 Upsets Homeostatic Equilibrium in the Coronary Bed

A. Juhász-Nagy, V. Kékesi

Dept. of Cardiovascular Surgery, Semmelweis University, Budapest, Hungary

Introduction: Endothelin-1 (ET-1) the most aggressive endogenous vasoconstrictor may elicit a lasting vasospasm, and this contradicts the well known propensity of the coronary vessels for immediate compensatory responses.
Methods: Experiments were performed on the *in situ* heart of open chest dogs (n=36) to analyze the background of this phenomenon. Intraarterial (i.a.) ET-1 boluses (10-1000 pmol) were given directly into the LAD. Coronary blood flow was measured with ultrasonic probes. Myocardial release of purine nucleosides (adenosine and inosine) was measured with HPLC and expressed as A-V difference times flow. Glibenclamide (1 micromol/min i.a.) was employed to block ATP-sensitive potassium channels. Nitric oxide (NO)-dependent vasodilation was tested by i.a. acetylcholine infusions (0.5-5.0 nmol/min).
Results: ET-1 elicited dose-dependent coronary vasoconstriction. By attaining a critical ET-1 dose (>300 pmol) the response turned into a long lasting spasm without any signs of secondary dilation. Myocardial purine release, however, was markedly augmented. Dose-response relationships of reactive hyperemia-induced stimulated purine nucleoside formation (flow plotted against release) were shifted to the right by nearly two orders of magnitude. ATP-sensitive potassium channel blockade potentiated the release and further reduced the flow. Blocking of NO-dependent vasodilation was obtained even by threshold (>10 pmol) ET-1 doses.
Conclusion: The data suggest that ET-1 reduces adaptive coronary capacity due to decreased vascular responsiveness and not to the lack of compensatory mediators. Contrary to the classic tenets of homeostasis, such a response pattern, involving positive feedback elements, may increase flow inhomogeneity and may lead to pathologic consequences.

126

Increased Concentrations of Pericardial Cathecholamines Affect Cardiac and Circulatory Function and Pericardial Levels of Endothelin-1

V. Kékesi, A. Nagy, I. Toma, L. Losonczi, M. Rusvai, A. Juhász-Nagy

Semmelweis University, Dept. of Cardiovascular Surgery, and Szent István University, Dept. of Microbiology and Infectious Diseases, Budapest, Hungary

Introduction: It has recently been shown that pericardial fluid may accumulate several endogenous regulatory agents which can exert their characteristic cardiovascular effects. Such agents are the catecholamines and endothelins, and their myocardial and/or pericardial concentrations are significantly elevated in different cardiovascular diseases. Although these agents seem to be important regulators of the cardiovascular function, very little information is available on the intrapericardial effects of catecholamines and their interaction with endogenous endothelins.
Methods: The cardiovascular effects of intrapericardially (i.p.) administered dopamine (12-60-300-1500 microgram/kg DA, n=8) were studied in the *in situ* canine heart. The closed pericardial sac was cannulated for the administration of DA and for the removal of the pericardial infusate samples. During subsequent DA bolus incubation periods (15 minutes each) systemic blood pressure (BP), heart rate (HR), left ventricular dP/dt, and standard ECG were recorded and compared with the effects of norepinephrine boluses (1.2-6-30-150 microgram/kg NE i.p., n=7). Following each drug administration two pericardial samples were obtained and endothelin-1 levels were measured by ELISA method.
Results: The intrapericardial DA elicited dose-dependent increases of HR (+11±1, +40±2, +38±2, +38±3 beats/min respectively, *p<0.05-0.01*) without changes in dP/dt and BP at lower doses. Only the highest dose of DA resulted in marked and significant elevation in both contractility and arterial pressure (+132±10% and +54±4 mmHg, *p<0.05*, respectively.). DA elicited moderate but significant increases of i.p. ET-1 levels (control vs. DA1500: 14.3±0.1, vs. 26.1±0.1 pg/ml/100g myocardial tissue, *p<0.001*). Similar changes were observed with increasing doses of i.p. NE with more parallel individual effect-components of the agent and more characteristic dose-response relationship than that of the DA.
Conclusion: The results confirm, that the i.p. administered cathecholamines can exert their cardiovascular effects, however, the strength and distribution of the individual effect-components of these agents are characteristically different from the intravascular ones. Such a difference could be explained by inhomogeneous tissue distribution/elimination of the agents or by the modulating effects produced by the released endothelin-1.

127

Role of Endothelin-1 in Tachyarrhythmias Developed during Myocardial Ischemia and Reperfusion

H. Vágó, G. Szűcs, P. Soós, E. Zima, T. Andrási, L. Gellér, A. Szűcs, V. Kékesi, A. Juhász-Nagy, B. Merkely

Dept. of Cardiovascular Surgery, Semmelweis University, Budapest, Hungary

Introduction: Electrophysiological effects of endothelin-A receptor antagonists during myocardial ischemia and reperfusion has not yet been studied. The aim of this study was to investigate the role of endogenous endothelin-1 (ET-1) in the development of ventricular tachyarrhythmias during myocardial ischemia and reperfusion using endothelin-A receptor antagonist LU 135 252 (LU) in a canine model.
Methods: LU (1 mg/kg, n=10) or saline (control, n=10) bolus was injected intracoronary into the left anterior descending coronary artery (LAD) before the onset of ligation of this vessel for 30 minutes followed by a 90-minute reperfusion period. Left and right ventricular monophasic action potentials (MAP) were registrated. Serum ET-1 and big-endothelin levels were determined from coronary sinus.
Results: There was no difference in hemodynamical parameters and in the left ventricular ischemic mass between the two groups. There was no significant difference in the incidence of sustained tachyarrhythmias (VT/VF) and nonsustained VT-s and in the number of ventricular premature beats between the two groups. During ischemia, MAP duration at 90% of repolarization (MAPD90) decreased significantly, while during reperfusion a significant prolongation of MAPD90 was observed in LAD region similar in both groups. During reperfusion, especially in the later phase, ET-1 and big-endothelin levels were increased in both groups. ET-1 level increased significantly during ischemia in dogs with ventricular fibrillation compared to dogs surviving ischemia and reperfusion (survival vs. VF: control: 15.1±1.3 vs. 15.2±1.3 fmol/ml; ischemia 30 min: 17.6±1.2 vs. 22.0±1.6 fmol/ml, *p<0.05*).
Conclusion: However, endothelin level was increased during ischemia-reperfusion, LU did not affect the repolarization changes and did not have antiarrhythmic effect during either ischemia or reperfusion probably due to their multifactorial origin.

128

The Effect of Intestinal Lengthening on Adaptation in a Piglet SBS-model: A Pilot Study

G.I. Koffeman[1], I.G. Schoots[2], D.C. Aronson[1], J.A.J.M. Taminiau[3], P.B. Bijlsma[3], T.M. van Gulik[2], H.A. Heij[1], W.G. van Gemert[1]

Pediatric Surgical Centre Amsterdam[1], Emma Children's Hospital-AMC/VUMC, Surgical Laboratory[2], Pediatrics Department Academic Medical Center[3], Amsterdam, The Netherlands

Introduction: Conservative therapy for short bowel syndrome (SBS) remains troublesome showing high morbidity and mortality. The Bianchi longitudinal intestinal lengthening and tailoring procedure (LILT) could potentially lead to development of a greater surface area, reduced bacterial overgrowth, and better peristalsis and transit time. This pilot study seeks to test the use of a piglet SBS model, and ascertain the feasibility of the LILT in this model.
Methods: Six piglets (Sus scrofa, aged 8 weeks) are included after one week acclimatization. Bianchi group (5 piglets): 75% small intestinal resection (day 1), followed by LILT (day 14) and termination (day 42). Control piglet (1 piglet): 75% small intestinal resection (day 1), followed by sham laparotomy (day 14) and termination (day 42). Peri-operatively, the following parameters were measured: body weight, intestinal length, -diameter, - wet weight, fat and protein absorption, biochemical parameters, amino acids (citrulline), D(-)-lactate (serum/urine), intestinal biopsies for microscopy, dsDNA, and electrophysiological measurements (Ussing Chamber).
Results: One Bianchi group piglet was terminated prematurely due to suture leakage. After resection there was significantly retarded growth, thinner faecal consistency, and reduced fat absorption. Citrulline was reduced following resection (23.32 ±7.93 µmol/l vs 53.34 ±8.46 in healthy animals). After intestinal lengthening the Bianchi group demonstrated improvement in these parameters compared to the control piglet. Villus growth was greater in Bianchi compared to control (42% vs 10%) and crypt depth was decreased in Bianchi group (11 vs 24% growth). Ussing Chamber measurements showed minimally decreased glucose uptake in the Bianchi group (short circuit current [Isc] change -1.5 $\mu A/cm^2$) and increased uptake in the control (Isc change 17.3 $\mu A/cm^2$). Crypt chloride secretion was reduced in the Bianchi group compared to control (Isc change -10.6 $\mu A/cm^2$ vs -2.3 $\mu A/cm^2$).
Discussion: Short bowel syndrome generates a complex intestinal adaptive process with clinical, biochemical, and anatomical changes. Surgical therapy (LILT) appears to induce variations in this model to aid adaptation. With the demonstrated feasibility of surgical intervention in this SBS-model further study will be conducted to clarify these effects.
Conclusion: This piglet model is appropriate to study the pathophysiology of SBS and the effect of intestinal lengthening. Preliminary results suggest a beneficial effect of intestinal lengthening on intestinal adaptation.

129

The Effects of Selective Neuronal NOS Inhibition during Acute Experimental Colonic Obstruction

Z. Palásthy[1], J. Kaszaki[2], L. Szalay[2] Á. Balogh[1], M. Boros[1]

Department of Surgery[1], Institute of Surgical Research[2], University of Szeged, Szeged, Hungary

Introduction: Nitric oxide (NO) produced by the isoforms of nitric oxide synthase (NOS) plays central role in the pathophysiology of large bowel diseases. It has been demonstrated that although all 3 types of NOS are constitutively expressed in the gastrointestinal tract, the predominant form is neuronal NOS (nNOS). The supposed main function of nNOS in the intestine can be the mediation of the neuronal signal transmission in the non-adrenerg non-cholinerg system and regulating gut motility. Our aims were to investigate the effects of selective nNOS inhibition on motility and haemodynamic changes during colonic obstruction.
Methods: Laparotomy and complete obstruction of the transverse colon was performed in dogs under Na-pentobarbital anaesthesia. Hemodynamic parameters were observed for 7 hr following bowel obstruction. Large bowel motility changes were measured with strain-gauge technique and analysed with computerised data acquisition system. Group 1 served as a sham-operated control (n=5), in Groups 2 (n=8) and 3 (n=5) colonic obstruction was performed. Group 3 was treated with the selective nNOS inhibitor 7-nitroindazol (7-NI) (10 mg/kg) 3 hr after the obstruction. At the end of the experiments, tissue biopsies were taken from the oral and aboral parts of the colon to determine the constitutive and inducible NOS (cNOS; iNOS) (measured by the conversion of ^{3}H-arginine to ^{3}H-citrulline) and to quantify granulocyte accumulation (myeloperoxidase assay - MPO).
Results: Acute large bowel obstruction decreased significantly the total peripheral resistance (TPR) and 7-NI treatment did not influence this effect. The motility significantly increased at the aboral part of the colon, which was inhibited by 7-NI treatment. The obstruction caused a significant increase in iNOS activity but there was no significant difference in respect of constituve isoforms of NOS activity as compared to the sham-operated group. The administration of 7-NI significantly decreased the cNOS activity and significantly increased the obstruction-induced elevation in MPO activity in both parts of the colon.
Discussion: Our results demonstrate that inhibition of nNOS decreased the aboral colon motility and induced significant granulocyte accumulation in the oral and aboral part of the large bowel.
Conclusion: Nitrergic mechanism may play an important role not only in the neurotransmission but in leukocyte-mediated inflammatory processes during colonic obstruction. Supported by research grant OTKA T035275.

130

Effect of Cholic and Deoxycholic Acid Treatment on Colonic Mucosa in Rats

P. Sipos[1], K. Hagymási[2], E. Fehér[3], A. Blázovics[2], P. Ondrejka[1]

2nd Dept. of Surgery[1], 2nd Dept. of Internal Medicine[2], Dept. of Anatomy, Histology and Embryology[3], Semmelweis University, Budapest, Hungary

Introduction: Bile acids play an important role in the lipid metabolism. Absence and excessive presence of bile acids are equally unfavorable in the colon. A surgical model was developed to study the direct effects of cholic and deoxycholic acid on the colon mucosa in normo- and hyperlipidemic rats. The aim of this experiment was to determine the free radical scavenger ability of colonic mucosal homogenate. Free SH-group concentration, proton donor activity and reducing power property of mucosal homogenates were measured and compared with the electronmicroscopical observations.
Methods: 150-200 g young male Wistar albino rats were treated with lipid rich diet (plus 2% cholesterol and 20% sunflower oil added to the normal chock) and 0.5% cholic acid or 0.5% deoxycholic acid for 10 days. Ductus choledochus was cannulated and bile was collected into plastic tube in deep narcosis (1 g/kg Nembutal). Bile samples were injected into the lumen of the proximal and distal part of the colon. Its blood supply was intact.
Results: A significant decrease was observed in the free SH-group content (0.1132±0.034/0.0956±0.065 mmol/l) and the reducing power (1169.49±97/871.25±157.61 nmol AS) of colon homogenate in fat rich diet and cholic acid treated animals compared to control. Deoxycholic acid made less pronounced alteration in the redox state parameters. Bile from deoxycholic acid treated rats given to control rat bowel caused significant decrease in the proton donor activity (0.334±0.016%) compared to bile from control animals (0.237± 0.042%). The electronmicroscopical alterations of epithelial cells both enterocytes and goblet cells - decrease of the goblet cells and disruption or necrosis of the enterocytes - caused by bile from hyperlipidemic rats were significantly greater than those of controls.
Conclusion: The present study justify that the bile acids and alimentary modified bile can influence the structure and redox state of the colon mucosa. The study was supported by the National Research Foundation (F029252) and Ministry of Health ETT 250/2000.

131

Effect of Colloid Solution Ladpulin on the Blood Coagulation System during Hemorrhagic Shock in Dogs

I.V. Kremenevskiy, V.N. Gapanovich, N.I. Melnova, A.L. Uss, P.T. Petrov, V.M. Tsarenkov, O.K. Kuzuk, A.S. Cheholskiy

Institute of Hematology and Blood Transfusion, Minsk, Belarus

Introduction: Hemorrhagic shock (HS) is a clinical syndrome, which is caused by tissue hypoperfusion and results in multiple organ failure and death. Disseminated intravascular coagulation (DIC) is a major pathophysiologic manifestation of HS. The aim of the present work was to study the effect of fluid resuscitation with colloid solution ladpulin (6% solution of natural polymer slowly hydrolyzed by plasma amylases; mean molecular weight 62500±10.000 Dalton) on DIC induced by experimental HS in dogs.
Methods: The experiments were performed on ten adult dogs of both sexes of average weight 20-25 kg which were bled to maintain mean arterial pressure at 50 mmHg for 60 minutes and then were administered with 6% ladpulin at volume equivalent to the withdrawn blood. Blood samples were collected at six different time points: before HS (baseline or control, immediately after HS, and 0.2, 2. 4 and 24 h after the resuscitation. The following coagulation parameters were measured: partial thromboplastin time (PTT, sec), prothrombin time (PT, sec), thrombin time (TT, sec), fibrin concentration (F, g/L), fibrin split products D-dimers concentration (D-dimers, mg/L), qualitative determination of the fibrin monomers dissoluble complexes (ethanol test).
Results: Infusion of ladpulin resulted in complete restoration of normal PTT at 0.2-24 h after the fluid resuscitation. At this time, the soluble fibrin monomer complexes (negative ethanol test) were absent in the blood of ladpulin-infused animals and the reduction of the prothrombin factor complex activity was observed. PT was increased by 54%, 37% and 38% at 0.2, 2 and 4 h post-infusion, respectively. At these time points, fibrin concentration was reduced by 35%, 62% and 61%, respectively.
Discussion: Analysis of obtained data showed that the experimental hemorrhagic shock within an hour resulted in hypercoagulation state of DIC. There were the fibrin monomer dissoluble complexes, the fibrin split product D-dimers in blood after finishing of hypotensive shock. We observed the reduction of PTT and the decrease of fibrin concentration after the colloid fluid resuscitation in HS.
Conclusion: The present results showed that the colloid solution ladpulin attenuates the development of DIC during hemorrhagic shock in dogs.

132

In Vitro Antineoplastic Activity of a Novel Steroidal Ester of Chlorambucil in Breast Cancer Cells

M. Kontos[1], P. Karamanakos[1], D. Trafalis[1], C. Menenakos[1], M. Nikolopoulou[2], C. Camoutsis[3], E. Bastounis[1]

1st Dept. of Surgery[1], University of Athens, "Laiko" Hospital, Athens, Dept. of Immunology and Histocompatibility[2], "Evagelismos" Hospital, Athens, Faculty of Pharmacy[3], University of Patra, Patra, Greece

Introduction: Homo-aza-steroidal esters of alkyliative agents comprise a group of experimental drugs presenting increasing interest in chemotherapy of solid tissue cancers. The aim of this study is to investigate the *in vitro* activity of a D-homo-aza (lactam) steroidal ester of chlorambucil namely 13a-amino-13,17-seco-1,5-estratrien-17-oic-13,17-lactam 4-[p-bis (2-chloroethyl) aminophenyl] butyric acetate (ESBL) in breast cancer cells and to compare it to a known antineoplastic agent that is chlorambucil (CBL).
Methods: 18 women with grade I ductal breast cancer (46-80 years of age, 8 pre- and 10 postmenopausial, 7 with stage I and 11 with stage II disease) were investigated in this study. Fresh tumor sections

sized 10-20 mm^3 were taken during operation and was incubated with a trypsin-collagenase protelytic system for 4-6 hours in 37°C in order to obtain single cell cultures. After proper infiltration and cultivation the single cell culture was divided in 48 parts and each of them was incubated with a different concentration of ESBL or CBL for 48 hours. Using a MTT assay cytotoxicity curves of ESBL and CBL were made and the concentration that achieved the death of the 50% of the cells (ID50) was calculated for each agent. Results were related with the menopausal status and the ER and PR positivity.
Results: ESBL demonstrated antineoplastic activity superior to CBL among both premenopausal and postmenopausal women. Moreover ESBL was more active at a ER/PR positive background compared to ER/PR negative while CBL activity showed little or no correlation to the ER/PR status.
Discussion: Breast cancer is one of the most common diseases in females and in most cases surgery must be accompanied by chemotherapy in order to achieve optimal results. ESBL demonstrates strong *in vitro* activity possibly due to its molecular structure and lipophilic properties which allows it to enter the tumor cell easier and thus increase its inracellular concentration.
Conclusion: ESBL is a novel steroidal ester of chlorambucil with strong *in vitro* activity. *In vivo* activity, toxicity and combined therapy still have to be investigated.

New Techniques

133

Sonodynamic Treatment of Cancer Cell Lines - A New Method in Tumor Therapy?

R. Grützmann[1], T. Zimmermann[1], S. Albrecht[2,1], H.D. Saeger[1]

Dept. of Surgery[1], Dept. of Gynaecology[2], Technical University Dresden, Dresden, Germany

Introduction: The effect of porphyrin excited by laser on tumor cells has been known and applied *in vivo* as photodynamic therapy for years. Sonoluminescence (SL) was first described by Harvey 1939 as emission of light out of fluids after excitation with ultrasound (US). The mechanism of sonodynamic action was suggested to involve photoexcitation of the sensitizer by sonoluminescent light, with subsequent formation of singlet oxygen. Sonodynamic therapy seems to be a new modality for cancer treatment based on synergistic effects on tumor cell killing by combination of a photosensitizer and US. In this study we examined, if porphyrins and its analogues are excitable with US and if yes, if there are antitumor effects *in vitro*.
Methods: We used the Luminometer Nightowl® from Berthold. This luminometer is equipped with a CCD-camera housed in a large chamber. As ultrasound source we used the HiFUS3 (high intensity focused ultrasound) produced by Siemens (HiFU-frequency: 1.8 MHz, focal intensity: 0-1000 w/cm^2, focal size: 1x1x6 mm, max. focal depth: 55 mm) connected to the amplifier ENI 3100L by Siemens. As photosensitizer Photofrin® (Porfimer-sodium), haematoporphyrin and magnesium-phtalocyanin were used for the experiments with the tumor cell lines: HeLa (cervix carcinoma) and HT29 (colon tumor). For intra- and extracellular ATP-determination we used the ATP-Bioluminescence-Kit from Roche/Boehringer.
Results: First the 3 porphyrin-analogues were tested in different concentrations and with ultrasound-energy up to 1000 w/cm^2. Luminescence response was measured inside the Luminometer Nightowl®. All 3 tested substances showed a clear luminescence response ("sonodynamic response" - measured as photons/pixel * s). The effect seemed to be dependent from the US energy and the concentration of the photosensitizer. In *in vitro* tests we could induce a tumor cell death in up to 95%. The combination of US and C lead to strong cell destroying effect as described above. The effect is dependent from Photofrin® concentration and US energy.
Conclusions: The preliminary results showed a tumor-destroying effect which might be used for effective and gentle therapy of tumors located within parenchymatous tissue. The exact mechanisms of "sonodynamic response" on tumor cells has to be interesting to test new generation of photosensitizers including phtalocyanines, which show an increased photodynamic efficiency and reduced phototoxic side effects in animal models.

134

Effects of Different Physical Barriers in Prevention of Adhesions to Intraperitoneally Placed Polypropylene Mesh in Rabbits

S.G. Sajjadi, G. Wéber, J. Baracs, I. Takács, M. Vajda, G.M. Giorgion

Department of General Surgery, Faculty of General Medicine, University of Pécs, Pécs, Hungary

Introduction: Prosthetic materials that are usually used in clinical practice often must be placed in direct contact with the visceral peritoneum. The prosthesis-peritoneum interface is the site of adhesions, causing ileus, erosions of intestinal loops and fistulas. This investigation was designed to compare the behaviour of four prosthetic material when placed in contact with the visceral peritoneum.
Methods: Defects of about 3x4 cm were created on both sides of the abdominal wall of 12 white rabbits weighing approximately 2500 g. The defects involved the aponeurotic and muscular planes and the parietal peritoneum. The rabbits were divided into 3 study groups according to the material covering the side of the prolene mesh that was put in contact with the visceral peritoneum. As a control in all the rabbits the right side defect was covered by a prolene mesh. In the first group the left side defect was covered by a prolene mesh covered with a silicon. In the second group the prolene mesh was covered with Op-Site foil and the in third group the prolene mesh was covered with hyaluronic membrane. The left side defect was covered in a way that the material covering the prolene mesh was put in contact with the visceral peritoneum. The prostheses were secured to the edges of the defect by 2-0 prolene continuous sutures.
Results: The presence and grade of adhesions to the repair were recorded on the 30th, 60th and 90th day. There was no post implant mortality, and no animal had signs of infection or rejection of the implant. Dense adhesions developed on all of the defects repaired by polypropylene mesh alone. Firm adhesions were detected in the silicon and foil covered prosthesis. Significant seroma and perigraft reactions were revealed also in these two groups. The hyaluronic

membrane decreased adhesions significantly and histopathological examinations supported these macroscopic observations.
Conclusion: These findings support the idea that hyaluronic membrane is a suitable physical barrier in rabbits against adhesion formation, but long-term results are necessary and these findings also need to be supported in humans.

135

The Use of a Suturing Task As a Measure of Technical Competence

M.S. Khan, S.D. Bann, A. Darzi, P.E.M. Butler

Academic Surgical Unit, St. Mary's Hospital, London, UK

Introduction: The acquisition of surgical competence and dexterity is a fundamental part of good surgery and must be one of the main objectives in a surgeon's training. The teaching of plastic surgeons during their training, although vital does not guarantee the transference of clinical skill. There must exist a system by which the technical skill of a trainee can be evaluated. When choosing a technical skill to be assessed one must start with basic skills such as suturing.
Method: We asked trainees to suture a 4 cm wound on a latex skin pad. Three independent observers, using the OSATS scoring system, consisting of a task specific scoring sheet, measuring specifics of the task, and a global scoring sheet measuring their general instrument and tissue handling ability, scored the candidates. They were also motion tracked using an electromagnetic motion-tracking device.
Results: Forty-three plastic surgeons were divided into four groups dependent on grade and assessed. Forty-six general surgeons were also similarly assessed. The difference in scores amongst the plastic surgeons gave a value of $p<0.001$, whereas the general surgeons gave a value of $p=<0.023$. However when similar grade but different specialties were compared, plastic surgeons scored significantly higher down to SHO level, mean p value = 0.019. Inter rater reliability was also high, Cronbach's alpha = 0.92.
Discussion: This task has shown that technical ability can be objectively assessed. The use of objective, structured assessment with feedback allows the deficiencies of the trainee to be highlighted early and therefore corrected early. It can therefore be seen that the task gives us the ability to not only measure the suturing competence of an individual, but also to allow instruction on the technique and then the ability to see an improvement in their technique and level of competence. The task also exhibits face, construct and concurrent validity.
Conclusion: This is a valid and objective measure of suturing ability. This has important implications for the future of surgical training, in that it allows us to identify whether the fundamentals of surgical technique have been passed on to the trainee, and to continually monitor their progress.

136

Heart Rate Variability Analysis as a Tool for Quantifying the Stress of the Surgical Team During Laparoscopic Versus Open Surgeries

L. Hejjel, I. Gál

Heart Institute, Medical Faculty, University of Pécs, Pécs, Hungary

Introduction: Laparoscopic surgery offers great advantages for the patient compared to open method, however, it is much more demanding for the surgical team. Quantitative assessment of this extra stress has remained challenging. Heart rate variability (HRV) closely reflects the current autonomic balance. HRV reduction has been found in several cardiovascular and other pathologies, as well as in various mental and physical stress situations. The authors addressed the preliminary investigation of HRV changes in comparing the mental load of laparoscopic versus open procedures.
Methods: Two surgeons, aged 54 and 28 were investigated during routine thyroid gland operation and laparoscopic Taylor procedure. The single-channel ECG-signal was digitized at 500 Hz by a Sound Blaster 16 soundcard and stored on the hard disk of a PC. Twelve-minute long records were achieved alternately. Following off-line RR-interval detection, filtering, and chopping to 5-minute long segments (n=5 in each group); the mean RR-interval (ms), its standard deviation (SDNN, ms) and coefficient of variation (CV, %), the root mean square of successive RR-differences (RMSSD, ms), and the percentage of consecutive RR-differences greater than 50 ms (PNN50, %) were computed. The entire system has been developed by the first author. The parameters were compared by paired t-test, $p<0.05$ was considered statistically significant.
Results: In the older surgeon (operator) laparoscopic/open: mean RR*: 680.2±18.1/739.4±11.8, SDNN: 23.31±2.39/25.85± .09, CV: 3.43±0.42/3.50±0.45, RMSSD*: 10.88±1.84/15.10±3.27, PNN50: 0.27±0.48/0.43±0.73. In the younger surgeon (assistant) laparoscopic/open: mean RR*: 690.6±38.8/753.5±26.3, SDNN*: 35.64±6.02/53.81±8.58, CV*: 5.14±0.66/7.15±1.19, RMSSD*: 15.59±3.29/24.77±5.4, PNN50: 0.77±0.99/3.38±2.10. (*$p\leq 0.05$)
Discussion: In the younger surgeon all parameters, in the older surgeon the mean RR and RMSSD were significantly reduced during laparoscopy compared to open surgery. The reduced basal HRV (related to age) can be a limit of such measurements. The authors selected contrasting operations in difficulty for the preliminary studies in order to get more diverse results.
Conclusion: HRV analysis can become an effective method to quantitatively compare the mental load of different surgical procedures, thus further studies are encouraged on a greater number of participants to get the real value of HRV analysis in these purposes.

Nutrition/Glutamine

137

Enteral Glutamine Reverses Th1/Th2 Shift In Severe Trauma Patients. A Randomised Double-Blind Controlled Study

P.G. Boelens, A.P.J. Houdijk, J.C.M. Fonk, B.M.E. Blomberg, S. Meijer, H.J.T.M. Haarman, P.A.M. van Leeuwen

VUMC, Departments of Surgery and Pathology, Amsterdam, The Netherlands

Background: Severe trauma leads to a Th2 immune response, which is associated with an impaired cellular immune response and subsequent increased susceptibility for infectious complications. Glutamine is the preferred fuel for immunocompetent cells. This study was designed to investigate the effect of enteral glutamine-enriched nutrition (>5 days) as compared to an iso-caloric, iso-nitrogenous control feeding on the Th1/Th2 response towards primary antigen KLH following severe trauma (ISS>20).
Methods: Trauma patients were sensitised with KLH (within 12 hours) and received enteral nutrition within 48 hours after the trauma. Cellular and humoral immune responses were determined. Healthy subjects were used to determine the reference values.
Results: IFN-gamma production of stimulated PBMCs (PHA) was significantly reduced after trauma on day 1 in both study groups. On day 14 the IFN-gamma production was significantly increased in the glutamine group as compared to the control group ($p<0.018$). IL-4 production was significantly depressed ($p<0.045$) following trauma in the control group while the glutamine group had an intact IL-4 production on day 1 and 14. Significantly less KLH specific IgG, IgG2 on day 9 was measured in the glutamine fed patients. Specific IgM, IgA, IgG1 and IgG3 were similar in both study arms.
Conclusions: Trauma caused a suppressed cellular immune response, as was observed by an impaired IFN-gamma production (day 1). Glutamine partially restored IFN-gamma production (day 14), preserved IL-4 production and part of the humoral immune response to KLH was less, suggesting a shift to Th1 by glutamine. Enteral glutamine might therefore play an important role in reversing the trauma-induced Th1/Th2 shift.

138

Butyrate and Glutamate Mucosal Metabolic Substrate Utilization in Normal Colon and Colon Cancer Tissue

D. Adawi, B. Jeppsson

Department of Surgery, Lund University, Malmö University Hospital, Malmö, Sweden

Introduction: Intestinal mucosal cells metabolize both circulating and luminal metabolic substrates. In the small bowel the preferred fuel substrate is glutamine. luminal short-chain fatty acids (SCFAs), the end product of bacterial fermentation of dietary carbohydrate, provide the principle substrates for oxidation by colonic mucosal cells and butyrate appears to be the major energy source for colonic mucosa. The aim of this study was to determine the metabolic substrate utilization of butyrate and glutamate in human healthy colonic and colon cancer tissue.
Methods: Tissue biopsy was obtained from resected human healthy colonic and colon cancer tissues. Using a closed microculture technique, biopsy utilization of ^{14}C-labelled butyrate and glutamine was measured as [^{14}C] carbon dioxide production.
Results: The metabolic flux of butyrate in the normal colonic tissue increased significantly compared to colon cancer tissue and it increased more than glutamate in the normal colonic tissue. In the right colon butyrate metabolic flux show a tendency to be increased in the normal colonic tissue compared to butyrate in colon cancer tissue and to glutamate in the normal colonic tissue. In the left colon the metabolic flux of butyrate increased significantly in the normal colonic tissue compared to colon cancer tissue, while it shows a tendency to be increased compared to glutamate in the normal colonic tissue.
Conclusion: It seems that healthy colonic tissue utilizes more butyrate than glutamate. In colon cancer tissues the utilization of butyrate is less compared to healthy colonic tissue and this could reflect decreased luminal substrate availability with down regulation of enzymatic pathways involved in butyrate metabolism.

139

Comparison of the Effects of a Glutamine-Rich and Glutamine-Free Diet in Patients with Esophagectomy

J. Hallay[1], G. Kovács[1], Gy. Kovács[1], S. Sz. Kiss[1], Z. Szentkereszty[2], P .Sápy[1], G. Lakos[1], S. Sipka[2]

University of Debrecen, Medical and Health Science Center, 2nd Department of Surgery[1] and 3rd Department of Internal Medicine[2], Debrecen, Hungary

Introduction: The aim of this study was to compare the effects of glutamine-rich and glutamine-free diet on nutritional and immunological laboratory parameters of 20 patients with esophagectomy.
Methods: 10 patients with esophagectomy were nourished jejunaly with Stresson Multi Fibre (glutamine 1.3 g/100 ml, Nutricia) and 10 patients with Nutrison Multi Fibre (Nutricia) for 10 days through a jejunal tube. The daily dose of food was increased from 500 to 2000 ml during the treatment. The daily protein intake elevated from 0.8 to 2.5 g/kg with Stresson Multi Fibre. In the group of Nutrison Multi Fibre we changed protein intake from 0.4 to 1.3 g/kg/day. The laboratory parameters were measured before the operation and on the 1st, 4th, and 10th postoperative days: serum total protein, albumin, prealbumin (PRA), retinol binding protein (RBP), immunoglobulins, complement factors and acute phase protein levels were measured by laser nephelometry, lymphocyte subsets by flow cytometry, while the activity of phagocytes were tested by luminol-amplified zymosan-induced chemiluminescence.
Results: After the decreases of the serum protein concentrations observed already on the 1st postoperative day there were significant differences in the increases of the levels of certain proteins according to the different types of nutrition. In the group nourished by Stresson Multi Fibre the recovery of the preoperative levels of serum total protein, RBP, IgG and PRA were faster and greater than in the patients with glutamine-free nutrition during the 10 days of treatment. The

mean of the protein levels are the following: In the first postoperative day with Stresson Multi Fibre (g/l): serum total protein: 44.5; RBP: 0.017; PRA: 0.101; IgG: 6.02. With Nutrison Multi Fibre (g/l): serum total protein: 41.9; RBP: 0.036; PRA: 0.083 IgG: 7,21. In the 10th postoperative day with Stresson Multi Fibre: serum total protein: 61.2**; RBP: 0.029**; PRA: 0.138**; IgG: 10.03*. With Nutrison Multi Fibre: serum total protein: 62.6**; RBP: 0.048; PRA: 0.116; IgG: 10.72*. (*$p< 0.05$; **$p<0.005$ - 10th day's result versus 1st postoperative day's result).

Conclusion: The laboratory measurements showed that glutamine-rich jejunal postoperative nutrition of patients with esophagectomy could result in a better recovery of serum protein levels than glutamine-free diet.

140

Does the Addition of Glutamine to Total Parenteral Nutrition Have Beneficial Effect on The Healing of Colon Anastomosis and Bacterial Translocation after Preoperative Radiotherapy?

M. El-Malt, W. Ceelen, T. Boterberg, G. Claeys, B. de Hemptinne, W. de Neve, P. Pattyn

Ghent University Hospital, Ghent, Belgium

Introduction: Glutamine administration stimulates mucosal growth and preserves the morphology of the intestine. Therefore, it could improve colonic anastomotic healing after radiotherapy (RT) induced epithelial damage and mucosal atrophy induced by total parenteral nutrition (TPN). We investigated this issue in a rat model.

Methods: The rectosigmoid colon in male Wistar rats was irradiated to a total dose of 25 Gy (5 Gy daily for 5 consecutive days). Five days after the end of RT, side-to-side anastomosis was performed between the irradiated rectosigmoid and the non-irradiated caecum. Postoperatively, animals were divided randomly into 3 groups; group I was fed orally (lab chow), group II received TPN and group III received TPN enriched with 2% glutamine (Gln-TPN). One week after surgery animals were sacrificed.

Results: All animals decreased in weight during RT and after surgery. Weight regain postoperatively was better in the orally fed animals in comparison to the parenterally fed animals (I versus II & III; $p<0.01$). Colonic anastomotic bursting pressure (BP) and bursting wall tension (BWT) were significantly less in group II in comparison to group I and group III (II versus I & III; $p<0.01$). BP and BWT were comparable in the animals that received Gln-TPN (group III) and the orally fed animals (group I). No significant differences were found between all the groups in gut bacterial translocation to the blood or to the mesenterical lymph nodes.

Discussion: McCauley et al (J. Parent. Enteral. Nutr. 1991; 15:437-439) reported that the healing of colonic anastomoses, assessed by the BWT, was not influenced by the administration of 1.2% Gln-TPN in malnourished rats. With a higher dose of glutamine (2.0%), in the present experiment, the colonic anastomotic BP and BWT were significantly higher in comparison to TPN alone and were comparable to the orally fed animals. Experimentally, Karatzas et al (Clin. Nutr. 1991;10:199-205) reported a decreased incidence of bacterial translocation to the MLN only, and not to the portal vein and aorta, after abdominal RT (11 Gy) and the provision of 3% oral glutamine. In the present study, where the animals were subjected to multiple stress factors (RT with a total dose 25 Gy, surgery and TPN), the supplementary glutamine did not reduce gut bacterial translocation either to the MLN or to the blood. Bark T. et al (Eur. J. Surg. 1995;161:3-8) reported also that supplementation of an enteral diet with 4% glutamine failed to prevent bacterial translocation after non-lethal haemorrhage in rats.

Conclusion: Glutamine-enriched TPN counteracts the negative effect of food deprivation on colonic anastomotic healing. Postoperative Gln-TPN does not influence gut bacterial translocation in this rat model.

Tissue Repair

141

Phospholipids Reduce Adhesions in the Uterine-Horn-Model

S.A. Mueller, K.H. Treutner, L. Tietze, M. Anurov J. Conze, A.P. Oettinger, V. Schumpelick

Department of Surgery, Medical Faculty, Rheinish-Westphalian Technical University, Aachen, Germany

Introduction: Adhesion formation following gynecologic or visceral surgery is a major cause of female infertility. Further sequelae are recurrent and chronic abdominal complaints and pain. Adjuvant therapy is needed to prevent adhesion formation as an important reason for postoperative morbidity and mortality. Previously published data proved the efficacy of phospholipids (PL) for this indication. This study was designed to access the ability of intraperitoneal phospholipids to reduce adhesions in a standardized model for gynecologic operations.

Methods: A total of 33 female Chinchilla rabbits were included in this study. After lower midline incision a 5 cm segment the uterine horns was abraded circularly and ischemia was induced by removal of the collateral blood supply. The operation was completed by intraperitoneal administration of 5.0 ml per kg body weight of phospholipids (75 mg/kg bw) or the same volume of Ringer's lactate solution. In animals assigned to the surgical control group, the abdomen was closed without additional treatment. After 10 days the animals were sacrificed and adhesions were examined and scored concerning severity and tenacity. The force of adhesions measuring larger than 25 mm^2 were assessed using a spring scale (values in Newton). After subtle dissection the areas of adhesions (mm^2) were measured using a digitizer board and a custom-made software on a personal computer.

Results: The mean area of adhesions in the surgical control group amounted to 394.0 mm^2±41.9 mm^2 (median 392.2 mm^2) in comparison to 384.2 ± 67.0 mm^2 (median 323.8 mm^2) in the Ringer group and 110.3 mm^2 ± 25.1 mm^2 (median 102.1 mm^2) in the phospholipid (PL) group. The comparison of the control group and the Ringer group versus the PL group were significant ($p< 0.05$). The differences in the severity score and the degree score according to Leach between surgical controls and PL as well as Ringer and PL were significant ($p<0.05$). The differences of the force to tear apart the adhesions were significant ($p < 0.05$). Statistical analysis of the force correlated with the area of the measured adhesions revealed no significant difference.

Discussion: The uterine horn model originally described by Nishimura induces consistent adhesion formation. Several substances have been proven capable in this model. A reduction of adhesion scores between 44 and 78% could be achieved with different substances. The results of the current study are in the line with previous experiments with phospholipids. Ar'Rajab achieved a reduction of adhesions by 79% after one week. In a cecum and sidewall abrasion / small bowel anastomosis model we achieved 72% (5 days) and 86% (10 days) reduction of adhesion areas after single intraperitoneal administration of phospholipids (PL) compared to the controls (NaCl).

Conclusions: These results prove the efficacy of phospholipids in the double uterine horn model. Future clinical studies are recommended.

142

Diphenhydramine and Hyaluronic Acid Derivatives Reduce Adnexial Adhesions and Prevent Tubal Obstruction Following Pelvic Operations

F. Avsar, F. Avsar, M. Sahin, H. Vatansev

ZTB Dogumevi-Ankara, ANH General Surgery-Ankara, SUTF General Surgery and Biochemistry-Konya, Turkey

Materials and Methods: 40 female rats of Sprague-Dawley type were used in the study. The rats were divided into 4 groups, each comprising of 10 subjects. After all rats were anaesthetized with 50 mg/kg ketamine-HCl, their abdomens were opened with a lower midline incision. Injury was induced on the right pelvic peritoneum and on the peritoneal surface of left uterine tube. No additional procedure was applied to the first group. 10 mg/kg diphenhydramine HCl was given to the second group intravenously. In the third group, 0.25 mg/kg "Orthovisc", a Na-hyaluronat derivative, was diluted with 2 ml serum physiologic and poured into the abdomen. For the forth group, "Seprafilm", a Na-hyaluronat derivative, layer of 0.7x3 cm was covered over left uterine tube. After 14 days, the rats were anaesthetized with Ketamin HCl again, and 5 ml blood sample was taken with cardiac puncture. The Abdomen was opened with an incision transverse to the upper end of the midline incision, and presence of adhesion was investigated. Detected adhesions were staged according to Mazuji classification. Tubal patencies were inspected by injecting metyhlene blue from uterus corpus into the lumen using an injector. A piece of abdomen wall of 4x4 cm was removed by extending the incision in the reverse U shape. Tensile strength and bursting pressure of suture line were determined using Peacock method. 1 g tissue was taken from the incision line, and hydroxyproline levels were determined by Bergman-Loxley method. AST levels were measured.

Results: All the rats completed the study. AST levels, tissue hydroxyproline levels and tensile strength and bursting pressure test results were found similar in all groups. While adhesion rates in the groups were respectively 100%, 40%, 40% and 30%, adhesion stages were found to be respectively as 2.1±1.7, 0.6±0.67, 0.6±0.67 and 0.5±0.85. Adhesion stages in the study groups were significantly lower ($p < 0.05$). Tubal obstruction rates were found to be 70%, 30%, 30% and 20% respectively.

Conclusion: Diphenhydramine, "Orthovisc" and "Seprafilm" reduce significantly postoperative peritoneal adhesion development, and they keep uterine tubes open.

143

Expression of Apoptosis and Cell Cycle-Related Proteins in Epidermis

H. Galkowska, W.L. Olszewski, U. Wojewodzka, J. Mijal, E. Filipiuk

Dept. of Surg. Res. and Transplant, Medical Research Center, Polish Acad. Sci., Warsaw, Poland

Introduction: The majority of studies dealing with cutaneous wound healing have focused on granulation tissue remodeling. Comparatively, little attention has been paid to the question of epidermal regeneration. During the processes involved in epitelialization keratinocytes at the wound margin undergo a series of changes, including cell migration, proliferation and differentiation. Keratinocytes become activated, they produce and respond to growth factors and cytokines and they express cell survival and cell cycle regulatory proteins. Apoptosis-regulatory proteins include those that block (bcl2) and promote (bax) apoptosis and DNA fragmentation (caspase3). Cell cycle regulatory proteins include p53 and PCNA. Differentiating keratinocytes undergo apoptosis (DNA fragmentation/TUNEL$^+$ nuclei).

Aim: In order to evaluate the role of apoptosis- and cell cycle releated proteins in the pathogenesis of protracted re-epitelialization in chronic leg ulcers we have characterized immunohistochemically the expression of these proteins in epidermis of diabetic foot and venous leg ulcers.

Materials and Methods: Studies were carried out in 12 patients with diabetic foot ulcer and 10 patients with varicous ulcers of the calf. Skin biopsies were obtained under local anesthesia from the border area of ulcers and from corresponding sites of normal subjects (orthopedic patients). The specimens were divided and one-half was snap frozen in a dry ice cold acetone and stored at -70 °C until processed, whereas the other was fixed in 4% formalin and paraffin embedded. Immunohistochemical detection was based on biotin-avidin-peroxidase complex technique (LSAB, Dako) using specific primary antibodies: PCNA, p53, bcl2, bax, caspase3, cytokeratin 10, 16 and 17. DNA fragmentation was assayed by TUNEL assay.

Results: Keratinocytes at the edge of ulcers and in the distal area expressed cytokeratin 16 and 17, both in diabetic and venous ulcers. There was no expression of cytokeratin 10. The expression of PCNA and p53 protein was elevated in keratinocytes at the ulcer edge, compared to control epidermis, both in diabetic and venous ulcers. These keratinocytes showed reduced expression of TUNEL positive nuclei than keratinocytes present in distal and normal epidermis. The expression of bax protein was unchanged compared to normal epidermis. There was higher expression of bcl2 protein in epidermis of diabetic ulcer compared to normal tissue, whereas in venous ulcers the expression of bcl2 by keratinocytes at the edge of ulcer was decreased compared to distal area of epidermis. Also expression of caspase3 was elevated in keratinocytes at the ulcer edge in diabetic ulcers and decreased in venous ulcers.

Conclusion: The expression of cytokeratin 16 and 17 as well as the presence of PCNA$^+$ and TUNEL$^-$ keratinocytes at the edge of both ulcer types points that epidermal proliferation is not a limiting factor in the healing process. The reduced expression of bcl2 and caspase3 at the edge of venous ulcers may reflect the persistence of inflammation, compared to diabetic foot ulcer, affecting keratinocyte differentiation.

144

Increased Keratinocyte Motility in Hypoxic Wounds is Via an Integrin-Dependent Up-Regulation of MMPs

P.F. Ridgway, P. Ziprin, D.H. Peck, A.W. Darzi

Dept. of Surgical Oncology and Technology, Imperial College Faculty of Medicine, St. Mary's Hospital, London, UK

Background: Human keratinocytes have been shown to demonstrate increased motility in hypoxic wounds correlating with the success of semi-occlusive hypoxic dressings, although the underlying mechanism remains unknown. The authors propose that the αv subgroup of integrins, suggested to have an inherent modulatory function in migration, as well as a regulatory role in Matrix Metalloprotease (MMP) activation, is a key step in re-epithelialisation of hypoxic wounds.
Methods: Sub-confluent Human keratinocyte cell monolayers were exposed to hypoxia for 24 hours. Reoxygenation studies were performed up to 72 hours. Control cells were left in normal growth conditions. Cellular αv subunit and αvß6 expression was measured by flow cytometry. Migration scratch assays on fibronectin (αvß6 substrate) post-hypoxic exposure were performed over 24 hours. Relative MMP-2,9 secretion was estimated using gelatin zymography. Inhibition studies were performed using a specific blocker to αvß6 (MAB10D5) and gelatinises (MMPI). ANOVA and Mann-Whitney U tests were used as indicated.
Results: Cell viability was not affected up to 72 hours post-hypoxic insult. Sustained increases in αv and αvß6 were demonstrated up to 48 hours in reoxygenation studies ($p< 0.001$). Standardised scratch assay confirmed increased migration in the hypoxic group ($p< 0.05$). This effect was attenuated by the addition of a specific inhibitor to αvß6. MMP-2,9 secretion was up regulated post-hypoxic exposure ($p< 0.001$; $p< 0.05$). Increased MMP expression was attenuated by addition of an αvß6 inhibitor ($p< 0.05$). Increased migration of keratinocytes is attenuated by the addition of MMPI ($p< 0.001$).
Conclusions: These results indicate that αvß6 dependent MMP-2,9 up-regulation is an integral feature of increased migration in hypoxic human keratinocytes thus identifying potential therapeutic targets for those with non-healing wounds.

145

The Effect of a Thermoreversible Gelatin Polymer (TGP) on Liver Regeneration in Experimental Hepatic Wound

M. Nagaya, S. Kubota, A. Isogai, K. Akashi

St. Marianna University, Kawasaki, Kanagawa, Japan

Introduction: It has been demonstrated that the loss of 30% or more of the liver tissue is required to start the liver regeneration. The result of our previous study clearly showed that hepatic tissue loss in less than 10% of volume was only replaced by fibrous tissue without liver regeneration in mongrel dog. For liver regeneration, the three factors, liver cells, growth factors and extracellular matrix, may play an important role in the process. We have developed a thermoreversible gelatin polymer (TGP) as an artificial extracellular matrix. The TGP composed of Poly-N-isopropylacrilamide (PNIPAAm)-based copolymer has characterization of dynamic viscoelastic properties as a functional of temperature. The TGP is water soluble below the lower critical solution temperature (LCST, 22 °C) and water insoluble upon heating over 22°C, and turns back into soluble upon cooling. The aim of our study was to experimentally investigate the efficacy of TGP for extracellular matrix in liver regenerating process, and to determine whether liver regeneration occurs in the loss of 10% or less of liver tissue.
Methods: Six adult mongrel dogs weighing 8.5 to 12 kg were used. All six dogs were fashioned 2×2 cm diameter and 1 cm deep defect in the section of the medial portion of the left lobe of the liver. Liver specimens were harvested 4 weeks after surgery for histological analysis. These dogs were divided into two groups. Group 1 consisted of 3 dogs. The liver defect was open without using any materials. Group 2 consisted of 3 dogs. The TGP was poured into the liver defect and the converted into a gel state due to the temperature of the wound surface. The gel state of the TGP was observed and the area of the wound healing was measured by taking photographs at interval 2 weeks. Photological examinations were performed at 2, 4, 6, 8 and 12 weeks.
Results: Hepatic wound defect was adhered by peritoneum severely in group 1. The defect was healed a little. HE and Masson Trichrome stain showed severe fibrosis. On the other hand, in group 2, the defect was almost completely healed without signs of demarcation. Adhesion was not observed. Intra-abdominal abscesses, necrosis and signs of peritonitis were absent. The wound was completely filled with TGP and proliferating neovascular channels contained within the liver like capsule "organoid".
Discussion: Our experimental results with TGP in hepatic wound show that TGP has good compatibility and provides a good healing environment to the regeneration process of the liver.
Conclusion: The liver regeneration was found in the presence of TGP, as an extracellular matrix, in the loss of 10% or less liver tissue. TGP may be an ideal artificial extracellular matrix which provides good environment in liver cells and growth factor for liver regeneration.

VP1

A New Technique for Radical Esophagectomy: Hand-Assisted Thoracoscopic Esophagectomy Using an Anterior Phreno-Mediastinal Approach

T. Nishikage, T. Kawano, K. Nagai, K. Ami, Y. Nakajima, K. Kawada

Department of Surgery, Tokyo Medical and Dental University, Tokyo, Japan

Introduction: We devised a new technique for thoracoscopic radical esophagectomy using a new supportive approach called hand-assisted thoracoscopic surgery using an anterior phreno-mediastinal approach (HATS / APMA esophagectomy) and applied to 15 cases of esophageal cancer.
Techniques: After preliminary abdominal and neck procedures in the supine position, the anterior right diaphragm and right-side mediastinal visceral pleura are cut several centimeters under left side uni-ventilation. The assisting surgeon inserts the left hand through the anterior phreno-mediastinal route during esophagectomy in the hemi-left lateral position. The main dissecting procedures are performed with the surgeon standing to the right of the patient. Sometimes the assisting surgeon on the left side of the patient performs right-handed dissecting procedures with intra-thoracic left hand assistance. After radical esophagectomy, esophageal reconstruction using a stomach tube through the retrosternal or posterior mediastinal route is completed.
Discussion and Conclusion: These procedures reduce stress on the surgeons, the number of thoracic ports, and costs compared with simple thoracoscopic thoracic esophagectomy, and may also reduce the operating time.

VP2

Kidney Transplantation in Rats. How I Do It

T. Karatzas[1] , S. Santiago[2] , C. Vagianos[1] , W. DeFaria[2] , C. Gandia[2] , S. Salgar[2] , A.G. Tzakis[2].

Department of Surgery[1], University Hospital of Rion-Patras School of Medicine, Patras, Greece, Department of Surgery[2], Division of Liver/GI Transplantation, University of Miami, Jackson Memorial Hospital, Miami-FL, USA

Introduction: This study describes a technique of kidney transplantation (KTx) in rats, involving an extravesical approach of ureter implantation to bladder, that is sewn in from the outside creating an antireflux mechanism, similar to human transplantation.
Materials and Methods: Allografts from adults males DA(RT1a) 15 rats, to LEW(RT11) 15 rats, weighing 200 to 250 g, were used as donors and recipients respectively. Immunosuppression was based on cyclosporine (CyA). A daily amount of 15 mg/kg/d intramuscularly was given, in two divided doses. Anesthesia was administered through a machine inhalation with isoflurane in 100% O_2.
Surgical Procedure: Donor surgery and kidney transplantation procedures were performed using microsurgical technique. Donor nephrectomy, on the left side, started with blunt dissection of the ureter down to bladder. The superior mesenteric artery (SMA), celiac axis, and adrenal are ligated close to the aorta and divided. The inferior vena cava (IVC) is dissected free following ligation and transection of the superior mesenteric vein. The right side renal vessels were ligated and divided. Complete dissection of the aorta and IVC were carried out. A 5-0 silk ligatures were placed around the aorta and IVC below the diaphragm and tied. The aorta was cannulated distally to flush the kidney with 1% heparin in ice-cold lactated Ringer's solution and the IVC was vented at the same level to aorta. The kidney was then mobilized by placing 5-0 silk ties to the upper and lower pole connective tissues and was removed including vascular segments from aorta and IVC in continuity to renal vessels. Kidney transplantation. The host animal aorta and vena cava, below the renal bifurcation, were dissected free from the fibrous structures and were both clamped. The anastomoses were performed in end-to-side fashion between distal donor aorta to recipient aorta and distal donor vena cava to recipient IVC, using prolene 10.0 continuous suture. Reperfusion of the kidney graft was followed. The ureter of the donor was brought down to the bladder taking care the vasculature of the ureter was well straightened so as not to twist or kink after the uretero-vescical anastomosis. A small opening into the bladder was done and sew the ureter in from the outside with prolene 10.0 isolated sutures. A purse string suture around the anastomosis, tied loosely, completed ureter implantation, that functioned as uretero-vescical valve creating at the same time an antireflux mechanism. To this model, bilateral recipient nephrectomy was performed one week after kidney transplantation.
Results and Discussion: Technical complications, such as renal vascular thrombosis and urinary leaks have not been observed in our series, neither at the time of recipients bilateral nephrectomy, nor on completion of the experiment. Survival of the recipients depends on the function of the transplanted kidney, whereas complete allograft failure results in death of the animal.

VP3

A New Method of Appendectomy for Complicated Acute Appendicitis

M. Farima, V. Saban, A. Gorea

Republican Hospital of Department of Penitentiary Institutions MJ RM, Chisinau, Republic of Moldova

Introduction: Every pathological process in the ileocecal area of intestines, including the ones caused by technical maneuvers of surgical intervention, exerts a great influence on the quality of life as a whole, and postoperative rehabilitation, particularly after appendectomy. This forces the search and elaboration of new methods of appendectomy. This is especially important, when it is performed under purulo-necrotic forms of complicated appendicitis.

Methods: In the Department of General Surgery 6 appendectomies were carried out to men between 21 and 38 years old, regarding acute appendicitis: phlegmonous form: 4, gangrenous: 1, chronic: 1. The first two forms were complicated by purulent diffusive peritonitis: 1, purulent-fibrinous local peritonitis: 3, serous local peritonitis: 1, as well as acute secondary inflammation of cecum cupola: 5, and chronical commissural process: 1. In all cases a new method of appendectomy elaborated in clinical conditions was used. It consists in application of a single-layer interrupted precision suture on the cecum cupola, after appendix excision at the base level. During this, an average of 8 single-knot stitches were applied on the cecum wall using atraumatic nonabsorbable monothreaded material of 6/0 dimension, microsurgical instruments and a x4 operating magnifier. In all cases the abdominal cavity was closed layerwise after inspection and sanation without external drainage.

Results: During the postoperative period, both early and late, there were no complications specific to intestinal suture. Peristalsis restored during the 1-3 days after operation. The enteral feeding began after several hours after the anaesthesia wore off. The medication provided for use of anti-inflammatory drugs and antibiotics for 3 to 7 days and of local treatment of the laparotomy wound.

Discussion: The vulnerable side of the existing appendectomy methods is the method of cecum restoration. It should provide physical and mainly biological impermeability, without disturbing the ileocecal valve functioning. The fulfillment of these requests is practically impossible if the cecum is involved in the inflammation, because any attempt of suture application using traditional methods ends up with failure. As an adequate barrier function may be performed only by a viable mucous tunic, the correct direction of research would be the elaboration of a physically hermetic suture that minimally affects microcirculation in the zone of congruous confrontation of the intestine wall layers.

Conclusion: Analyzing the obtained clinical results of the use of the new method of appendectomy, we can assume, that the single-layer interrupted precision suture, even under a complicated acute appendicitis, with the cecum cupola involved in the inflammation, and purulent peritonitis, provides a sufficient physical and, mostly important, biological impermeability, during both early and late postoperative period.

VP4

New Organ-Preserving Pancreatic Head Resection in Chronic Pancreatitis

G. Farkas, L. Leindler

Department of Surgery, University of Szeged, Faculty of Medicine, Szeged, Hungary

Introduction: Twenty to thirty per cent of patients with chronic pancreatitis (CP) develop enlargement of the head of the pancreas in a consequence of inflammatory alterations which leads to complications such as obstruction of the pancreatic duct, common bile duct stenosis and duodenal compression. All of them represent an indication for surgical treatment consisting of different types of pancreatic head resection i. e. pylorus-preserving pancreaticoduodenectomy, duodenum-preserving pancreatic head resection (Beger procedure). Resective procedures give an effective control of complications of CP but these operations increase the exo- and endocrine insufficiency as a consequence of removing an average of 35-40% of the whole gland. A new safety procedure has been developed for organ-preserving pancreatic head resection, and this video demonstrates the important steps of operation.

Method: The surgical procedure consists in a wide local resection of the inflammatory tumour in the region of the pancreatic head without division and cutting of the pancreas over the portal vein. Reconstruction, with drainage of the secretion from the remaining pancreas into the intestinal tract, takes place through a jejunal Roux-en-Y loop. In icteric case, prepapillary bile duct anastomosis is also performed with the jejunal loop.

Results: This new procedure was performed in 50 patients and no morbidity or mortality was noted in the postoperative period. Duration of the hospitalisation ranged between 7 and 12 days, with a median of 8.5 days. In the median follow-up period of 10 months (range 6 to 14), all patients became complaint-free, and the body weight increased by a mean of 8.9 kg (range 4-20). No change was noted in the preoperative endocrine function.

Conclusion: The results clearly demonstrate that the new organ-preserving pancreatic head resection is a safe and effective procedure for definitive control of the complications following the inflammatory alterations of CP.

VP5

Endoscopic Ultrasonography Using Sonoprobe for Early Esophageal Carcinoma

K. Kawada, T. Kawano, K. Nagai, T. Nishikage, K. Ami, Y. Nakajima

Department of Surgery, Tokyo Medical and Dental University, Tokyo, Japan

Background: Almost all cases of superficial esophageal carcinoma are curable by endoscopic mucosal resection (EMR), but a precise diagnosis of the depth of tumor invasion is necessary to assess the indication for EMR. Although endoscopy has a high rate of accuracy for the diagnosing the depth of tumor invasion, it is based on the experience of the examiner in interpreting surface information of the lesions. Today, endoscopic ultrasonography (EUS) is one of the most powerful techniques for obtaining objective tomographic images of a tumor. The high frequency ultrasound probe is appropriate for EUS in cases of superficial esophageal carcinoma due to its excellent near field resolution that provides precise ultrasound images under direct control of the endoscope.

Method: We performed EUS using the Sonoprobe System™ (Sonoprobe) in 85 cases of superficial esophageal carcinoma before treatment, and evaluated the resected specimens histopathologically. We interpreted the depth of tumor invasion based on our fundamental studies of ultrasonograms taken with a 20 MHz probe.

Results: The clinical usefulness of the Sonoprobe with linear and radial scanning modes exists in its capacity to differentiate between mucosal and submucosal carcinoma by means of analyses of the muscularis mucosae. Although a clear assessment of micro-invasion and lymphoid hyperplasia surrounding the tumor of interest remains speculative, the diagnostic accuracy rate for 96 lesions of superficial

esophageal carcinoma reached 93% in terms of differentiating between mucosal from submucosal carcinoma.
Conclusion: EUS by the Sonoprobe can play an important role in the pre-treatment diagnosis of superficial esophageal carcinomas.

VP6

Analysis of the Quality and Efficiency in Learning Laparoscopic Skills

D. Bordos, F. Lazar, F. Miculit, C. Duta, M. Miclaus, M. Ionac, S. Pantea, S. Vascu, M. Groza

Surgical Clinic 2, "Pius Branzeu"; Center for Laparoscopic Surgery and Microsurgery, "Victor Babes" University of Medicine and Pharmacy, Timisoara, Romania

Introduction: The rapidly growing field of minimally invasive surgery will made laparoscopic surgery to become an integral part of the general surgery training. Now, there are two aspects of training for laparoscopic surgery that require consideration. First the education of surgeons who are out of residency and in practice and secondly incorporating laparoscopic training into surgical residency.
Discussion and Conclusion: As in laparoscopic surgery it is necessary a special training of the surgeons, it is recommended that the medical universities should train the surgeons and residents in postgraduate courses. At the local level, each training program should have a director of surgical endoscopy, designated to supervise laparoscopic teaching. In this way surgical residents benefit from all the available teaching methods, which include: educational courses, training boxes, experimental animal work and finally, the laparoscopic operative experience itself. For this purpose we started laparoscopic courses in our modern laparoscopic training center, including laparoscopic surgery in live tissue. At the same time the medical scientific societies should establish the steps for obtaining the competence in the field.

Gastrointestinal Surgery

PP1

Evaluation of Usefulness of Enteral Nutrition for Three-Field Radical Surgery and Palliative Surgery of Esophageal Carcinoma

M. Ohara, M. Ishizaka, N. Iwashiro, K. Saito, H. Hashida

National Hakodate Hospital, Hakodate, Japan

Introduction: Three-field radical surgery of esophageal carcinoma is relatively safe in Japan, but the loss of physical ability is not low. On the other hand, palliative surgery of esophageal carcinoma has high risk of post-operative complication or hospital death. We have used enteral nutrition to decrease post-operative death.
Method: From January 2000 to December 2001, 36 patients with esophageal carcinoma received esophagectomy in our hospital. Three-field radical surgery was performed for 14 cases, and palliative esophagectomy was performed for 4 cases. For these 18 cases, we inserted feeding tube from stomach or colon to jejunum.
Results: There was no operative death or hospital death. 5 patients had the mechanical support by respirator because of pneumonia or respiratory failure, 10 patients got sepsis by intravenous catheter. Enteral nutrition was effective even if the patients had mechanical support by respirator with sedative. Enteral nutrition assisted the recovery of the general conditions after the patients were discharged. Most of the patients had the feeding tube removed about three months after the discharge.
Conclusion: Enteral nutrition is useful for the patients who have three-field radical surgery and palliative surgery of esophageal carcinoma.

PP2

Roux-Y Reconstruction after Distal Gastrectomy Reduces IL-8 in the Gastric Remnant

K. Fukuhara, H. Osugi, N. Takada, M. Takemura, S. Lee, M. Ueno, Y. Tanaka, Y. Fujiwara, S. Nishizawa, Y. Hashimoto, H. Kinoshita

Department of Gastroenterological Surgery, Osaka City University Graduate School of Medicine, Osaka, Japan

Introduction: Remnant gastritis deteriorate the quality of life of the patients who had distal gastrectomy for gastric cancer. Effects of biliary diversion on reducing remnant gastritis were evaluated with concentration of IL-8 in the tissue.
Patients and Methods: Eighty-two patients who had curative distal gastrectomy for gastric cancer during these two years were subjected and classified into Group A (n=22), B (n=40), and C (n=20) by reconstructive procedures of Roux-Y, Billroth I, and Billroth II, respectively. Endoscopies were performed twelve weeks after surgery and biopsy specimens were taken from the anal site of gastric remnant. Supernatants of homogenates were measured for IL-8 levels by ELISA. The presence of *H. pylori* infection was assessed by H-E staining, immunostaining and urease activity. When none of these three tests was positive, patients were judged to be uninfected. Mann-Whitney U-tests and Kruskal-Wallis test were used for detecting difference between two groups, and among three groups, respectively.
Results: The incidence of *H. pylori* infection was 68, 48, 45% in Group A, B, and C, respectively ($p=0.22$). The IL-8 concentration was 141.1 pg/mg protein in patients with *H. pylori* infection and 56.9 pg/mg protein in patients without *H. pylori* infection ($p<0.01$). In patients with *H. pylori* infection, the IL-8 concentration was 61.1, 160.6, 233.6 pg/mg protein in Group A, B, and C, respectively ($p<0.01$). In patients without *H. pylori* infection, the IL-8 concentration was 12.7, 55.7, 87.3 pg/mg protein in Group A, B, and C, respectively ($p<0.01$).
Conclusion: *H. pylori* infection increased the IL-8 concentration in the gastric remnant. Furthermore, there were significant differences in IL-8 concentration in the gastric remnant by reconstructive procedures. Roux-Y reconstruction prevented remnant gastritis more effectively than Billroth I or II reconstructions.

PP3

Etiology and Prevention of Stomal Prolapse in Loop Stoma

K. Maeda, M. Maruta, T. Utsumi, H. Sato, H. Aoyama

Department of Surgery, Fujita Health University, Toyoake, Japan

Purpose: Stoma prolapse of covering stoma is one of the most frequent complications after stoma surgery, however, its etiology and prevention are still unclear. The aim of this study is to investigate the mechanism and the way of prevention of stoma prolapse in loop stoma of the colon.
Methods: Three patients with reducible prolapse of the loop stoma in the transverse colon were entered in the study. Barium was stained on and in the prolapsed colon and the colon was reduced once. Non-prolapsed transverse colon was filled with barium and the patient was forced to prolapse the stoma again. After reduction of prolapsed stoma, colonic wall was pressed by finger to the abdominal wall (fascia level) and the patient was forced to prolapse again. The movement of the colon was documented under the X-ray by video.
Results: All prolapses occurred in the distal part of the covering stoma and distal part of the transverse colon was redundant in all cases. All prolapses started around the anastomotic site of the colon. The colon around the anastomotic site ballooned in accordance with

an increase of abdominal pressure and the prolapse proceeded. Prolapse did not occur by pressing the colonic wall to the abdominal wall.

Conclusions: Stoma prolapse of loop stoma in the transverse colon started by adding the abdominal pressure between the colon and the anastomotic site of the stoma and proceeded under the redundant colon. Stoma prolapse did not occur after fixation of the colonic wall to the abdominal wall.

PP4

Treatment of Fecal Incontinence and Defecatory Disturbances

K. Maeda, M. Maruta, T. Utsumi, H. Sato, Y. Koide

Department of Surgery Fujita Health University, Toyoake, Japan

Purpose: Fecal incontinence and defecatory disturbances are often difficult to treat. The aim of this study is to assess the clinical results of pelvic floor repair for the pathology.

Methods: 16 patients underwent pelvic floor repair for fecal incontinence and defecatory disturbances. Mean age was 62 year-old and male to female ratio was 1 to 15. For patients' selection, defecograpy, transit study and anorectal manometry were performed after excluding the organic diseases. Surgery was done only when symptom was associated with the pathology. The pathology included rectocele in 6 cases, rectal prolapse in 5 cases, birth injury in 3 cases, idiopathic incontinence in one case and total sphincter defect after anal operation in one case. Anterior levatorplasty or total pelvic floor repair with or without sphincter plication were performed as pelvic floor repair in addition to the surgery for the initial diseases.

Results: Incontinence, defecatory disturbances and other associated symptoms disappeared in all cases except in one case with sphincter defect. Anatomical abnormality improved in cases with rectocele.

Conclusions: Pelvic floor repair is a useful treatment modality for fecal incontinence and defecatory disturbances in case proper patients' selection is performed. Pelvic floor repair is not indicated for cases with total sphincter defect.

PP5

Contrast Radiography for Anastomotic Integrity Prior to Reversal of Defunctioning Stoma - Does it Change Management?

A.A. Warsi, A. Woodward, M.E. Foster

Royal Glamorgan Hospital, Llanttrisant, S. Wales, U.K.

Introduction: Results of our audit for rectal cancer showed that the APER rate decreased from 72 % in 1991 to 19 % in 1997 as a result of increased subspecialisation, resulting in a concomitant increase in Anterior Resection (AR). However, most surgeons have resorted to formation of temporary covering loop ileostomies designed to protect from the effects of leak resulting from a primary anastomosis. The aim of this study was to assess if the results of routine pre-operative Gastrograffin enemas (GGE) defer reversal of defunctioning stomas designed to protect the primary anastomosis, following Anterior Resection.

Methods: Data was collected from pathology reports for all histologically proven rectal cancer between January 1995 to December 1997. Data were collected retrospectively from operation notes and clinical case records for all patients who underwent Anterior Resection (AR) for rectal cancer between 1995-97.

Results: A total of 55 patients underwent AR between 1995-97. 35 (64%) of the patients had covering loop ileostomies to protect the anastomosis. Prior to reversal all except 2 patients had gastrograffin enemas to assess the integrity of the primary anastomosis, one died 18 days other died 35 days post-operatively. 8 (14.5% of total) patients had leak varying from small to definite leaks and therefore the reversal of the stoma was postponed. It was delayed by an average of 9 months (range 3 -18) They subsequently underwent repeat gastrograffins at 3 monthly interval until the anastomosis healed before reversal. The average duration of closure of cases with leak was 12 months as compared to 6 months in those that did not leak ($p< 0.05$). Air insufflation test was normal in all cases of leak. There were 6 incomplete doughnuts of which 3 leaked. 13 patients did not have covering loop ileostomy and only 3 patients had GGE of which only 1 leaked and eventually died.

Discussion: Our data suggests that the routine use of GGE significantly delay the reversal of the covering loop ileostomies. Stomas have been known to be reversed commonly from as early as 45 days to 145 days. However, reversal of stomas without prior knowledge of its anastomotic integrity may be dangerous and potentially life threatening if the stoma was to leak. Moreover, as shown in our data patients can die from anastomotic leak leading to peritonitis as they have no covering ileostomiés to minimise the effect of anastomotic leak.

Conclusion: Contrast studies are useful in planning the reversal of loop ileostomies and it does alter the management of such patients. A negative air insufflation test is not a reliable prognostic indicator of potential cases liable to leak.

PP6

Prevention of Permanent Colostomy

V. Sulyma

Medical Academy, Dnipropetrovsk, Ukraine

Introduction: Patients with cancer of the distal ampullar part of the rectum are subject to a greater risk of carrying out of the operation Quenu-Mails and decreased quality of life after surgical treatment with forms of permanent colostomy. We recommend a new surgical intervention: the in-suture of anal anastomosis with a device for its performance - for prevention of permanent colostomy and preservation or increase the quality of life of the patients after the treatment.

Methods: From 1994 to 2001, 8 patients with cancer of the distal ampullar part of the rectum were treated with surgical intervention and in-suture of anal anastomosis. Dissection of the rectum with cancer of the distal ampullar part must be done immediately adjacent to the external rectal wall to avoid injury of the autonomic nerves responsible for normal sexual and urinary function. Posterior dissection must be in the plane of pararectal fat. Bleeding can be reduced by in-continuity ligation of the superior rectal artery. Anterior dissection is most difficult in young males with narrow pelvis. Great care must be taken to avoid injury of *nervi erigentes*. Abdominal dissection of the rectum is performed circumferentially at the level of levator muscles to facilitate the perineal phase: the dissection is carried out in the submucosal plane from the anal verge to the anorectal ring, preserving the internal and external sphincters and the levators. The dissection of the circular and longitudinal muscles of the rectum is carried out over the anorectal ring. The dissection is deepened circumferentially in the submucosal plane with dissection of the muscles of the rectum until the abdominal cavity can be entered posteriorly to guide the removal of the specimen at the level of the anal verge with a special device in the sigmoid pushed down.

Results: From the 8 patients with cancer of the distal ampullar part of the rectum in whom in-suture of anal anastomosis was carried out, a temporary colostomy was applied in two cases (closed from 3 to 6 months).

Discussion and Conclusion: We recommend the in-suture of anal anastomosis for prevention of permanent colostomy. This new surgical intervention may be used for removal of the rectum tumor and prevention of permanent colostomy with preservation or increase the quality of life of the patients after treatment.

Surgical Pathophysiology

PP7

Progenitor-Like Cells of Islets from Pancreatic Ductal Tissue Fragments in Three-Dimensional Culture System

A. Isogai, M. Nagaya, K. Akashi, S. Kubota

Department of General Surgery and Emergency Critical Care Medicine, Kawasaki, Japan

Introduction: Because pancreatic ductal cells include progenitor cells of the islets of Langerhans, we examined the pancreatic ductal tissue fragments of beagles for evidence of islet endocrine cells in three-dimensional culture system using thermoreversible gelation polymer (TGP) as a culture material. TGP is characterized by dynamic viscoelastic measurement as a function of temperature. The characteristics of viscoelasticity below the soluble gel transition temperature and of thermoreversibility, the water-soluble state below this temperature changing water insoluble upon heating, contributed to simplifying the culture technique. Our previous experiments showed that there was no growth of fibroblasts in TGP.

Method: Adult beagles (10 kg b.w.) were used. The right limb of the pancreas was removed under sodium pentobarbital anesthesia. A guidewire was inserted through the pancreatic duct and its tip was advanced into the peripheral region. Pancreatic tissue was carefully removed along the guidewire and pancreatic duct was isolated. The pancreatic duct was minced in a mechanical chopper into fragments with an average diameter 0.5 mm. The minced tissues were resuspended in 10 ml of cold RPMI-1640 containing of 10% TGP, 10 ng/ml keratinocyte growth factor, 100 mg/ml HGF and 10 mM nicotinamide, which was in fluid state because of below the LCST. 1 ml of culture medium included 2 or 3 tissue fragments were poured into each well of plates on the hot plate at 37°C and then turned into hydrogel. They were incubated at 37°C for 12 weeks. Morphological observation was performed with a phase contrast microscope. They were stained by the immunocytochemical technique with specific antiserum to insulin, glucagon, and somatostatin.

Result: At three days, proliferation in the ductal cell population occurred and was followed by budding from the ductal structures. Clusters which consisted of small rounded cells grew to size of 100-150 micrometer on 4 weeks. A significant number of immature, and non-differentiated cells were present. After 6 weeks culture these cells were not expanded and differentiated to form islets of endocrine cells.

Discussion and Conclusions: Recently, progenitor cells or stem cells have been identified in the pancreatic duct cells that are capable of differentiating into islet endocrine cells. In our experiments we were able to generate progenitor-like cells from ductal tissue fragments *in vitro* but they did not show any signs of the differentiation of islet endocrine cells. These immature cells (progenitor-like cells) could differentiate into islets endocrine cells, if the appropriate external stimuli were applied in our culture system. The external stimuli except HGF, KGH, and nicotinamide contained in our culture medium include VEGF, TGF-alpha, beta-cellulin and activin-A. Creating an *in vitro* environment using combination of these factors will accelerate the process to differentiate and proliferate into islet endocrine cells.

PP8

The Effect of Mycophenolate Mofetil on Liver Fibrosis in an Experimental Model

N. Sikas, K. Patsiaoura, G. Imvrios, F. Karasavidou, I. Antoniadis, S. Papaemanouil, A. Antoniadis

Transplantation Department, Hippokration Hospital, Thessaloniki, Greece

Introduction: It is well established that liver fibrosis remains a significant problem in patients undergoing liver transplantation. Chronic rejection, recurrent cholangitis and biliary complications may result in fibrosis. Mycophenolate mofetil, an immunosuppressive agent, has been found to have antifibrotic effect as well, especially in fibrosis associated with chronic inflammation with lymphocytes and monocytes being involved. This study explored the effect of mycophenolate mofetil on liver fibrosis secondary to biliary obstruction.

Methods: Forty male Wistar rats were studied. In all of them the bile duct was ligated and divided. Following this, rats in the study group were given mycophenolate mofetil 40 mg/kg i.d. by gavage and the control group equal volume of vehicle. The rats were sacrificed after 28 days. Liver function tests (ALT, AST, γ-GT, bilirubin) were performed. Liver samples were subjected to immunohistochemistry for desmin, alpha-smooth muscle actin and cytokeratins. The expression of TGF-β1 was determined by PCR.

Results: All the animals developed extensive fibrosis due to biliary obstruction. There was no significant difference between the two groups regarding the level of liver function tests. Immunohistochemistry results showed profound proliferation of bile ducts and increased activation of hepatic stellate cells. The difference, however, was not substantial. Increased expression of TGF-β1 was found in both groups, but again the difference was not considerable.

Conclusion: Lymphocytes and monocytes play a minor role in this experimental model of fibrosis. Mycophenolate mofetil does not seem to affect progression of this type of fibrosis, which is mainly the result of proliferation of bile duct epithelial cells.

PP9

The Mid-Term Effectiveness of Branched Chain Amino Acid Supplement in Cirrhosis

H. Nozaki, T. Inoau, T. Takano, Y. Kuroki

Department Surgery Towa Hospital, Tokyo, Japan

Introduction: To clarify which branched chain amino acid granules (BCAA-G) dosing may improve the protein nutritional state of cirrhosis, we performed nutritional therapy using BCAA-G. While Fisher ratio (BCAA/AAA) is well known as the evaluative index for plasma albumin synthesis in cirrhotic patients, BCAA/tyrosin ratio (BTR) is cost effective measurement and correlates with Fisher ratio. The nutritional states can be monitored by BTR measurement.
Methods: Fourteen patients (9 males, 5 females, mean age 61.2 years) of cirrhosis with their initial serum albumin level less than 3.5 g/dl were subject of this non-controlled prospective study. The causes of cirrhosis were hepatitis C in 11 patients; hepatitis B, non B non C and idiopathic portal hypertension one each. Their cirrhotic state were 7 in Child B, 4 in A and 3 in C. The composition of BCAA-G (Livact granules, Ajinomoto Co., Inc.): 1p include 4g BCAA (ratios, Lle:Leu:Val = 1.0:2.0:1.2), 1p = 16 kcal. Patients were given orally BCAA-G in a daily dose of 12 g over a 3 years period. Monitored BTR (by rapid enzymatic assay, Ono Pharmaceutical Co., Ltd.), serum albumin, ALT, total cholesterol and platelet count were analyzed. Clinical symptoms were observed especially whichever disappear or not cramp of sural region by medical interview.
Results: A comparative analysis was done using before, months 12, 24 and 36 as comparative points. At months 36, BTR and albumin were significantly increased statistically (Wilcoxon test, $p=0.0003$, and $p=0.015$). BTR was markedly elevated in most cases, while albumin was slightly improved. The other laboratory data were not improved significantly. Before the therapy, symptoms of cramps were observed in 9 cases, but those disappeared or ameliorated in 7 cases.
Conclusion: BCAA powder is effective to improve both malnutrition and cramp of sural region in cirrhosis on mid-term follow-up. However larger and double blind prospective study is needed to determine this effectiveness.

PP10

The Role of Predicting Factors in Progression and Response of Patients with Oesophageal Cancer Undergoing Neoadjuvant Therapy (An Immunohistochemical Study)

G. Bognár[1]; A. Imdahl[2]; G. Ledniczky[1]; G. István[1]; P. Ondrejka[1]

2nd Department of Surgery, Semmelweis University, Budapest, Hungary[1], Surgical Dept. of Albert Ludwigs University, Freiburg, Germany[2]

Purpose: Analysis of so called predicting factors related to proliferation, vascularization and cellular apoptosis of oesophageal cancer in patients undergoing praeoperative radio-chemotherapy followed by surgical resection, with special regard to the responder group.
Materials and Methods: The records of 56 patients with oesophageal cancer undergoing radio-chemotherapy according to the Neuheim protocol followed by surgical resection within 4 weeks at Albert Ludwigs University in Freiburg were evaluated, between 1994 and 1999. Histological analysis of praeoperative biopsy was followed by immunohistochemical workup by VEGF (vascular epithelial growth factor), Ki-67 Ag, CD34 and anti-bcl-e antibodies. The biologic response to neoadjuvant therapy was evaluated by comparison of surgical findings and tumor-staging established by praeoperative histologic, clinical and CT examinations. Three patient groups were established: responder group with full remission of the disease, a group of partial responders with downstaging, (smaller tumor size and fewer lymph nodes at operation), and a group of non-responders including those with progression of disease. (MIB-1 proliferation factor was determined in all patients whose survival was also recordable, while in 21 out of 56 patients treated between 1997 and 1999 all other factors were evaluated).
Results: The male/female distribution was 48 to 8, with a median age of 62 years. Out of 42 planocellular cancer and 14 adenocarcinomas we found 14 (25%) responders, 19 (34%) partial responders and 23 (41%) non-responders. The proliferation index (PI) was significantly higher than 40% in the group of responders, in which the VEGF-index showed significant negative correlation with PI. The MIB-1/VEGF ratio was higher than 6:1 ($p<40\%$).
Conclusion: 25% of patients undergoing neoadjuvant therapy become responders, with a MIB-1 index higher than 40% and a PI:VEGF ratio higher than 6:1. These factors prove to be valuable tools in determining prognosis with further prospective immunohistochemical analyses to refine prediction of survival.

PP11

Histochemical Appearance and Prognostic Significance of *Maackia amurensis* Leukoagglutinin-Positive Glycoconjugates in Human Gastric Cancer

W. Tang[1], M. Nakata[2,3], K. Mafune[1], T. Konishi[4], N. Kokudo[1], M. Usuda[3], N. Kojima[2,3], T. Mizuochi[2,3], M. Makuuchi[1]

Department of Surgery[1], Graduate School of Medicine, University of Tokyo, Bunkyo, Tokyo, Institute of Glycotechnology[2], Department of Applied Biochemistry[3], Tokai University, Hiratsuka, Kanagawa, Department of Surgery[4], Kanto Medical Center, NTT EC, Japan

Introduction: Cell surface glycosylation changes dramatically during oncogenesis. Among the many types of carbohydrates, sialic acid is extremely important in cancer, since enhanced sialylation is thought to play an important role in tumor metastasis and progression. *Maackia amurensis* leukoagglutinin (MAL) is a sialic acid-binding lectin with a carbohydrate-binding specificity defined as NeuAcα2,3Galß1,4GlcNAc/Glc. This study involved histochemical analysis of human gastric cancer tissues using MAL to investigate the relationship between sialylation of glycoconjugates and clinicopathological characteristics of the tumor.
Methods: Tissue samples prepared from 71 patients were subjected to histochemical staining using biotinylated MAL and the MAL staining index (MI; the percentage of MAL-stained tumor cells in the total tumor cell population in 10 random microscopic fields) was

determined. The relationships between the MI level and clinicopathological characteristics of tumors and between the MI level and prognosis were statistically analyzed.
Results: The cancer regions of all 71 tissue samples stained positive for MAL, although the population of MAL-positive tumor cells varied among the samples. In contrast, the corresponding non-cancer regions of all of the samples had no MAL staining. The distribution of MI values clearly showed two distinct populations, high and low levels of MI, with a cut-off level of 40% of MI. High MI levels were significantly frequent in cases of lymph node metastasis, lymphatic vessel invasion, and venous invasion, as well as in cases of advanced tumors. In analysis of survival, patients having tumors with a high MI level displayed a significantly poorer prognosis than those having tumors with a low MI level. Furthermore, multivariate analysis showed that a high MI level is an independent factor in a shorter survival together with the depth of invasion and the venous invasion.
Discussion: The present results indicate that MAL-positive glycoconjugates appear in gastric tumor tissues and suggest that the abnormal glycosylation detected using MAL closely related to unfavorable behavior of gastric cancer. Therefore, MAL would be an effective tool used to determine the prognosis of patients with gastric cancer.
Conclusion: MAL-positive glycoconjugates appear in gastric tissues and their high level of expression is related to a poorer prognosis among patients with gastric cancer.

PP12

Expression of Cell Cycle Control Proteins in Colon Cancer and Their Correlation in Prognosis

G. Kouraklis, D. Mantas, S. Theoharis, A. Glinavou, C. Vagianos, G. Karatzas

2nd Department of Propedeutic Surgery, University of Athens, Athens, Greece

Introduction: Cell cycle control proteins play major role as potential contributors to the multistep process of oncogenesis, nevertheless their prognostic significance in colon cancer has been examined in a few studies.
Methods: One hundred and eleven patients who underwent colonic surgical resection due to colon cancer constituted the group of our study. The immunohistochemic expression of Cyclin D1 and E, Rb, p16, p21 and Ki-67 proteins was examined in this study.
Results: The 5-year survival rate of patients presenting positive tumors of each of the cell cycle control proteins, even though was shorter, the difference was not statistically significant. Multivariate survival analysis revealed statistical significance for stage, grade, lymph node, hepatic metastasis and vessel invasion, while there was no any significance for Cyclin D1 and E, Rb, p16 and p21. Univariate analysis showed worse survival in patients presenting advanced stage and Cyclin D1 positivity ($p=0.025$). Additionally, the survival of patients aging less than 70 years old significantly correlated to Cyclin D1 positive expression ($p=0.009$).
Conclusions: The importance of expression of cell cycle control proteins seems to be complex and different between tumors. Cyclin D1 expression may be a predictor of patients presenting in advanced stage and of patients of young age.

PP13

Analysis of K-Ras and P53 Gene Mutations in Human Colorectal Carcinoma: Relationship to Clinicopathological Variables

L. Zajac[1], J. Polanski[1], J. Dluzniewska[2], B. Interewicz[3], J. Stanislawska[3], E. Szyter[3]

3rd Surg. Dept.[1], Med. Fac., Med. School, Mol. Biol. Dept.[2], Med. Res. Ctr. Inst., Pol. Ac. Sci., Surg. Res. Transpl. Dept.[3], Med. Res. Ctr. Inst., Pol. Acad. Sci., Warsaw, Poland

Introduction: Molecular pathogenesis of human cancer is due to structural and/or functional changes of specific genes whose normal function is to control cellular growth and differentiation. Colorectal tumorigenesis is accompanied by accumulation of genetic alterations, involving activation of oncogenes (ras) and inactivation of tumor suppressor genes (APC, p53 and DCC). Mutation of K-ras and p53 genes are the most common genetic abnormalities present in colorectal cancer. Such mutations are presumed to promote the clonal proliferation of affected cells with more aggressive growth properties. The aim of the study was to prospectively evaluate the prognostic significance of K-ras and p53 gene mutations in colorectal carcinoma.
Material and Methods: Twenty four patients undergoing surgical resection for colorectal adenocarcinoma with no liver metastases were studied. Primary tumors and paired nonadjacent areas of normal colonic mucosa were collected as fresh specimens, snap frozen and then stored at -80°C. After the extraction of DNA PCR amplification was performed with specific primers to detect K-ras point mutation at codon 12 followed by digestion with MvaI. Mutations at p53 gene (exons 5-9) were detected with three sets of primers and characterized by SSCP. Products were run on acrylamide gels, silver stained and scanned.
Results: Histological grading of tumor specimens revealed 12 Dukes'B grade and 12 Dukes'C grade adenocarcinoma. The median follow-up was 20 months (range 12-34 months). Metastatic disease was found in 4 patients (66.6%) and local recurrence was noted in 2 patients (33.3%), 2 patients died due to recurrent disease. Tumors from 17 patients (70.8%) contained K-ras and p53 mutations, K-ras mutation was detected in 8 (47%), p53 mutation in 13 (76.4%) specimens, 4 tumors (23.5%) were positive in both. K-ras mutation was more frequent in tumors with Dukes' stage C (41.6%) than in Dukes' stage B tumors (25%). All patients with Dukes'C and K-ras mutation developed liver metastasis during 12 months follow-up period. Out of 12 patients with Dukes'B grade, 3 patients showed K-ras mutation but none of them developed metastasis to the liver during 25 months follow-up. p53 mutation was identified in 13 patients (54.2%). The prevalence of p53 mutation occurred equally in tumors with Dukes'B and Dukes'C grade and was not linked with progression of the disease.
Conclusion: The current study indicated that detection of K-ras mutation at codon 12 in patients with Dukes'C but not with Dukes'B grade was associated with the metastatic potential of colorectal carcinoma in the liver. The presence of K-ras mutation may predict clinical outcome and help to define the type of therapy in patients with Dukes'C grade colorectal carcinoma.

PP14

Copper-Transporting P-Type Adenosine Triphosphatase (ATP7B) is Expressed in Human Gastric Carcinoma

K. Ogawa

Department of Surgery, Tokyo Women's Medical University Daini Hospital, Tokyo, Japan

Introduction: The ATP7B gene, mapping to 14q14.3, has been cloned and encodes a copper-transporting P-type adenosine triphosphatase (ATP7B). ATP7B is expressed in human liver, kidney, and placenta. ATP7B protein includes the ATP-binding domain to the transmembrane segment and is a member of a class of heavy metal-transporting, P-type ATPases that pump copper, cadmium, zinc, silver, or led. The recent search for new marker of chemoresistance has identified that ATP7B was involved in cisplatin-resistance, and the induction of ATP7B was observed by exposure to cisplatin in human prostate cells. In this study, we investigated the hypothesis that ATP7B is expressed in certain gastric carcinomas.
Methods: To test this hypothesis, ATP7B expression level was examined in 51 gastric carcinoma patients by immunohistochemistry using fresh frozen surgical specimens.
Results: ATP7B protein could be detected in 41.2% (21/51) of gastric carcinoma by immunohistochemical analysis. In ATP7B-positive tumors, adjacent non-neoplastic tissues was similarly analyzed, revealing that ATP7B is upregulated in gastric carcinoma. ATP7B expression in poorly-differentiated/undifferentiated carcinoma was significantly higher than that in well-/moderately-differentiated carcinoma ($p=0.0278$).
Conclusion: These findings suggested that ATP7B expression might be a chemoresistant marker against cisplatin in some patients with poorly-differentiated/undifferentiated gastric carcinoma.

Hepatobiliary and Pancreatic Surgery

PP15

Consideration of Detection of *Helicobacter Pylori* in the Gastric Mucosa as a Respective Factor for Occurrence of Acute Attack of Cholecystitis at a Glance of Asymptomatic Cholecystolithiasis

N. Ueno, H. Haranomura[1], S. Matsuoka, M. Terada, Y. Makino, M. Fujikura[2], Y. Fujio[1]

Department of Surgery[1] and Internal Medicine[2], Kita-Osaka Hospital, Osaka, Japan

Introduction: In management of cholecystolithiasis, asymptomatic cases will regularly be followed up conservatively and symptomatic ones will be converted to surgery. During the follow up of asymptomatic cases, patients are always exposed to some risk of acute attack of cholecystitis, but there is no predictive factor at the moment. Now we have considered possibility of detection of *Helicobacter pylori* in the gastric mucosa as the predictive factor of acute attack and performed a retrospective study in cases of cholecystolithiasis.
Methods: 83 cases which were followed up from 1st of January to 31st of December, 2001 with cholecystolithiasis (symptomatic: 35, asymptomatic: 48), entered this study. Additionally 31 cases with gallbladder polyp were also entered as control. Stones and polyps in gallbladder were detected with abdominal ultrasonography. Upper gastrointestinal scope was performed for 24, 16 and 18 cases in each group. Detection of *Helicobacter pylori* was created by H-E staining for samples of biopsy from the antrum through gastrointestinal scope.
Results: *Helicobacter pylori* was detected in the gastric mucosa in 71.4% and 50.0% of cases with symptomatic cholecystolithiasis and gall-bladder polyp, on the other hand in 14.3% of ones with asymptomatic cholecystolithiasis, which is a significantly lower incidence than ones in the other groups.
Discussion: There have been some papers reporting the possibility that *Helicobacter pylori* is associated with gallstone formation. In this study there was no significant difference in the detection of *Helicobacter pylori* in the gastric mucosa between the group of cholecystolithiasis (both symptomatic and symptomatic cases included) and the control (42.9% vs 50.0%).
Conclusion: Detection of *Helicobacter pylori* in the gastric mucosa might help us to follow up cases with asymptomatic cholecystolithiasis. The lack of *Helicobacter pylori* may indicate fewer occurrence of acute attack of cholecystitis.

PP16

Liver Regeneration and Angiogenesis in Mice Deficient for Plasminogen

J.M. Vogten, T.A. Drixler, I.H.M. Borel Rinkes

Department of Surgery; University Medical Center, Utrecht, The Netherlands

Introduction: Degradation and remodeling of the extracellular matrix (ECM) is an important process in angiogenesis as well as in the regenerating liver, e.g. following partial hepatectomy. Our previous studies have shown that urokinase plasminogen activator is needed for normal liver regeneration, but is not essential for vessel growth during regeneration. In this study we expand on this observation by analyzing the regenerating liver of mice deficient for the key component of the plasmin system: plasminogen (Plg). We hypothesize that deficiency of plasminogen leads to impaired liver regeneration and angiogenesis.
Methods: Mice deficient for Plg (Plg-/-) were subjected to 70% partial hepatectomy. Liver regeneration was assessed by measuring wet liver weight (WLW) on days 2 (POD2), 7 (POD7) and 14 (POD14) post-hepatectomy and by bromodeoxyuridine (BrdU) incorporation assay. Formation of neovasculature in the liver was assessed by determining microvessel density (MVD) in the liver after staining for CD-31. In addition, the ability of these mice to form new bloodvessels was analysed in the cornea neovascularisation assay.
Results: Plg-/- mice showed reduced angiogenic response in the cornea neovascularisation assay. Liver regeneration after partial hepatectomy as measured by WLW was delayed in Plg-/- mice by 26.9% and 19.1% (POD2 and POD7, respectively) compared to WT mice. The BrdU incorporation peak was delayed and reduced in Plg-/- mice (peak at 96 hrs post hepatectomy, 9.5%±1.7 labeled cells)

compared to WT mice (peak at 48 hrs post hepatectomy, 22.8%±3.0 labeled cells). Finally, Plg-/- mice showed reduced microvessel density after PH compared to WT mice (65±2 and 68±1 vs 85±3 and 86±3 vpf on POD 7 and 14, respectively).
Discussion and Conclusion: Deficiency for Plg induces a delay in murine liver regeneration as measured by liver mass and BrdU labeling index. This effect appears to be due to inhibition of microvessel growth during physiological angiogenesis.

PP17

Anterior Liver Resections for Surgical Treatment of Primary and Secondary Liver Tumours

I. Takács, A. Vágvölgyi, M.G. Boland, P. Sápy

University of Debrecen, Medical and Health Science Center, School of Medicine, 2nd Department of Surgery, Debrecen, Hungary

Introduction: Authors evaluate the experiences of the anterior major liver resections performed without previous dissection and clamping of the hilar vessels between 1992 and 2001.
Methods: 10 of 55 major resections were operated in this manner. This method was used in cases where the portal vessels could not be dissected safely due to tumour enlargement, or cirrhotic and fragile liver. The mean age of the patients was 54 years. The proportion of men to women was 5:5. The indication of the resection was primary liver carcinoma in 3 cases, secondary tumour in 4 cases, focal benign disease in 3 cases. The operations were performed using CUSA ultrasonic equipment. Resections were initiated at the diaphragmatic surface of the liver without dissection and ligation of the hilar vessels. During the surgery, simultaneous resection of 4 or 5 liver segments occurred after the incision of the Glisson capsule using the CUSA ultrasound dissector. The average operation time, blood consumption and survival data were compared to the results of the other, 'non-anterior' operational procedures. Student's t-test was used in the statistical analysis where a significant result was $p< 0.05$.
Results: There was no mortality in the postoperative period. Complications were the following: fever in 3 cases, leakage of bile in 2 cases, biloma in 1 case, seroma in 1 patient. The average operation time was 165 (45-200) minutes, which was less than the time used in liver resections started with dissection and ligation of the hilar vessels [178 minutes (90-290)]. However, this difference was not significant. The mean volume of transfusion was 560 (0-2000) ml, which is not more than the blood needed for the major resections with previous selective vessel ligation [938 (0-4000) ml]. The median survival time is 26.5 (7-37) months in the cases of anterior resections and 29 (1-108) months for non anterior resections. This difference is not significant.
Conclusion: According to their results the authors believe that anterior resections can be performed safely. The number of perioperative complications is low. Regarding to the operation time, use of blood transfusion, and survival time, the authors did not find better results significantly comparing to the major resections (those started with dissection of the hilar vessels) - in contrast to the literature. The authors recommend this procedure in cases where the hilus can not be safely isolated due to any reason. Using this technique, the ratio of liver resectability can be well increased.

PP18

Surgical Impact of Liver Resections with Microwave Tissue Coagulator

S. Satoi, Y. Matsui, H. Kitade, M. Kaibori, H. Yamada, T. Hijikawa, N. Terakawa, S. Takai, A.H. Kwon, Y. Kamiyama

First Department of Surgery, Kansai Medical University, Osaka, Japan

Background: Hepatocellular carcinoma (HCC) is a major health concern worldwide, with an incidence of approximately 1 million cases per year. Liver resection is the most effective form of treatment for patients with HCC. The use of microwave tissue coagulator (MTC) has been reported to reduce blood loss and to enable limited liver resection for the patients with poor hepatic reserve. We have routinely performed liver resection with MTC for the patient with HCC. We report results of 185 liver resections for the patients with HCC.
Methods: Between 1992 and 2000, the data of 185 patients with HCC who underwent liver resection with MTC was collected from the prospective HCC database in Kansai Medical University Hospital. Liver resection was done without Pringle's maneuver following liver tissue coagulation by repeatedly insertion of a monopolar MTC needle along the intented resection line. Tumor was resected with a margin of about 1 cm. The clinical characteristics of the patients were evaluated, and postoperative complication incidence, operative mortality, overall patient survival and disease free survival were calculated. All of data were expressed as mean ± SD.
Results: Eighty percent of all patients were male and age was 63±8 years old. Operative time and amount of blood loss were 284±110 minutes and 1674±2213 ml, respectively. The retention rate of indocyanine green dye at 15 min was 19.1± 9.6 % and exceeded 30% in 13% of all patients. PIVKA showed 1586±6065 and tumor size was 3.9±2.7 cm in diameter. Seventy-three percent of the patients had solitary tumors and 27% had multiple. Forty-four percent of patients had microscopically liver cirrhosis. TNM classification showed stage 1 (19%), 2 (47%), 3 (19%), and 4 (15%). Overall patient survival rates were 91, 72 and 56% at 1, 3 and 5 years, respectively. Disease-free survival rates were 75, 50 and 29% at 1, 3 and 5 years, respectively. The most common cause of death was cancer, but liver failure and variceal bleeding were included among the causes of death. The follow-up period ranged from 1 to 100 months and the median follow-up period was 25 months. Postoperative complication incidence was 35% and operative mortality was 1%.
Conclusion: The liver resection with MTC was a safe and technically easy procedure, and the results in this study appear partially acceptable.

PP19

Experimental Model of Intraoperative Radiotherapy on Ischemic Rat Liver

O. Hahn, A. Szijártó, P. Kupcsulik

1st Department of Surgery, Semmelweis University, Budapest, Hungary

Introduction: The aim is to create a model of a liver resection combined with intraoperative irradiation for micrometastases. This combined ischemic-reperfusion and radiation injury of the liver has not been investigated yet.
Methods: Wistar male rats (300-350g) were used for the experiment. Under aether and ketamine anaesthesia plasma ALP, GOT, GPT, GGT, LDH, bilirubin, and TNF-α tests were performed before and at various times after the ischemia, and liver radiation. The liver microcirculation was continiously monitored by Laser-Doppler-flowmeter. During the 30, 45, 60, and 90 minute normothermic liver ischemia the rat liver was exposed intraoperatively to graded doses (0-25-50 Gy) of 137Cs gamma-radiation, centered to the I, II, IV lobes of the liver. The remaining lobes, and the other organs were shielded by lead. Liver histology was done on animals sacrificed 7 days after irradiation.
Results: Any group of longer ischemia, or higher dose irradiation showed significant histological abnormalities (parenchymal necrosis, fibrosis, bile duct proliferation) and liver injury, as measured by increased TNF-α and elevated liver enzymes.
Discussion: Survival is rather determined by the length of the ischemic period, than the irradiation dose. Low dose irradiation (25 Gy) with short-term ischemia (30 min) did not result in increased liver enzymes and resulted only in minimal histological changes.
Conclusion: The group of low dose irradiation (25 Gy) with normotherm, short-term ischemia (30 min) seems to be tolerable for the tumor-free liver. Further investigations are to be done with tumor-inoculated liver.

PP20

Pattern and Risk of Postoperative Recurrence in Solitary Hepatocellular Carcinoma

Y. Takada, M. Otsuka, T. Todoroki, K. Fukao

Department of Surgery, Tsukuba University, Tsukuba, Japan

Introduction: A high recurrence rate after hepatic resection adversely influences the postoperative prognosis of patients with hepatocellular carcinoma (HCC). Although it is known that patients with solitary HCC have a better survival after hepatic resection than those with multiple ones, pattern and risk of recurrence in solitary HCC cases have not been fully described. In the present study, long-term results and prognostic factors were evaluated in patients who underwent hepatic resection for solitary HCC.
Methods: The records of 105 patients who underwent hepatic resection for HCC were retrospectively reviewed. In 61 patients with solitary HCC who survived the curative operation, the prognostic significance of 11 clinicopathological parameters was investigated by univariate and multivariate analyses. The median postoperative follow-up period was 48 months (range 2-172).
Results: After curative resection, the cumulative survival rate at 5 years in these 61 patients with solitary HCC was significantly better than in 25 patients with multiple HCC (44% vs. 25%, *p=0.012*). However, even in the solitary group, the cumulative recurrence-free survival rate at 5 years was only 32%, and 27 (75%) of 36 patients, in whom recurrence was confirmed within 5 years, recurred within 2 years. In 28 of the 36 patients, the site of recurrence was liver alone. The diameter of the primary lesion in these 36 patients (median 3.1 cm, range 0.5-17.0 cm) was not significantly different from that of 13 patients who survived without recurrence more than 5 years (median 3.2 cm, range 1.7-7.0 cm). On the other hand, both the univariate and multivariate analyses disclosed that only accompanying liver cirrhosis was a variable having prognostic significance for recurrence-free survival.
Discussion: It is generally agreed that tumor size as well as the number of tumors is one of the greatest prognostic factors. However, in the present study, tumor size had no significant value in predicting overall or recurrence-free survival. On the other hand, underlying cirrhosis was indicated as a unique risk factor for postoperative recurrence. Since a number of studies have shown that the presence of cirrhosis is closely associated with postoperative recurrence and that liver fibrosis may be related to multicentric carcinogenesis, it is speculated that multicentric cancer may contribute considerably to intrahepatic recurrence in the present solitary HCC cases.
Conclusion: It is suggested that hepatic resection can be indicated in patients with a solitary HCC, irrespective of its size. Though the postoperative recurrence associated with underlying cirrhosis is still frequent, long-term survival can be expected if the recurrent tumors are successfully treated by a strategy using multiple modalities.

PP21

Hepatocyte Growth Factor Level in Liver and Blood and Post-Operative Liver Cell Proliferation in Patients with Benign and Malignant Liver Tumors Undergoing Partial Hepatectomy

B. Lukomska[1], J. Dluzniewska[2], J. Polanski[3], L. Zajac[3], D. Sitkiewicz[4]

Surg. Res. Transpl. Dep.[1], Med. Res. Ctr. Inst., Pol. Acad. Sci., Mol. Biol. Dept.[2], Med. Res. Ctr. Inst., Pol. Acad. Sci., 3rd Surg. Dept.[3], Med. Fac., Med. School, Clin. Bioch. Dept.[4], National Institute of Cardiology, Warsaw, Poland

Introduction: The liver constitutes a conditional renewal system in which hepatocytes may be induced to proliferate following surgical resection. Partial hepatectomy initiates the release of various cytokines and growth factors that result in proliferation of all hepatic elements. One of the main molecules involved in proliferation of normal hepatocytes is hepatocyte growth factor (HGF) produced by nonparenchymal liver cells and cells in different extrahepatic sites. Vascular complications and ischemic injury in hepatectomized patients could result in adequate regeneration leading to hepatic insufficiency or liver failure. Moreover, regeneration of human liver is influenced by coexisting liver diseases. The aim of the present studies was initiated to determine the expression of HGF in blood and liver tissue in relation to hepatocyte proliferation and liver regeneration in patients with benign and malignant liver tumors who underwent partial hepatectomy.

Methods: Twenty five patients undergoing partial hepatectomy (PH) for colorectal adenocarcinoma liver metastases (ACC) (15 cases) and benign liver tumors (10 cases) were studied. Immunohistochemical examination for the presence of HGF, cMET/HGF-R and proliferating cell nuclear antigen (PCNA) was performed on formalin fixed sections of liver tissue using MoAbs (Novocastra, UK). Circulating HGF in patient sera was determined with ELISA kit (R&D System, UK).

Results: No difference in the intensity of HGF and cMET/HGF-R expression was detected between liver samples in malignant and benign liver tumor patients during liver regeneration. HGF expression was found in 60% (9 of 15) and cMET/HGF-R in 33% (3 of 15) of colorectal carcinoma liver metastatic tissue samples. Serum level of HGF in patients with colorectal liver carcinoma metastases was higher compared with those with benign liver tumors (618.3±145.2 vs 366.6±127.9 pg/ml before operation; 1045.2±494.0 vs 343.9±99.4 pg/ml 30 min after PH; 750.5±326.1 vs 422.6±159.9 pg/ml 7 days after PH, $p<0.02$, respectively). In malignant liver tumor patients serum HGF level increased 30 min after PH compared with preoperative value (1045.2±494.1 vs 618.3±145.2 pg/ml, $p<0.02$). This was not observed in benign liver tumor patients. PCNA labeling index in liver specimens taken 7 days after PH from colorectal liver metastatic patients was higher than in benign liver tumor group (42.4±10.2 vs 23.0±7.4, $p<0.05$).

Conclusion: Proliferation rate of hepatocytes was higher in patients with metachronous colorectal liver metastases than in patients with benign lesions undergoing PH. The presence of HGF in carcinoma cells suggests that this growth factor derived from residual tumors remaining in non-resected liver fragments may support the proliferation of liver cells in these patients.

PP22

Antireflux Effectivity of Various Porto-Enterostomas

T. Cserni, I. Csízy, I. Furka, T. Józsa, J. Papp Szekeres**, T. Lesznyák*, I. Mikó**

Department of Pediatric Surgery, Department of Operative Techniques and Surgical Research, Medical and Health Science Center, University of Debrecen, Debrecen*, Bács-Kiskun County Hospital, General Surgical Department, Kecskemét**, Hungary

Introduction: The main problem of the Porto-enterostomy (PE) in children with extrahepatic biliary atresia is the ascending cholangitis. There are many modifications of PE to avoid the cholangitis. Lengthening of the Roux-Y inserting an antireflux valve using the ileocoecal segment (Bauhin valve) for PE. In our study we compared the antireflux effetivity of these various conduits. The question was how long the invaginated antireflux valve should be created to reach enough antireflux effectiveness without high anterograd resistance and without damaging the wall of the intestine.

Method: We performed the maneuver in dogs under general anesthesia, fulfilling the requirements of the Animals Protection Act. We isolated 30 cm long gaps of the intestine, inserted Foley balloon catheter on one end and begun the retrograd filling the intestine gaps with X-ray contrast fluid or methylene blue. The opening of the valves was observed on X-ray monitor or endovideo.

Results: The conduit without valve filled up at 10 cm high fluid column pressure. The Bauhin valve opened at 25 cm high fluid column. The 4 cm long antireflux valve opened at 60 cm high fluid column. The 7 cm long valve did not open.

Discussion: The intestine without valve filled up very easily. The Bauhin valve had significant antireflux effectivity. The 4 and the 7 cm long invaginated valve had surprisingly high antireflux resistance.

Conclusions: The Bauhin valve may be enough to prevent ascending cholangitis if we consider the mean pressure in the intestine. A short invaginated valve has good antireflux effectivity. There is no need to create longer valves.

PP23

The Effect of Intraductal Corticosteroid Treatment on the Experimental Acute Pancreatitis of Dogs

L. Kerekes, S. Sipka Jr., B. Dezső, A. Furka, K. Pető, E. Bráth, I. Mikó, I. Furka, P. Sápy

2nd Department of Surgery, Department of Operative Techniques and Surgical Research, Medical and Health Science Center, University of Debrecen, Debrecen, Hungary

Background/Aims: We have compared the effects of intravenous and intraductal applications of glucocorticosteroid (GCS) treatment on the experimental acute pancreatitis in 14 adult mongrel dogs.

Methods: Experimental acute pancreatitis were induced by olive oil injected to the main pancreatic duct. Soluble methylprednisolone was applied intravenously and intraductally after the oil. Serum amylase and lipase measurements were monitored daily. The macroscopic and histological evaluations of the pancreases took place on the 4th day of experiments.

Results: Although the amylase and lipase elevating effects of intraductal treatments (with various doses of GCS) were found less than those of intravenous application, even the 0.15 mg/kg dose of intraductal GCS resulted in significant increases in the serum levels of amylase and lipase.

Conclusions: Though there are efforts for the clinical use of smaller doses of GCS in the autoimmune forms of pancreatitis and for the prevention of ERCP-induced pancreatitis, we suggest to avoid all the forms of glucocorticosteroid treatment in pancreatitis (including the intraductal type of application) and to look for new anti-inflammatory protocols in this disease.

PP24

Clinicopathological Evaluation of Long and Short-Term Survivors Treated for Pancreatic Carcinoma

S. Takai, S. Satoi, H. Yanagimoto, Y. Koike, H. Toyokawa, H. Araki, A.H. Kwon, Y. Kamiyama

1st Department of Surgery, Kansai Medical University, Osaka, Japan

Background: Even with the recent advances in diagnostic and therapeutic methods, clinical course of patients with pancreatic cancer remains very poor. Between April 1992 and December 2001, 169 patients with invasive ductal cancer of the pancreas underwent operation in Kansai Medical University. Of these patients, we experienced only 6 patients who survived more than 5 years after surgery.
Methods: The clinicopathological findings of 10 short-term survivors and 6 long-term survivors were reviewed to reveal the factors which produce the opposite clinical course. We defined short and long-term survivors as follows. Short-term survivors: non-surviving patients following tumor recurrence within 1 year after the curative resection. Long-term survivors: surviving patients for 5 years or more after pancreatectomy.
Results: 1. Significant differences were not found in the clinicopathological features between short- and long-term survivors. 2. Clinical staging did not always appear to be a prognostic factor in these long-term survivors. 3. Most long survivors were treated with postoperative chemotherapy of low dose cisplatinum (CDDP) and 5-fluorouracil (5FU). 4. Liver metastasis was most frequently observed in both groups.
Conclusion: 1. For improvement of the prognosis of pancreatic cancer patients, it is probably worthwhile treating those patients with chemotherapy of low dose CDDP and 5-FU, and developing the reliable regimen to control liver metastasis. 2. In order to eradicate locoregional recurrence after pancreatectomy for invasive ductal adenocarcinoma of the pancreas, aggressive protocols of the preoperative chemoradiation therapy are ongoing for patients with locally advanced pancreatic cancer in our department.

Sepsis and Inflammation

PP25

The Effects of Dimethylsulfoxide and Pentoxifylline on Plasma Malondialdehyde Levels and Tissue Damage in Sepsis

S. Tekin, M. Sahin, H. Alptekin, M. Avunduk, M. Gürbilek

SUTF General Surgery, Pathology and Biochemistry, Konya,Turkey

Objective: Scavenging or inhibiting of occurrence of free oxygen radicals (FOR) during sepsis by antioxidants may lessen tissue damage and reduce morbidity and mortality.
Background: Tumor necrosis factor alpha (TNF-α) released after endotoxin stimulation leads to activation of neutrophils and enable their adherence to vascular endothelium. It also stimulates degranulation and free oxygen radicals formation.
Methods: 40 Wistar Albino rats were divided into four groups. Sepsis was induced by cecal ligation and perforation method in the first three groups. Nothing was used in the first group, in the second group, 15 mg/kg pentoxifylline (PTX), in the third group 300 mg/kg dimetylsulfoxide (DMSO) was given, and in Sham group nothing was given. Blood and tissue samples were taken 24 hours after the induction of sepsis and then animals was sacrificed. The plasma malondialdehyde (MDA) levels were measured as an intermediate product of FORs, and the histopathological damages in lungs, liver and kidneys were evaluated.
Results: The plasma MDA levels of sepsis group in comparison to the other 3 groups was higher and statistically significant ($p<0.05$). The neutrophil infiltration, interstitial edema and alveolar basal membrane damage in the lungs of PTX group, compared to the sepsis group, were less and statistically significant ($p<0.05$). Increase in distance of Bowman's capsule was much less in PTX group than sepsis group. PTX and DMSO prevented the hydrophic degeneration in the liver ($p<0.05$).
Conclusions: PTX is more effective than DMSO in decreasing plasma MDA and preventing the end organ damages of sepsis.

PP26

The Effects of Selective iNOS Inhibitory Aminoguanidine on Plasma NO Levels, Tissue Damage and Organ Function in Sepsis

M. Sahin, M. Belviranli, M. Gölcük, F. Avsar, H. Pasaoglu, S. Hücümenoglu

Selcuk Univ. Medical Faculty Konya, ANH General Surgery Ankara, Gazi Univ. Biochemistry Ankara, SSK Hospital Pathology, Ankara, Turkey

Aim: The aim of this study is to investigate the effects of aminoguanidine, L-arginine and pentoxyfillin on plasma nitric oxide levels, tissue damages and organ functions in sepsis.
Methods: Sixty Wistar albino rats were included, and the rats were divided into 6 groups. Sepsis was induced by cecal ligation perforation methods into the all rats except sham group. Group I: Sham procedure, Group II: Sepsis only, Group III: Sepsis + L-arginine 10 mg/kg, Group IV: aminoguanidine 15 mg/kg, Group V: L-arginine + aminoguanidine together, Group VI: pentoxifillin 15 mg/kg. At 24th hour of the experiment; blood samples were taken, for the measurements of plasma NO, MDA, AST, ALT, BUN, CRE, blood gasses and WBC. Tissue samples of liver, kidney and lungs were taken for histopathological evaluation of tissue damages.
Results: L-arginine caused a significant increase in NO levels in plasma, and tissue damage. Aminoguanidine caused a significant decrease in NO levels in plasma and tissue damage in liver, kidney and lungs, and no change in organ functions.
Conclusion: Aminoguanidine, a selective iNOS inhibitor, may prevent tissue damage and organ failure in sepsis.

PP27

Pirfenidone Ameliorates Endotoxin-Induced Liver Injury after Partial Hepatectomy in Rats

H. Tsuchiya, M. Kaibori, N. Yokoigawa, A.H. Kwon, T. Okumura, Y. Kamiyama*

First Department of Surgery, Department of Medical Chemistry*, Kansai Medical University, Osaka, Japan

Introduction: Extended hepatectomy is performed for radical resection of hepatobiliary tract malignancies. Hepatic failure is a major contributor to mortality after extensive liver resection, with the pathophysiology being similar to that of sepsis. Pirfenidone (PFD), 5-methyl-1-phenyl-2(1H)-pyridone, is a compound that can prevent extracellular matrix accumulation in several organs, as shown by experimental studies on pulmonary fibrosis. PFD also has been reported to inhibit both TNF-α induction and subsequent endotoxin shock. We investigated the effect of PFD on endotoxin-induced liver injury following partial hepatectomy.
Methods: Male Sprague-Dawley rats underwent a 70% hepatectomy. Two days after surgery, LPS (1.5 mg/kg) was injected intravenously. 300 mg/kg of PFD or 0.5% carboxymethylcellulose (control) was administered peroral either 2.5 h and 0.5 h before the LPS injection. After the LPS injection, we determined the following: (1) survival rate (2) serum AST, ALT, and LDH levels (3) inflammatory cytokine levels in serum and liver tissue (4) iNOS protein in liver tissue, and (5) tissue necrosis and neutrophil infiltration by histological analysis.
Results: The survival rate was significantly increased by PFD administration. Values for serum AST, ALT, and LDH and for TNF-α, IL-1ß, IFN-γ, IL-6, and CINC were significantly lower in the PFD-treated group. PFD markedly inhibited the induction of iNOS protein, hepatic necrosis and the number of infiltrating neutrophils.
Conclusion: PFD had a protective effect against endotoxin-induced liver injury following partial hepatectomy, through inhibiting the induction of inflammatory cytokines, iNOS protein, and infiltrating neutrophils.

PP28

The Influence of Probiotics in Bacterial Translocation

K. Kotzampassi, E. Tsiakiri, D. Paramythiotis, N. Charlaftis, G. Metaxas, A. Zatagias, E. Eleftheriadis*

Departments of Surgery and Microbiology*, University of Thessaloniki, Greece

Objective: Probiotics are non-pathogenic microorganisms exerting beneficial effects, when ingested, by maintaining intestinal microfloral balance and the integrity of the host. They modify the microflora ecology of the gut, prevent the adhesion of pathogenic bacteria, enhance the production of antimicrobial substances and stimulate the host immune defense. Since commensal flora and mucosal barrier consist the principal structures responsible for bacterial translocation, the present study was designed to investigate whether *Lactobacillus reuteri* would be effective in reducing bacterial translocation in zymosan-induced non-septic peritonitis in the rat.
Method: Forty male Wistar rats received *Lactobacillus* [10^7 CFU/day] or placebo for 5 days, in drinking water. On day 5, half of the rats of each group were subjected to intraperitoneal injection of 500 mg/kg b.w. of Zymosan for non-septic peritonitis induction, while the remaining received normal saline. Mesenteric lymph nodes were collected, under aseptic conditions, 18 hrs later for evaluation of bacterial translocation, by means of culture, as well as a specimen of cecal content for identification of indigenous bacterial flora.
Results: Control rats treated by either *Lactobacillus* or placebo revealed no evidence of bacterial translocation to mesenteric lymph nodes in relation to placebo-treated, Zymosan-injected group ($1.5x10^6$ CFU/g tissue). On the contrary *Lactobacillus* treatment in Zymosan-induced peritonitis group resulted in a significant reduction of the amount of translocated bacteria ($2.5x10^5$ CFU/g, $p=0.001$) in relation to placebo-treated Zymosan-group.
Conclusion: In this placebo controlled trial, modification of enteric flora by means of *Lactobacillus* reuteri seems to be effective in reducing bacterial translocation in Zymosan-induced peritonitis in rats.

PP29

Diagnostic Value of Urine "Biopyrrins" (Bilirubin Oxidative Products) in Severity of Acute Abdomen

Y. Tsuji, M. Misumi, T. Takahashi, K. Kaai R. Hirayama

Department of General and Gastroenterological Surgery, Saitama Medical School, Saitama, Japan

Introduction: It has been clarified that bilirubin plays an important role as an antioxidant in oxidative stress. We investigated that hyperbilirubinemia in surgical stress such as severe panperitonitis is correlated with antioxidative effect against oxidative stress. So we examined the levels of urine "Biopyrrins" (bilirubin oxidative products) in patients of acute abdomen.
Methods: 20 urine samples from patients with acute abdomen were measured. Urine Biopyrrins values were measured by the enzyme linked immunosorbent assay (ELISA) method using the home-made anti-bilirubin monoclonal antibody (24G7).
Results and Conclusions: Almost all of patients in SIRS tended to show high levels of Biopyrrins. In addition, two patients (strangulation ileus and severe panperitonitis) demonstrated the high levels of Biopyrrins, nevertheless they did not show the SIRS criteria. So we thought that the levels of urine Biopyrrins reflect the severity of acute abdomen.

PP30

Effect of Octreotide on the Oxidative Stress of Acute Experimental Pancreatitis

K. Kotzampassi, A. Makedou, D. Paramythiotis, G. Metaxas, K. Kourti*, E. Eleftheriadis*

Department of Surgery & Biochemical Lab.* of 2nd Pediatric Clinic, University of Thessaloniki, Greece

Objective: Since there is a lack of information about the influence of octreotide on the oxidative stress induced during the outcome of acute pancreatitis, we investigated its possible action, in a rat model of this disease.
Method: Acute pancreatitis was induced in 16 male Wistar rats by injection of 5% sodium taurocholate into the duodenal loop, which remained closed for 60 sec, while 16 animals served as controls. A dose of 4 μgr/kg octreotide or placebo was injected subcutaneously immediately after the procedure and 12 hrs later, creating 4 groups. At 24 hrs blood was obtained from the abdominal aorta for MDA, as well as SOD and Gpx estimation.
Results: The pancreatitis group exhibited a statistically significant ($p=0.01$) elevation of MDA levels (9.7±3.8) in relation to the control (4.1±2.2) or to control plus octreotide (4.2±2.5) groups. On the contrary, a significant ($p=0.001$) decrease of SOD and Gpx levels was prominent (1.01±0.01 and 2299±114, respectively) in relation to control (2.23±0.3 and 4103±72) or to control plus octreotide (2.15±0.3 and 4143±144) groups. Octreotide treatment after pancreatitis induction resulted in a significant ($p=0.01$) suppression of MDA levels (4.4±2.5) and a significant ($p=0.001$) diminution of SOD (1.59±0.33) and Gpx (2979±169) expenses versus placebo treatment pancreatitis group (9.7±3.8, 1.01±0.01 and 2299±114 respectively).
Conclusion: The results obtained from this rat model indicate that the widely accepted beneficial effects of octreotide in the development of acute experimental pancreatitis could be partly explained by its ability to reduce oxidative stress.

PP31

Tissue Factor in the Pathophysiology of Patients with Major Trauma - Role of NF-κB and AP-1

G. von Gagern[1], T. Zimmermann[1], M. Kotzsch[2], H. Zwipp[3], H.D. Saeger[1]

Department of Surgery[1], Institute of Pathology[2], Department of Traumatology[3], Technical University Dresden, Germany

Introduction: Tissue Factor (TF) is a cell surface glycoprotein in human cells. Together with Tumor Necrosis Factor alpha (TNF-α) are characterized as early immediate genes. TF is responsible for initiating the extrinsic pathway of coagulation that has been shown to have a role in the pathophysiology of sepsis. Investigations in animal models have shown that TF is involved in reaction after trauma.
Aims: Activated transcription factors (NF-κB and AP-1) were measured: we were looking for a link between TF levels and the outcome of patients with major trauma. Are the transcription factors activated? Are there differences between the *jun*- and the *fos* group?
Methods: We took blood samples from 50 polytraumatized patients during a period of 28 days after trauma. We measured TNF-α and IL-6 and the binding capacity of AP-1 and NF-κB. The patients were divided into survived and non-survived groups. The patients were scored with APACHE II and MOF-scores.
Results: A difference of more than 26 pg/ml in the TF levels divided the patients into surviving and non-surviving groups (Kaplan-Meier-Curve $p=0.03$). There were significant differences between NF-κB levels in both groups (2nd day $p=0.005$; 3rd day $p=0.05$). We measured higher AP-1 binding capacity in non-survived patients.
Conclusion: Non-surviving patients showed significant differences in TF levels and NF-κB binding capacity. The outcome of this patient group seems to be connected with transcription factors and the specific target genes. Further investigation will reduce the lethality of patients with major trauma.

PP32

ATP Synthase and Keratinocyte Growth Factor Gene Expression in Experimental Gastroesophageal Reflux Disease

K. Szentpáli[1], M. Széll[2], J. Kaszaki[3], G. Lázár[1], L. Kemény[4], A. Dobozy[4], Á. Balogh[1], M. Boros[3]

Department of Surgery[1], Dermatological Research Group of the Hungarian Academy of Sciences[2], Institute of Surgical Research[3], Department of Dermatology[4], University of Szeged, Szeged, Hungary

Introduction: We recently published our data on the effects of bile in a large animal model of acute esophageal reflux disease (GERD) and we have shown that bile, but not hydrochloric acid (HCl), evoked a significant (40%) decrease in the ATP level of the esophageal tissue (Szentpáli et al.: Scand. J. Gastroenterol. 36, 2001). With the next set of experiments we aimed to investigate the effects of bile alone, HCl, and combined bile/HCl treatments on ATP synthase gene expression changes. We were also interested in keratinocyte growth factor (KGF) gene expression changes induced by the above treatments, since the elevation of this epithelial cell-specific mitogen has been reported in inflammatory bowel disease (Finch, 1996) and in the intestinal mucosa as an adaptive response after malnutrition (Estivariz, 2000).
Methods: Tissue biopsies were obtained from saline-treated control; bile-treated (exposed to canine bile for 4 hr), HCl + bile, or HCl-treated animals, respectively. Approximately 1 cm^2 pieces of the canine esophagus were separated to mucosal and muscle layers and total RNA was isolated from them. Semi-quantitative reverse transcriptase polymerase chain reactions (RT-PCR) were carried out for the ß subunit of the ATP synthase gene (ß-ATPase) and KGF mRNAs, respectively.
Results: Bile, HCl and combined bile/HCl treatments induced more pronounced changes in the ß-ATPase gene expression in the muscle layer of the esophagus than in the mucosa. Bile treatment alone had the least effect on the ß-ATPase gene expression level in both tissue types (5% decrease in the mucosal layer and 35% decrease in the muscle layer as compared to the control treatment). HCl and bile/HCl treatments caused more severe decreases in both layers: the combined bile-HCl treatment resulted in a 46% decrease in the mucosa and 93% decrease in the muscle layer, while HCl alone decreased the ß-ATPase gene expression by 49% in the mucosa and 91% in the

muscle layer. Both bile and combined bile/HCl treatment caused significant decrease in KGF gene expression (40% and 12 % as compared to control tissues, respectively). However, HCl treatment alone almost completely abolished KGF mRNA from the tissue specimens.
Discussion: These data suggest that the level of ß-ATPase gene expression is more sensitive to external noxious stimuli in the muscle layer (characterized by very active metabolism) than in the resistant/ defensive mucosal layer. Our results show that the primary step of bile-induced ATP depletion is not the transcriptional down-regulation of ß-ATPase gene expression. In contrast with previous reports on elevated intestinal KGF gene expression in chronic mucosal inflammation and malnutrition we demonstrated that KGF mRNA level is decreased in the esophageal mucosa after acute bile or HCl treatment.
Conclusion: We conclude that bile, HCl and the combined bile/HCl treatment-induced necrotic processes are coupled with down-regulation of ß-ATPase and KGF gene expression in the esophageal mucosa in acute experimental GERD.

PP33

Pathophysiology of Decrease in Erythrocyte Deformability in Acute Pancreatitis

B. Chmiel, R. Grabowska-Bochenek, L. Cierpka, K. Zagalski

Clinic of General and Transplantation Surgery, Medical University of Upper Silesia, Poland

Introduction: Deformability of erythrocytes (RBC) is an important factor in maintenance of microcirculation. Reduced RBC deformability was found during sepsis and acute pancreatitis, too. The most common etiological factors of acute pancreatitis are ethanol and gallstones. Among determinates of severity of this disease hyperproteasemia, cytokines, platelet activating factor, oxygen free radicals and endotoxemia are cited. Hence the aim of this study was to examine the influence of most common etiological factors and determinants of severity of acute pancreatitis on erythrocyte deformability *in vitro*.
Methods: Washed erythrocytes obtained from five healthy volunteers were resuspended in phosphate buffered saline (pH 7.4, 290 mOsm) and incubated with addition of ethanol, acetaldehyde, bilirubin, sodium taurocholate, bovine trypsin (activity 3.5 IU/mg), lipopolisaccharide from *E. Coli* 0127:B8 (LPS), platelet activating factor (PAF), and free radical generating system hypoxantine+xantine oxidase. After 60 min erythrocyte deformability was measured by shear stress diffractometer Rheodyn SSD (Myrenne, Germany) and expressed as elongation index (EI) at shear stresses 0.3; 0.6; 1.2; 3.0; 6.0; 12.0; 30.0; 60 Pa.
Results: There were no changes in EI in any measured shear stresses after incubation with ethanol up to 2 promille, bilirubin up to 170 µmol or sodium taurocholate up to 2.7 mmol. After incubation of erythrocytes with 100 µg/ml trypsin an increase in elongation index at shear stresses between 1.2 and 12.0 Pa has been observed. Acetaldehyde in concentration up to 15 mmol, or 1 mmol hypoxantine + 0.2 IU/ml xantine oxidase caused decrease in EI of erythrocytes at shear stresses between 0.3-6.0 and 0.3-12.0 Pa, respectively, with no changes at higher shear stresses. Incubation with 100 µg/ml LPS or 10^{-7} mol PAF caused decrease in elongation index of erythrocytes at shear stresses 3.0-60 Pa and 6.0-60 Pa, respectively, with no changes in lower shear stresses.
Conclusion: Several factors which have significant contribution to the development of acute pancreatitis influence the erythrocyte deformability in different ways.

Shock and Ischemia-Reperfusion Injury

PP34

Formation of Peroxynitrite as a Result of Nitric Oxide-Superoxide Interaction in Ischemia and Reperfusion - A Clinical Trial

D. Ockert[1], T. Zimmermann[1], S. Kersting[1], S. Albrecht[2], H.D. Saeger[1]

Department of Visceral, Thoracic and Vascular Surgery[1], Department of Gynecology[2], Technical University Dresden, Dresden, Germany

Introduction: Peroxinitrite is one of the strongest oxidants formed in reperfusion after ischemia. It is produced from nitric oxide (NO) and reactive oxygen species and plays a crucial role in the damage of the capillary endothelium. In a clinical trial the authors investigated the role of the dynamic balance of NO and superoxide as an indirect marker of the peroxynitrite formation in the ischemia-reperfusion model.
Methods: In 40 patients undergoing a peripheral vascular reconstruction blood samples were taken pre-, intra- and postoperatively (1st - 7th POD). Levels of reactive oxygen species (O_2^-, H_2O_2) and NO were measured in the serum. These findings were compared to those in patients undergoing a liver resection with clamping of the hepatoduodenal ligament.
Results: In both groups of patients a biphasic curve for the measured parameters could be observed. It could be divided in an early onset phase after declamping and a late onset phase from 1st to 7th POD. In both groups the concentration of NO and superoxide reacted in an opposite sense. These findings were statistically significant.
Discussion and Conclusion: Ischemia-reperfusion models display a biphasic reaction which can be divided into an early and a late phase and does not depend on the type of the operation. There is a dynamic balance between NO and superoxide as an indirect sign of formation of peroxynitrite. Radical scavengers can be considered as therapeutic options using the protective effects of NO and a promotion of the sheltering mechanisms of the antioxidative properties of glutathion peroxidase which is dependent on selenium.

PP35

The Antioxidative Effect of DHEA-S *In Vitro* and *In Vivo* - Chemiluminometric Determination of Hydroperoxy-groups in Lipoproteins

T. Zimmermann[1], S. Albrecht[2], H.D. Saeger[1], W. Distler[2]

Department of Visceral, Thoracic and Vascular Surgery[1], Department of Gynaecology[2], Technical University Dresden, Dresden, Germany

Introduction: In order to clarify the mechanism of antiatherogenic action of several steroids, we investigated the effects of dehydroepiandrosterone sulphate (DHEA-S) on the photodioxygenation of human lipoproteins (LDL, HDL). First we found that up to 30 % of circulating DHEA-S in humans is located in lipoproteins which were separated by ultracentrifugation.
Methods: We have developed a new chemiluminometric detection method of hydroperoxy-groups in lipoproteins. The separated lipid particles were incubated with several amounts of DHEA-S (5-50 µmol/l) and treated for 30 min with UV light in presence of rose bengal and oxygen.
Results: The generated reactive singlet oxygen leads in a non-radical pathway to the formation of HOO-groups as primarily lipid peroxidation state. The chemiluminometric measuring signal was directly proportional to the concentration of HOO^- groups in the HDL and LDL fractions. We found a dramatic decrease in lipid peroxidation concerning both HDL and LDL in comparison to samples not incubated with DHEA-S. In cases of patients with aortic surgery we found a significant decrease of plasma DHEA-S and increase of androstendione. This effect could be verified by *in vitro* experiments. It was shown that one of the reaction products of the antioxidative pathway of DHEA-S is androstendione.
Conclusion: The protective role of DHEA-S may be caused by inhibition of lipid peroxidation via the singlet oxygen non-radical pathway *in vivo*.

PP36

Characterization of a Hemorrhagic/Traumatic Shock Model in Rats Mimicking Clinical Settings

L. Szalay[1,2], F. Umar[1], A. Khadem[1], C. Weber[1], M. Jafarmadar[1], H. Gasser[1], W. Fürst[1], H. Redl[1], S. Bahrami[1]

Ludwig Boltzmann Institute, Experimental & Clinical Traumatology[1], Vienna, Austria, Institute of Surgical Research[2], University of Szeged, Hungary

Background: Uncontrolled/controlled bleeding followed by adequate resuscitation are traditional models of experimental hemorrhagic shock. They do, however, not adequately reflect the clinical situations often associated with periods of low flow, which may alter targets for therapeutic strategies.
Aim: The present study was performed to establish and characterize a model of hemorrhagic/traumatic shock in rats, mimicking clinical settings.
Methods: Anaesthetized rats were bled to a mean arterial pressure (MAP) of 30-35 mmHg. After the onset of decompensation MAP was increased to 40-45 mmHg and maintained for 40 min (low flow state), followed by adequate resuscitation over 1 hr. In addition, the animals underwent a midline laparotomy at the onset of shock for 30 min. Groups of five animals each were sacrificed at the time of decompensation, end of low flow, and 3 and 24 hrs after resuscitation.
Results: Our data show a transient decrease in energy status during shock and low flow state, with restoration to the baseline values early after resuscitation. The characteristic infiltration of neutrophils into the lung starting already at the time of decompensation reached maximum levels early after resuscitation. An increased interleukin 6 (IL-6) mRNA gene expression in the lung tissue was found at the time of decompensation. However, tumor necrosis factor alpha (TNF-α) and inducible nitric oxide synthase mRNA increased after resuscitation reaching maximum levels at 24 hrs. Plasma IL-6 reached maximum levels at the end of low flow state, while TNF-α could not be detected at any time point. Metabolic parameters indicated abnormalities of liver and kidney function already at the time of decompensation.
Conclusion: The new hemorrhagic/traumatic shock model in rats, with a prolonged low flow state, proceeding adequate resuscitation, offers the opportunity to study more clinically adapted therapeutic measures.

PP37

Comparison of Granulocyte Activation and Leukocyte Adhesion Molecule Expression Through Acute Ischemia and Prolonged Reperfusion in Open and Closed Chest Dog Model

J. Lantos, G. Jancsó, M.T. Jaberansari, E. Rőth

Department of Experimental Surgery, Faculty of Medicine, Pécs University, Pécs, Hungary

Introduction: The role of leukocyte activation and migration during early reperfusion after myocardial infarction has been widely investigated and well documented. However, the extent and the time course of leukocyte function during late reperfusion, as well as the effect of applied model on this parameter is still unclear. The purpose of this study was to determine the time course of leukocyte adhesion molecule expression and the dynamism of granulocyte activation after myocardial ischemia followed by prolonged reperfusion in an open and closed chest model.
Methods: The left descending coronary artery (LAD) was occluded for 3 hours followed by 4-week reperfusion in dogs in an open chest (OC Group, n=9) and in a closed chest (CC Group, n=8) model. A left thoracotomy was performed and the left anterior descending coronary artery (LAD) was ligated just distal to the first diagonal branch by a suture thread in OC Group. LAD was occluded by a PTCA catheter in CC Group. Peripheral blood samples were collected before the operation, at the end of 3-hour ischemia, at the acute (5 and 60 min), subacute (1-3 days) and chronic periods (1, 2, 3 and 4 weeks) of reperfusion. Production of reactive oxygen species in whole blood was measured by luminol dependent chemiluminescence. Flow cytometry was used to measure CD11a expression of leukocytes in blood samples.

Results: The luminol dependent whole blood chemiluminescence started to increase during the acute reperfusion reaching its maximum (258.3±68.2%, $p<0.05$) on the second postoperative day in OC Group. In CC Group, however, it started to elevate only on the first day with a peak (288.2±85.9%, $p<0.05$) on the second postoperative day and normalised earlier than in OC Group. The elevation of CD11a expression was higher on all types of leukocytes in OC than in CC animals. The higher increase was observed on monocytes on the third postoperative day in both groups (241.9±61.3% vs. 203.6±31.4% ($p<0.05$)), and it remained on elevated level even after 4-week reperfusion (181.4±53.6% vs. 118.1±10.3%).

Discussion: Our results revealed that the oxidative burst preceded adhesion molecule expression in the phase of acute and subacute reperfusion. While the oxidative stress parameters normalised by the second postoperative week, the increased adhesion molecule expression during later reperfusion might indicate the prolonged healing of injured myocardium in which monocytes seemed to play a crucial role.

Conclusion: Similar changes in granulocyte activation and leukocyte adhesion molecule expression could be observed in OC and CC ischemia-reperfusion models. The greater surgical trauma in OC animals influenced the measured parameters mainly in the acute and subacute phase of reperfusion. (Supported by ETT 369-02 and OTKA-T3481)

PP38

Relative Antioxidant Activity in Relation with Renal Ischemia-Reperfusion Injury

K. Pető, V.A. Oláh, E. Bráth, I. Furka, I. Mikó*

Department of Operative Techniques and Surgical Research, Department of Pediatrics*, University of Debrecen, Medical and Health Science Center, Debrecen, Hungary

Introduction: In open renal surgery the renal artery is often clamped for different periods. Ischemia and the following reperfusion (I/R) may cause structural changes in the renal parenchyma. Allopurinol (AP) being an antioxidant can prevent tissue damage. In our experiment we evaluated the change in relative antioxidant activity (rAOA) to detect the renal damage and the effect of AP.

Methods: Experiments were performed on 34 mongrel dogs in intramuscular narcosis induced by Xylazine-Ketamine. The animals were divided into 3 groups. In the 1st group (Gr.1, n=13) the left renal artery was isolated and clamped for 45 minutes. In the 2nd group (Gr.2, n=12) 100 mg/kg AP was infused systematically 20 minutes before clamping. The 3rd was the sham-operated group (Gr.3, n=9) where only midline laparotomy was performed. Blood samples were taken preoperatively, at the beginning of the reperfusion, and also at 30, 60, 120 minutes, 1, 2, 3, 5, 7, 9 days after the reperfusion for determination of rAOA using a modified method of Stocks (by the inhibition of autooxidation of bovine brain homogenate). Statistical analysis was performed using the Student's t-test and the Mann Whitney Rank Sum test.

Results: In Gr.1 the mean value of rAOA decreased to 56% 120 minutes after the reperfusion and as an induction effect it began to increase 1 day later. After another 2 days it returned close to the initial range (79%). In Gr.2 and Gr.3 the tendency was similar but prolonged (Gr.2: decreased to 70% and returned to 94% on the 5th day, Gr.3: decreased to 73,5% one day after the reperfusion returning to 94% on the 9th day). The difference between the groups was not significant because of the high standard deviation. Statistically significant difference in the values was found only in Gr.1.

Discussion: The structure of enzymes and other antioxidants (SOD, catalase, GSH-Px) are damaged by free radicals formed during I/R. AP prevents the production of free radicals as it is a xanthin-oxidase inhibitor. The prolonged process of regeneration of AOA presented the harmful effect of I/R in Gr.1 and Gr.2. During regeneration of AOA the protective effect of AP can be observed. The mild decrease in rAOA in the control group can be explained by the effect of the surgical intervention.

Conclusion: The rAOA is a sensitive indicator of tissue damage caused by ischemia-reperfusion and is suitable for the demonstration of the protective effect of antioxidants. (This study was supported by research grants ETT 6003/1/2001 and OTKA T 032571/2000.)

PP39

Follow-Up of Red Blood Cell Deformability after Short Hindlimb Ischemia in Rat

N. Németh, T. Lesznyák, G. Ács, E. Bráth, I. Furka, I. Mikó

Department of Operative Techniques and Surgical Research, University of Debrecen, Medical and Health Science Center, Debrecen, Hungary

Introduction: Since the article of Reid and Dormándy (1976) the measurement of red blood cell (RBC) deformability is a well-known procedure to detect the effect of different hereditary and acquired diseases and injuries on erythrocytes. Although the relation between the ischemia-reperfusion injuries (IRI) and the RBC deformability is also well-known, the follow-up of these changes in small animals is raising new problems.

Methods: Our experiments were approved by the Committee of Animal Research of the University of Debrecen. 24 male CD outbred rats were subjected to unilateral hindlimb ischemia for 1 h (IR, n=6) by microvascular clips on femoral vessels, or to the same procedure with Allopurinol pretreatment (50 mg/kg) (AIR, n=8), or to sham operation (Sham, n=6) and to an absolute control (n=6). Measurement of erythrocyte deformability with FT-1 type Filtrometer by a special setting of measuring hematocrit (1%), and determination of hematological parameters were performed on every day during the survival period of one week. The Filtrometer determines two parameters: Relative Cell Transit Time (RCTT) in msec and Initial Relative Filtration Rate (IRFR).

Results: The RCTT parameter shows an increased level on 1st and 2nd postoperative days (8.15±3.15; 14.61±11.29 msec), which was not observable in the control, Sham or the AIR groups. The differences among the experimental groups are significant (on 1st postoperative day: IR vs control: $p=0.002$; IR vs Sham: $p=0.0091$; IR vs AIR: $p=0.0036$; on 2nd postoperative day: IR vs control: $p<0.0001$; IR vs Sham: $p=0.0003$; IR vs AIR: $p=0.0025$). Hematological parameters has been changed in the different groups similarly with the exceptions of Mean Corpuscular Hemoglobin (MCH) and Mean Corpuscular Volume (MCV) parameters. MCV and MCH values changed much more in both of the IR and the AIR groups than in the control or in the Sham groups.

Discussion: The special setting on measurement of RBC deformability gave possibility to follow up the changes in rats. A relative short ischemic period (1h) and the following reperfusion induced a decreased RBC deformability values on the 1st and 2nd postoperative days which could be prevented with Allopurinol probably through the free-radical pathways. These results are well correspondent to previous data of ours in the aspects of kidney, bowel and spleen surgery or amputate model in dogs. The background of the changes in MCV and MCH parameters in the IR and AIR groups may be found out in the fluid balance of the body, or in deviance of ion-shift caused by the IRI.
Conclusion: This study suggests that hemorheological status and its changes have great importance during the injuries, on the treatment and prospectively also in the rehabilitation. (This study was supported by The Ministry of Welfare Research Grant No. 6003/1/2001/ETT.)

PP40

Special Adaptation of Different Measuring Methods on Experimental Animals in the Aspect of Ischemia-Reperfusion Injuries

N. Németh, G. Ács, T. Lesznyák, G. Szabó, E. Bráth, K. Pető, A. Dán, J. Tumpek*, I. Furka, I. Mikó*

Department of Operative Techniques and Surgical Research, University of Debrecen, Medical and Health Science Center, Central Laboratory*, Kenézy Gyula County Hospital, Debrecen, Hungary

Introduction: Modelling of ischemia-reperfusion injuries (IRI) on experimental animals is a prominent part of surgical research. Free radicals and the different cascades induced by them result many changes in the tissues and in the hemorheological parameters. The follow-up of these deviations - in the view of the blood sample volume - and the physiological differences in the experimental animal species raise new problems. The purpose of our presentation is to summarize the adaptations of special techniques to measure the red blood cell deformability (RBCd), blood and plasma viscosity and the coagulation parameters in dogs, rats and rabbits.
Methods: 89 mongrel dogs, 22 rabbits and 52 rats were involved in the study and hindlimb ischemia for 1 and 3 hours was induced. FT-1 type Filtrometer was applied to determine the RBCd by Initial Relative Filtration Rate (IRFR) and Relative Cell Transit Time (RCTT) parameters. The system needs 600-700 μl erythrocyte suspension (by 2.1-2.5 ml blood) to set the measuring hematocrit to 5%. This relative large blood volume is not suitable for follow-up of changes in small animals day by day. We reduced the measuring hematocrit to 1%. In that case 0.5-0.6 ml blood is enough for the test. Hevimet-40 Capillary Viscosimeter was used to measure the whole blood and plasma viscosity. Hemostasis parameters was determined by Sysmex CA-530 Coagulometer (PT, APTT, TT, fibrinogen level). The proportion of the volumes of sample and reagent and buffer is different from the human practice. After the new settings we began to define a healthy control group among the dogs to determine the normalized ratio values later by PT.
Results: We found that the normal range of RCTT was 3.9-7.17 msec in dogs, 2.71-5.75 msec in rabbits and 1.6-4.31 msec in rats. RCTT parameter was increased on the 1st and 2nd postop. days in rat after 1 h ischemia and on 3rd and 5th postop. days in dogs after 3 h ischemia on hindlimb. The hindlimb ischemia increased the PT, APTI and TT and Fbg levels and the plasma viscosity in dogs from the 1st postoperative day to the 5th (normal value that we found: PT=6.1±0.76 sec; APTT=14.9±2.94 sec; TT=19.76±4.32 sec; Fbg=3.35±1.08 g/l).
Discussion: The results suggest that the relations among the IRI and the hemorheological and coagulation parameters are correspondent to each other and seem to be suitable for using in the experiments. The differences among the animal species suggest new questions to be answered in the future.
Conclusion: The special adaptations of these measuring techniques that we summarized are suitable to detect and follow up of changes caused by ischemia-reperfusion injuries. (This study was supported by OTKA No. T 032571/2000 and The Ministry of Welfare Research Grant No. 6003/1/2001/ETT.)

PP41

Endothelin-A Receptor Antagonism Reduces Torsion-Induced Aspermatogenesis and Microcirculatory Failure in the Rat

R. Varga[1], A. Szabó[1], M. Pákáski[2], Z. Bajory[3], L. Pajor[3], M. Boros[1]

Institute of Surgical Research[1], Department of Psychiatry, Alzheimer's Disease Research Centre[2], Department of Urology[3], University of Szeged, Szeged, Hungary

Introduction: Testicular torsion-induced germ cell loss represents an urology emergency of still high incidence. Regardless of the aggressive diagnostic and surgical management, biological function of the salvaged testes is often found to be considerably compromised. Previous investigations in laboratory animals demonstrated the role of endogenous endothelins in the pathogenesis of ischemia/reperfusion-induced tissue injury in other organs. The present study was undertaken to examine the early microcirculatory and late tissue protecting effects of endothelin-A receptor antagonism following experimental testicular torsion in anesthetized rats.
Methods: Early microcirculatory effects of testicular torsion were examined for 240 min after a one-hour testicular torsion. We used orthogonal polarization spectral imaging (OPS) technique to examine the changes in testicular capillary perfusion and fluorescence intravital microscopy to visualise the leukocyte-endothelial cell interactions. Germ cell-specific apoptosis was evaluated after 4 hr and 24 hr of reperfusion using the *in situ* TUNEL technique. Loss of the testis weight was used as a measure of torsion-induced atrophy 45 days after the ischemic insult. To examine the role of endogenous endothelin-1 in the pathogenesis of torsion-induced early microcircular and late biochemical reactions, rats received the selective endothelin ET-A receptor (ET-A) antagonist ETR-p1/fl peptide intravenously in a dose of 100 nmol/kg at the onset of reperfusion.
Results: Vasomotion / pulsatile microvascular flow, a characteristic feature of the intact testicular microcirculation, was eliminated by torsion and returned only in some of the experiments during the reperfusion period. Increasing number of primary and secondary leukocyte-endothelial interactions -rolling and sticking of leukocytes- was generally observed in subtunical venules. Although germ cell-specific apoptosis was not influenced by the ET-A antagonist, this treatment caused an earlier return of pulsatile microvascular flow, increased red cell velocity in the capillaries and significantly

reduced leukocyte rolling during the early post-torsion period. Long-term consequences of testicular torsion could also effectively be ameliorated by ET-A inhibition as evidenced by preserved testis weight values in response to this treatment.
Conclusions: The rescue of testis function provided by ET-A antagonism implicates the role of endogenous endothelin-1 in the pathogenesis of acute experimental torsion. The preserved flow and decreased local leukocyte activation may beneficially affect the long-term testicular function and ultimately fertility. (Supported by grant OTKA F 032069.)

PP42

Akt Activation Protects Rat Liver from Ischemia-Reperfusion Injury

N. Harada, E. Hatano, N. Koizumi, T. Nitta, M. Yoshida, N. Yamamoto, Y. Yamaoka

Department of Gastroenterological Surgery, Kyoto University, Graduate School of Medicine, Kyoto, Japan

Introduction: Mechanism of cell death during warm hepatic ischemia-reperfusion (I/R) is still controversial. We have shown that serine/threonine protein kinase Akt protects mouse hepatocytes from TNF-α and Fas-mediated apoptosis. The role of Akt during hepatic I/R is unclear. Our aims are to clarify the role of apoptosis and Akt activation and the effect of adenovirus-mediated expression of active Akt on hepatic I/R injury in the rats.
Methods: Hepatic I/R injury was induced by Pringle maneuver for 20 min followed by reperfusion in male SD rats. Replication-defective adenovirus encoding a constitutively active form of Akt (AdmyrAkt) or ß-galactosidase (AdLacZ) was injected through the tail vein at 72 hours before hepatic I/R.
Results: Western blots with phospho-Akt antibody demonstrated the activation of Akt 30 min to 2 hours after reperfusion, though there was no difference in the total Akt during hepatic I/R. Terminal deoxynucleotidyl transferase-mediated dUTP-biotin nick-end labeling (TUNEL) staining showed 3.2-fold increase in positive cells 2 hours after reperfusion, compared with those in control livers. Western blotting confirmed that the expression of the HA-tagged myrAkt construct and an increase in phosphorylated Akt at 72 hours after AdmyrAkt injection dose-dependently. HA immunostaining also showed myrAkt expression in both parenchymal and non-parenchymal cells in the rat liver 72 hours after AdmyrAkt injection. The number of TUNEL-positive cells decreased in AdmyrAkt-infected rats 2 hours after reperfusion (64% of control livers before ischemia, 20% of control livers 2 hours after reperfusion). Histological appearance of livers stained with hematoxylin and eosin demonstrated liver damage around the central veins observed in control and AdLacZ-infected rats was almost totally blocked in AdmyrAkt-infected rats. The increase in serum AST and ALT levels 2 hours after reperfusion was observed in control rats (1677±356 IU/L, 1761±671 IU/L, N=5) and AdLacZ-infected rats (1579±637 IU/L, 1528±671IU/L, N=4). However, adenovirus-mediated expression of myrAkt significantly attenuated the elevations of serum AST and ALT (666±438 IU/L, 297±131 IU/L, N=5, $p<0.05$).
Conclusion: Overexpression of myrAkt could inhibit apoptotic cell death and subsequent hepatic I/R injury in the rat. Akt may represent an important nodal target for prevention in hepatic I/R injury.

PP43

Lower Limb Ischaemia-Reperfusion Induced Remote Hepatic Injury Is Not Altered by Kupffer Cell Depletion

A. Lewis, D.W. Harkin, M. Hoper, F.C. Campbell, A.A.B. Barros D'Sa.

Department of Surgery, Belfast, Northern Ireland

Introduction: Limb ischaemia-reperfusion is associated with elevated levels of endotoxin in the portal circulation. We hypothesised that a resultant pro-inflammatory Kupffer cell response may contribute to hepatic injury.
Methods: Adult male Wistar rats were randomised to three groups (n=5); Control (anaesthesia only), 3 hours ischaemia followed by 2 hours reperfusion (I/R) and I/R with Kupffer cell ablation with gadolinium chloride ($GdCl_3$) 10mg/kg i.v., 24 hours prior to study. Serum aspartate aminotransferase (AST), alanine aminotransferase (ALT) and liver tissue´wet-dry ratio indicate remote hepato-cellular injury. Plasma IL-6 and TNF-α were measured by bioassay. Kupffer cell ablation was confirmed by immuno-histochemistry.
Results: I/R causes a significant rise in plasma AST 313 (257: 369) and ALT 100 (87: 139) compared to control AST 112 (98: 173) and ALT 80 (69: 86). ($p<0.05$) Treatment with gadolinium chloride did not alter the AST and ALT response, 291 (265: 359) and 125 (123: 134) respectively. Liver wet-dry ratio was unaffected after I/R with 3.56, (3.31: 3.60) or without 3.39, (3.28: 3.56) gadolinium chloride compared to control 3.28, (3.33: 3.41). Data represents median (1st quartile: 3rd quartile). Between group comparisons Mann Whitney U test was used.
Conclusion: Lower limb I/R is associated with remote liver injury. Depletion of Kupffer cells with gadolinium chloride does not alter this response.

Organ Transplantation

PP44

Urinary Trypsin Inhibitor (UTI) Exerts Protective Effects on the Hepatic Microvasculature in Hypotensive Brain-Dead Rats

T. Takahashi, K. Itabashi, Y. Ito, K. Sato, A. Kakita

Kitasato University Hospital, Dept. of Surgery, Sagamihara, Japan

Introduction: The use of liver allografts from brain-dead marginal donors has significantly increased recently, because of an increasing need for the organ and the decreasing number of donors. To utilize potential liver allografts from brain-dead donors, it is important to understand the pathophysiology of the brain-dead liver and to minimize the graft dysfunction during brain death. Thus, we examined protective effects of urinary trypsin inhibitor (UTI), a protease inhibitor, on the brain-dead liver associated with systemic hemodynamic instability.

Methods: Male rats (Lewis) were used in this study and were divided into the following 3 groups: 1) sham-operated rats, 2) untreated brain-dead rats, and 3) UTI-treated brain-dead rats. Brain-death was created by inflating a balloon catheter placed in the epidural space of the skull. UTI was i.v. administered at a dose of 100,000 units/kg/hr starting at the induction of brain death for 6 hours until the end of experiment. Hemodynamic parameters measured during the experiment included the mean arterial pressure (MAP: mmHg), heart rate (HR: beats/min) and hepatic tissue flow (HTF: ml/min/100g tissue). Biliary excretion rate as well as serum AST and ALT levels were determined, too. Serum levels of cytokine-induced neutrophil chemoattractant (CINC), TNF-α and IL-1β were also measured (ELISA). Furthermore, hepatic tissue specimens were subjected to neutrophil staining, immunohistochemical staining for ICAM-1, P-selectin and CINC, and transmission electron microscopy (TEM).

Results: The induction of brain death resulted in a significant decrease in both MAP and HTF (average 33% reduction from the baseline), and an increase in serum AST and cytokines such as TNF-α (1.8-fold) and CINC (4.2-fold). Also, an increased number of sequestered neutrophils (32.1±1.7/HPF vs. 10.8±0.8/HPF in sham-operated rats) and an enhanced expression of ICAM-1 and CINC were noted in the liver. Continuous intravenous administration of UTI to brain-dead rats significantly restored HTF to the basal level, without affecting the lowered MAP and the biliary excretion rate. Morphological examinations revealed that the UTI treatment decreased the number of sequestered neutrophils (20.1±1.7/HPF), and suppressed the expression of ICAM-1 and CINC in the sinusoids. It also decreased serum levels of TNF-α and CINC by 39.6% and 19.3%, respectively. TEM demonstrated that changes in Kupffer cells, such as cellular enlargement and a number of filopodia on the cell surface as well as phagosomes in the cytoplasm, were minimized to the degree comparable with those in sham-operated rats.

Conclusion: Intravenous administration of UTI is likely to attenuate insults to the hepatic microvasculature evoked by brain death, thereby effectively maintaining the functional integrity of liver allografts.

PP45

Diagnosis and Treatment for the Late Vascular and Biliary Complications after Living Donor Liver Transplantation

N. Kawagishi, N. Ohkohchi, S. Satomi

Division of Advanced Surgical Science and Technology, Tohoku University, Sendai, Japan

Introduction: As the number of LDLTx is accumulating, late-onset problems such as vascular and biliary complications should be recognized as important factors for the quality of daily life (QOL). In our institution we experienced 12 cases with late vascular and biliary complications out of 52 LDLTx patients and report the indication and outcome in this paper.

Methods: From July 1991 to December 2001, 52 cases of LDLTx were performed in our institution. Immunosuppression consisted of tacrolimus or cyclosporine, corticosteroids and in some cases azathioprine or mycophenolate mofetil. Late hepatic artery thrombosis (HAT) was defined as the complete disruption of arterial blood flow to the graft more than 1 month posttransplant and was identified by Doppler ultrasound and angiography. Late portal or hepatic vein stricture was defined as to have a narrow segment which congested the venous flow to or from the graft more than 1 month posttransplant and was identified by Doppler ultrasound, CT, angiography and histopathological findings. Late biliary stricture of the hepaticojejunostomy was diagnosed clinically, biochemically or radiologically after readmission. Ultrasonography was the initial radiologic investigation, followed by CT, biliary scintigraphy and percutaneous transhepatic cholangiography (PTC).

Results: One recipient was diagnosed as late HAT by angiography. She was asymptomatic and accidentally diagnosed. Her collateral circulation supplied enough arterial blood flow to the graft. Five recipients had late portal vein stricture and were treated by percutaneous transluminal angioplasty (PTA) or balloon dilatation through superior mesenteric vein operatively. They had symptoms such as intestinal bleeding and hypersplenism. Two recipients had late hepatic vein stricture and were treated by PTA. Five recipients had late biliary stricture and were treated by balloon dilatation and stenting in 2 cases, by revision of hepaticojejunostomy in 2 cases, by observation in 1 case.

Discussion and Conclusion: Although the mortality rate of late vascular and biliary complications are lower than that of early complications, they substantially influence the QOL after LDLTx. We need more intention on the diagnosis and treatment for late vascular and biliary complications.

PP46

Indication and Efficacy of Apheresis for the Liver Transplant Recipients - Experiences of 22 Cases in 52 LDLTx

N. Kawagishi, N. Ohkohchi, N. Koyamada, S. Sekiguchi, S. Tsukamoto, S. Satomi

Division of Advanced Surgical Science and Technology, Tohoku University, Sendai, Japan

Introduction: Apheresis has been recognized as the extracorporeal immunomodulation for the transplant recipients as well as the treatment of hepatic failure or hyperbilirubinemia. In our institution we experienced 22 cases with apheresis out of 52 LDLTx patients and report the indication and outcome in this paper.

Methods: I) Pre-Tx apheresis: Indications for the pretransplant apheresis were ABO incompatibility in 3 cases, crossmatch positivity in 2 cases, hyperbilirubinemia in 2 cases, acute renal failure in 1 case and hypercholesterolemia in 1 case. ABO incompatible recipients whose titer of IgM was more than 16 were the indication for apheresis. Plasmapheresis (PP) or double filtration plasmapheresis (DFPP) was performed on 3 consecutive days before transplantation for the recipients with ABO incompatibility and crossmatch positivity. They were also administered azathioprine 3 days before the transplantation followed by tacrolimus or cyclosporine, as well as methylprednisolone. II) Post-Tx apheresis: Indications for the posttransplant apheresis were graft, respiratory and cardiac failure in 12 cases, hyperbilirubinemia in 6 cases and acute renal failure in 2 cases.

Results: I) Pretransplant apheresis was performed in 9 cases, including PP in 7 cases, DFPP in 1 case, hemodialysis (HD) in 1 case, LDL apheresis in 1 case. All of the serum titers and scores were normalized and no adverse effect was observed such as septic episodes or coagulation disorders. II) Posttransplant apheresis was performed in

19 cases, including PP in 14 cases, continuous hemodiafiltration in 9 cases, plasma adsorption in 3 cases, extracorporeal ultrafiltration method in 2 cases, hemoadsorption in 1 case, continuous hemofiltration in 1 case and HD in 1 case. Survived case even with graft, respiratory and cardiac failure was only one of 12 patients. The most common reasons of liver failure in these recipients were vascular complications. For the patients of hyperbilirubinemia both PP and PA were effective and improved the critical condition.
Discussion and Conclusion: Preoperative reduction of preformed antibody titers by apheresis was successful. However, posttransplant apheresis is not the indication for the recipient who is under the condition of graft dysfunction with respiratory and cardiac failure.

PP47

Experimental Study on Hepatic Reinnervation after Orthotopic Liver Transplantation in Rats

I. Sakamoto, T. Takahashi, A. Kakita, I. Hayashi, M. Majima, S. Yamashina

Kitasato University Graduate School of Medical Science, Sagamihara, Japan

Introduction: The present study was conducted to examine whether or not extrinsic hepatic reinnervation occurred after orthotopic liver transplantation (OLT) in rats.
Methods: Inbred male Lewis rats were used as recipients and females as donors. Tissue specimens were obtained postoperatively until 6 months after OLT from the stump of recipients' hepatoduodenal ligament (A), the hepatic hilus (B), and the liver parenchyma (C). The specimens were subjected to immunohistochemical examination using growth-associated protein (GAP)-43 as axonal marker and transmission electron microscopy (TEM) for observing regenerating axons, as well as the polymerase chain reaction assay for detecting the rat sex-determining region Y (SRY) protein gene of the regenerating nerves.
Results: At site A, GAP-43-positive nerve axons were identified from 1 day to 1 month post-OLT, and SRY protein gene was expressed at and after 3 days post-OLT. At site B, GAP-43-positive axons were observed between 3 days and 1 month, and SRY protein gene was detected at 1 month post-OLT and thereafter. TEM confirmed the presence of regenerating axons at and after 3 days post-OLT.
Conclusion: The results demonstrate that extrinsic innervation occurs immediately after OLT and is likely to terminate in about 3 months in rat liver allografts.

PP48

Dual Kidney Transplantation in the Use of Marginal Donors

R. Cadrobbi, N. Baldan, M.L. Valente, S. Scapin, F. Marchini, L. Dall'Olmo, E. Ancona, P. Rigotti

Clinica Chirurgica IV, Dept. of Medical and Surgical Sciences, University of Padua, Italy

Purpose: With a view to extending the use of cadaveric donors with a poor organ function in the kidney transplantation setting, both kidneys can be transplanted into a single recipient as a dual transplant. We evaluated the outcome of our dual kidney transplant (DKT) program that started in 1999.
Methods: From October 1999 to December 2001 19 DKT were performed at our center. The eligibility criteria for marginal donors were: age >60 years, creatinine clearance 165 ml/min/1.73m^2 and/or long-standing hypertension and/or diabetes and/or proteinuria (>60 years, mean 66±5 years) transplanted in the same period (control group).
Results: After an average follow-up of 15 months (range 3-25), all DKT recipients are alive (patient survival=100%) and 18/19 have functioning grafts (graft survival=95%). In one patient one graft was immediately removed because of poor revascularization and the other graft never functioned. Acute tubular necrosis developed in 9 patient, requiring a mean of 3 hemodialysis sessions per patient. We observed 3 early surgical complications: one urinary leakage due to ureteral necrosis (requiring kidney removal) and two wound infections. Acute rejection was experienced by 3/19 patient and these episodes were steroid-sensitive. The mean hospital stay was 26 days. The average serum creatinine (S-Cr) was 183±102 μmol/L after 1 month, 149±59 μmol/L after 3 months and 152±63 μmol/L after 6 months. In the control group, patient and graft survival were 88 and 83%, respectively. Renal function was worse among controls after 1 month (S-Cr=269±21 μmol/L) and 3 months (S-Cr=170±56 μmol/L), but similar at 6 months (S-Cr=160±46 μmol/L).
Conclusions: Transplant function and survival of patients after DKT indicate that this procedure is suitable in the case of marginal donors, giving access to an expanded pool of cadaveric organs without exposing recipients to a major risk of acute rejection, surgical complications or worse renal function.

PP49

Omental Flap Harvesting for Free Transplantation. Preliminary Data on the Operative Technique in Dogs

J. Papp Szekeres[1], I. Furka[2], M. Svébis[1], T. Cserni[3], E. Bráth[2], N. Németh[2], I. Mikó[2]

Bács-Kiskun County Teaching Hospital[1], Department of General Surgery, Kecskemét, Department of Operative Techniques and Surgical Research[2], Department of Pediatrics[3], Division of Surgery, University of Debrecen, Medical and Health Science Center, Debrecen, Hungary

Introduction: The purpose of our presentation is to report initial experimental results on the development of an omental flap free transplantation technique by microsurgical methods for supporting the circulation of an extra abdominal segmental blood supplied organ (esophagus).

Methods: We performed operations on five dogs using adequate premedication and general anesthesia, adhering to the rules of the University of Debrecen Committee of Animal Research. A free omental graft based on the gastroepiploic vessels was harvested from the abdomen and was transferred to the lateral region of the neck. During the procedure the isolated vascular pedicle was irrigated with an experimentally developed solution containing pentoxyphillin (0.2 mg/ml), vitamin E (0.06 mg/ml), vitamin C (0.2 mg/ml), heparin (100 IU/ml) and cooled to 20°C. A microvascular running end-to-side anastomosis was performed between the graft vessels and common carotid artery, jugular vein at the recipient site.

Results: The optimal technique of obtaining the omental flap has been worked out with the development of adequate anastomosing and sewing methods and the preservation technique to avoid the ischemia-reperfusion damage. Our results compared with the data of the unique publication of Daren et al. indicate significant improvements in some of the most important factors. With the help of our method the duration of the operation was reduced from 4 hours to 2, and the anastomosing time from 1 hour to 30 minutes, respectively. The average graft ischemic time was reduced to 45 minutes.

Discussion and Conclusion: Omental flap free transplantation by microsurgical methods is feasible in dogs. The next stage of our experiment is to develop the appropriate method to control the viability and function of the transplanted omental flap. Further studies may result in a clinically useful technique for recovering the blood supply of the extra-abdominal organs. (This study was supported by OTKA No. T 034211/2001 and The Ministry of Welfare Research Grant No. 6003/1/2001/ETT.)

PP50

Histologic Findings in Small Bowel Tissue Following Pancreatico-Duodenal Allotransplantation with Venous Drainage into the Portal or Systemic Circulation

U.J. Hesse, D. Meester, R. Troisi, B. de Hemptinne, P. Pattyn, H. van Vlierberghe, M. de Vos, N. Lameire, C. Cuverlier

University Hospital, Department of Surgery, Ghent, Belgium

Introduction: Composite pancreatico-duodenal transplantation is performed with increasing success in type I diabetics with or without end stage renal failure and exceptionally in patients suffering from pancreatic exocrine insufficiency. Despite extensive knowledge on the historical pattern of pancreatic exocrine and endocrine tissue under various conditions there is only scarse information about the histological changes in the small bowel tissue compartment of these grafts following transplantation. It was the purpose of this study to analyse histological specimens of the intestinal tissue taken at various events to be correlated with the clinical course of the patients.

Patients and Methods: Between 5/1994 and 10/2001 a total of 47 [32 males (68.1%)/15 females (31.9%), age 42±7.5 years] transplantations of composite pancreatico-duodenal allografts were performed at our institution. Exocrine drainage was performed by duodenocystostomy in 12 (25.5%) and by duodenojejunostomy in 35 (74.5%) patients. 7 (14.9%) grafts had porto-portal venous drainage and the remaining were performed as porto-systemic drainage. Immunosuppression consisted of Neoral or Tacrolimus in combination with Mycophenolate mofetil and low dose steroids. All patients received induction therapy using monoclonal or polyclonal antibodies. Rejection was diagnosed by biopsy of the transplanted graft and on clinical grounds and treated appropriately. Histology was performed using HE and immunohistochemical staining with a panel of monoclonal antibodies to evaluate antigen presentation and the presence of immune cells.

Results: After a median follow up of 24 months (1-79) all patients 100% are alive. A total of 4 (8.5%) grafts had to be removed (3 thrombosis, 1 infection). 3 (6.4%) had to be treated for rejection, 3 (6.4%) patients underwent conversion from bladder to intestinal drainage. Histology showed necrosis in thrombosed grafts and inflammation in infected grafts. In the converted patients no histological signs of rejection were present correlating with the clinical course comparable with specimens taken after preservation and at reperfusion.

Conclusion: The histological findings (normal, rejection and infection) in the small bowel compartment of pancreatico-duodenal allotransplants under Tacrolimus/Cyclosporine therapy correlated well with the clinical course of the patients and graft function 1-79 months post transplantation indicating the usefulness of small intestinal biopsies in this subset of patients.

Circulation

PP51

Pharmacological and Ischemic Preconditioning of Pig Hearts in the Working Heart Model

W. Beierlein, A.M. Scheule, J. Haas, D. Jost, H.P. Wendel, G. Ziemer

Klinik für Thorax-, Herz- und Gefäßchirurgie, Universitätklinikum Tübingen, Tübingen, Germany

Introduction: Ischemic preconditioning increases the myocardial ischemic tolerance. Heat shock proteins (HSP) initiate this mechanism. Herbimycin A induces HSP *in vitro* in cardiomyocytes. The aim of this study was to examine in a big animal model whether this protective effect is inducible *in vivo* by Herbimycin A.

Methods: 21 piglets (10.6±1.2 kg) were divided into the groups no preconditioning (NP=control), ischemic preconditioning (IP), and pharmacological preconditioning (PP, n=7 each). Herbimycin A was given 16 h before cardiac donor explantation. In the ischemic group one diagonal branch was ligated three times for the duration of 3 min and in intervals of 5 min before preexplantation cardioplegia (5 min, cold, antegrade, blood). All hearts were explanted and stored for 90 minutes. After reperfusion with homologous pig blood stroke-work-index (SWI) was measured continuously in an *ex situ* working heart model for two hours. Samples for morphological and biochemical parameters were taken before ischemia, and two hours later (myocardial water content, light microscopy for hypercontraction bands and apoptotic cells, HSP70, Troponin-I).

Results: During the first 30 min working heart, the SWI was significantly higher in the IP-group (8.6±4.6 10^3dyn×cm×beats-1×g^{-1}) than in the other groups (PP: 6.4±4.6; NP: 6.3±3.6; $p<0.001$). Immediately after ischemia, the coronary venous Troponin-I levels were lowest in IP with a median of 2.3 ng/ml (interquartile range 1.8-2.7); PP: 7.7 (3.8-12.2); NP: 5.3 (3.6-11.9); $p<0.044$. All further parameters did not differ between groups.

Conclusion: Myocardial protection by ischemic preconditioning is effective. The agent Herbimycin A does not work for pharmacologic preconditioning *in vivo*.

PP52

Selective and Immediate Neuronal Injury during Cardiac Surgery in Domestic Pig

Z. Tóth, I. Győrimolnár, Á. Hevesi, L. Papp*

Department of Cardiac Surgery, University of Pécs and Institute of Diagnostic Imaging, Faculty of Animal Science, University of Kaposvár*, Hungary

Introduction: Cerebral complications constitute the leading source of morbidity and disability after cardiac operations. Air introduced into the cardiac chambers during open heart surgery can embolize to the brain. Since air requires a considerable time to dissolve in the blood, air embolism can be considered a form of transient ischaemia, where the duration of vascular obstruction is long enough to cause infarction. Using an appropriate pig model of cardiopulmonary bypass (CPB), we investigated the acute and chronic effects of open heart surgery on neuronal integrity and survival in the hippocampus, prefrontal and cerebellar cortex via molecular and neuroanatomical methods.

Methods: The overall strategy was to compare the presence of neuronal injury in three experimental groups: controls (n=3), sham-controls was maintain CPB without open heart surgery (n=3), CPB with open heart surgery in different survival time (n=9). Basic dye and special silver staining were used as a reliable method to demonstrate immediate neuronal injury. Determination of DNA fragmentation, biotinylated dUTP were used for nick-end labeling of apoptotic cells mediated by terminal deoxytransferase. Ultrathin sections were obtained from tissue blocks to those containing argyrophilic neurons and examined with transmission electron-microscope. Counting Nissl-stained neurons, sections were analysed with computer assisted semi-quantitative neuronal analysis.

Results: Sections from both of the control groups did not contain affected neurons. Ischaemia following open heart surgery resulted in numerous hyper-basophilic, argyrophilic, shrunken and hyper-electrondense neurons in discrete regions of the prefrontal and cerebellar cortex; within 1 hr of the surgery and can be detected 24 hrs after. In addition, a significant proportion of neurons in the hippocampal CA3 and CA1 pyramidal cell layer was affected. These morphopathological changes of neurons were not accompanied by *in situ* end-labeling. By 4 weeks after the surgery, no significant neuronal dropout in these regions was evident.

Discussion: Transient ischaemia following open heart surgery alters immediately the structure of selected neuronal populations in the hippocampus, prefrontal and cerebellar cortex. The injured neurons scattered among unaffected cells of the same type. The distribution of affected neurons provides the first reported topographical "map" of neuronal vulnerability to open heart surgery. In regions where the physicochemical changes induced by ischaemia are highly abundant, few neurons manifest apoptotic changes.

Conclusion: An appropriate approach to therapeutic and preventive strategies requires a fitting sense of proportion and an understanding of the mechanisms of neuronal injury during cardiac surgery. The goal of the current study was to investigate potential acute neuronal injury induced by open heart surgery during CPB, to define the topographical distribution of vulnerable neurons, and to determine whether immediate neuronal injury after CPB produces significant cell loss.

PP53

Microcirculatory Changes in Ischemia-Reperfusion-Induced Cystitis in Rats

Z. Bajory[1,2], J. Hutter[1], F. Krombach[1], K. Messmer[1]

Institute for Surgical Research[1], University of Munich, Klinikum Grosshadern, Germany, Department of Urology and Institute of Surgical Research, University of Szeged[2], Hungary

Purpose: The aim of the study was to determine the microcirculatory disturbances of ischemia-reperfusion-induced cystitis in a rat model using intravital fluorescence video-microscopy.

Methods: Sprague-Dawley rats were used for the experiments. After intraperitoneal pentobarbital anesthesia, a midline laparotomy was performed and the bladder was exteriorized. The urethra was ligated and the ureters were dissected. The intravesical pressure was monitored via a catheter inserted into the bladder dome. In ten animals, 60 minutes of warm ischemia of the bladder was induced by clamping both cystic artery branches. After 30 minutes of reperfusion, macromolecular leakage, leukocyte-endothelial cell interactions, venular red blood cell velocity, functional capillary density, as well as arteriolar and venular diameters were determined on the bladder wall by *in vivo* fluorescence (FITC, rhodamine 6G) video-microscopy. Macrohemodynamic parameters were assessed during the experiments. Sham-operated animals served as controls (n=10). A Mann-Whitney rank sum test was applied for statistical analysis. Mean values and standard deviations are given.

Results: Ischemia-reperfusion significantly increased the numbers of rolling and firmly adherent leukocytes in postcapillary venules by about 527% and 4637%, respectively. The venular red blood cell velocity and functional capillary density decreased from 1.16 mm/s and 145 1/cm to 0.42 mm/s and 41.2 1/cm, respectively. The arteriolar and venular macromolecular leakage was also significantly increased to about 133% of the control values. The arteriolar and venular diameters also were reduced by about 27%.

Conclusion: Ischemia-reperfusion caused inflammatory reactions and microcirculatory failure in the urinary bladder. This study targets the microcirculatory consequences of I/R-induced cystitis using *in vivo* fluorescence microscopy. Since the parameters investigated here are relevant not only for ischemia-reperfusion of the urinary bladder, but also for cystitis caused by other stimuli, this model represents a novel tool in the field of inflammation research in urology. (Supported by EUSP and OTKA: F 032069)

PP54

Strain and Physical Activity: Determinants of Lymph Drainage in Murines

M. Ionac, D. Bordos

'Pius Branzeu' Center for Laparoscopic Surgery and Microsurgery, Surgical Clinic 2, "Victor Babes" University of Medicine and Pharmacy, Timisoara, Romania

Introduction: Studies in immunology, pharmacology and haematology require the sampling of total lymph output of the thoracic duct (TD) in the awake and unrestrained rat. Since the first report by Bollman, several approaches have been used for cannulation of the TD in small laboratory animals. Some of them, however, are characterised by a modest reproducibility and a low lymph flow rate.
Aim of the study: We describe improved techniques for obtaining thoracic duct lymph (TDL) in both rats and mice.
Methods: The TD cannulations were done in 12 Sprague-Dawley rats and in 7 C57Bl/6 mice (average preoperative weight of 305 and 16 g, respectively). We used 0.9 mm and 0.6 mm outer diameter silicone tubing. Postoperatively, animals were not (rats) or only partially restrained (mice), allowing an increased mobility and consequently a constant lymph flow.
Results: Surgery ranged from 30 to 45 minutes. Intra- and postoperative mortality rate was zero. Rats yielded a mean of 45.6 ml/day TDL over 7 days (14.9% of the mean body weight), while the lymph output in mice reached unexpected volumes of 29.3 ml/day over 3 days (183.1% of the mean body weight).
Conclusions: The use of an operating microscope, silicone cannula and the maintaining of mobility of the animals during lymph collection prove to offer a reliable method for a high and constant output of TDL. Interestingly, we have detected strain dependent differences in the anatomy of the thoracic duct in the mouse, which have to be considered when cannulation procedures are attempted. Further aspects of the rat TD anatomy have been also described.

PP55

Effects of Extracellular Magnesium Concentration on Inflammatory Stimulus Induced Enhancement of Granulocyte MAC-1 Avidity and Affinity

H. Habazettl, A. Vogel, S. May, M. Gründel, W.M. Kuebler, H. Kuppe

Department of Physiology, Freie Universität Berlin and Department of Anesthesiology, Deutsches Herzzentrum Berlin, Germany

Introduction: Magnesium (Mg^{2+}) may protect cardiac surgery patients from myocardial reperfusion injury. However, post-operative outcome is also jeopardized by systemic inflammatory response syndrom (SIRS). Activation and endothelial adhesion via MAC-1 of polymorphonuclear granulocytes (PMNs) are considered to contribute to SIRS. While function MAC-1 (CD11b/CD18), is critically dependent on divalent cations such as Ca^{2+} or Mg^{2+}, suggesting a synergistic effect of both ions (Lundgren et al., J. Leukoc. Biol. 51:603-8, 1992), Mg^{2+} might also act as a Ca^{2+} antagonist that attenuates PMN adhesion. We, therefore, studied the effect of different Mg^{2+} concentrations on MAC-1 expression and binding affinity in cytokine stimulated PMNs.
Methods: 10 ml of peripheral venous blood from healthy volunteers (n=7) were centrifuged and the buffy coat was removed and washed in PBS. The cell pellet was resuspended in PBS containing 1.25 mM Ca^{2+} and 0.625, 1.25, 2.5, 5, or 10 mM Mg^{2+}. Cell suspensions were incubated at 37°C for 10 min, stimulated for another 10 min with the cytokine TNF-α (100 U/ml), the chemotactic peptide fMLP (25 pmol/ml), or the protein kinase C (PKC) activator PMA (5 pmol/ml). Reactions were stopped with 200 μl of 1% sodium azide, the cells were washed and incubated for 30 min at 4 °C with the respective antibodies: MAC-1 expression, Phycoerythrin labeled monoclonal mouse IgG anti-human CD11b (Becton Dickinson, San Jose, CA); MAC-1 affinity, monoclonal antibody CBRM1/5 (recognizes high affinity state of MAC-1, gift from TA Springer, J. Cell. Biol. 120:545-56,1983). Binding of antibodies to PMNs was then measured by FACS analysis.
Results: Stimulation induced increase in fluorescence units is given in percent of unstimulated control. All data are means±SEM; *$p<0.05$ by Repeated Measures ANOVA on Ranks. Mg^{2+} had no major effect on the TNF or fMLP induced increase of expression or affinity of MAC-1. In contrast, PMA induced increase in MAC-1 expression was concentration dependently reduced from 203±62 at 1.25 to 139±33 and 98±29 at 5 and 10 mM Mg^{2+}. Similarly, the PMA mediated increase in MAC-1 binding affinity was significantly attenuated by 5 and 10 mM Mg^{2+} from 139±42 at 1.25 mM to 93±37 and 68±28.
Discussion: Independently from mode of stimulation or Mg^{2+} concentration, MAC-1 avidity and affinity are altered concurrently. Mg^{2+} supplementation does neither exacerbate nor attenuate the cytokine induced activation of PMN.
Conclusions: The selective effect of Mg^{2+} only after direct PKC activation suggests alternative signalling pathways for receptor mediated PMN activation.

PP56

Effects of Celecoxib on the Synovial Microcirculation in Mouse Antigen-Induced Arthritis

H. Gebhard, H.J. Refior, K. Messmer, A. Veihelmann

Department of Orthopedics and Institute for Surgical Research, Ludwig-Maximilians-University of Munich, Munich, Germany

Introduction: Non-steroidal anti-inflammatory drugs (NSAID) are established in the treatment of rheumatoid arthritis. To minimize gastrointestinal side effects of NSAIDs selective cyclooxygenase-2 (COX-2) inhibitors such as Celecoxib have been developed. However, it has been shown *in vitro* that COX-2 also might play a protective role by limiting adhesion molecule expression (e.g. VCAM-1, ICAM-1). The aim of this study was to investigate the course of swelling and leukocyte-endothelial cell interaction of the synovium in mouse antigen-induced arthritis (AiA) *in vivo*.
Methods: Balb/c-mice were allocated to 4 groups (n=8). After induction of AiA in the left knee joint one group received Celecoxib (30 mg/kg BW in 0.3 ml solution) intragastrically by gavage twice per day, another arthritic group was treated the same way using saline.

Two more groups served as non-arthritic controls and were treated the same way as described above. On day 14 after AiA-induction, the patella tendon of the left knee joint was microsurgically resected under general anesthesia and measurements were performed by means of intravital fluorescence microscopy. Afterwards, animals were sacrificed and the knee joint was removed for histology.
Results: The arthritic animals treated with Celecoxib revealed a significant reduction of the rolling leukocyte fraction as well as of the number of leukocytes adherent to the endothelium of postcapillary venules (0.25±0.1 versus 96±34 mm^2) in comparison to the untreated animals with AiA (0.44±0.03 versus 206±22 mm^2). Furthermore, swelling of the arthritic knee joint was significantly reduced after treatment with Celecoxib.
Conclusion: Celecoxib effectively reduces swelling and leukocyte-endothelial cell interactions in mouse AiA. We found no evidence for a protective role of COX-2 in AiA.

PP57

Comparison of the Circulatory Effects of Different Hypertonic Colloid Volume Expanders

E. Eszlári, E. Csonka, J. Kaszaki, G. Molnár, A. Szabó, M. Boros*

Institute of Surgical Research, University of Szeged and Department of Surgery, County Hospital, Szentes*, Hungary

Introduction: Small volumes of hypertonic crystalloid-colloid fluids applied for resuscitation in circulatory disturbances effectively restore cardiovascular function and have a vasodilator effect. However, there are conflicting data on the myocardial effects of different types of colloid components. In the present study we compared the circulatory responses after hypertonic saline-dextran (7.5% NaCl-10% dextran; HSD) and hypertonic saline-hydroxyethylstarch (7.5% NaCl-6% hydroxyethylstarch; HES), central and peripheral hemodynamic parameters following thoraco-laparotomy in a large animal model.
Methods: The experiments were performed on pentobarbital-anesthetized, thoraco-laparotomized mongrel dogs. Mean arterial pressure (MAP), pulmonary arterial pressure (PAP) cardiac output (by thermodilution method) were monitored and total peripheral resistance (TPR) and heart rate (HR) were calculated. Myocardial contractility was estimated from the slope of the left ventricular end-systolic pressure-diameter relationship by monitoring left ventricular pressure and left ventricular diameter with a catheter-tip micromanometer and a pair of ultrasonic crystals sutured onto the myocardium, respectively. The animals were divided into three groups. Test solutions were infused 30 min after surgery. Group 1 served as the saline-treated control (n=5). Group 2 (n=7) and Group 3 (n=5) were given 4 ml/kg HSD or HES solutions i.v. for 15 min. Following the volume expander treatment hemodynamic parameters were monitored for 2 hrs. Non-parametric statistical tests were used, p values < 0.05 were considered significant.
Results: This major surgical procedure decreased cardiac output by approx. 30% in all groups. HSD and HES infusions caused a significant, 60-min elevation in MAP, cardiac output and PAP. In Group 2 myocardial contractility, TPR and HR increased significantly; while in HES-treated animals TPR stayed at baseline level but myocardial contractility and HR decreased significantly at the end of the resuscitation period as compared to the baseline.
Discussion: Our results demonstrate that HSD solution effectively restores cardiovascular function after surgical trauma while HES (containing 6% hydroxyethylstarch) can have unfavourable side-effects due to the depressed cardiac contractility.
Conclusion: We suggest that HES should be given after individual titration and not in a fixed dosage. (Supported by research grant OTKA T037835)

PP58

Co-Localization of the Vanilloid VR1 and Trka Receptors and Substance P in Neurons of the Cochlear and Vertebro-Basilar Arteries

Z. Vass[1,2], P.S. Steyger[2], D.R. Trune[2], A.L. Nuttall[2,3]

Department of Otolaryngology[1], Szeged University, Hungary, Oregon Health Sciences University[2] Portland, OR, USA, Kresge Hearing Research Institute, Department of Otolaryngology[3], University of Michigan, Ann Arbor MI, USA

Introduction: Evidence suggests the trigeminal ganglion innervates spiral modiolar artery (SMA), radiating arteriole and stria vascularis in cochlea. However, it is not known if the components of sensory fiber capsaicin (VR1), TrkA receptors, and substance P (SP) co-localize in cerebral blood vessels [e.g., basilar artery (BA)] or in vessels of the cochlea. Therefore the distribution of TrkA, SP and VR1 was investigated by triple immunolabeling to determine the anatomical and functional relationship between the cochlea, vertebrobasilar, and trigeminal sensory fiber system.
Methods: Immunolocalization of VR1, SP and Trka was demonstrated in albino guinea pigs. The BA, anterior inferior cerebellar arteries (AICA), SMA, radiating arterioles, were isolated, fixed and incubated with anti-VR1 antibody and visualized with Fluorolink Cy-5TM conjugated to streptavidin. Tissues were also incubated with anti-SP antibody and labeled with FITC conjugated secondary IgG; and with TrkA antibody and labeled with Alexa-568 conjugated IgG. Tissue labeling were analyzed with a Bio-Rad confocal laser microscope system.
Results: VR1, SP and TrkA co-localization occurred in axons within the adventitia layer of BA, AICA, SMA and radiating arterioles of the cochlea. The TrkA receptor immunolabeled fibers always co-expressed VR1 and SP. However, not all VR1 and SP-labeled fibers were labeled for TrkA receptors.
Discussion: That difference may demonstrate two subtypes of sensory neurons differentiated by trophic factor dependence. TrkA labeling in the adult cochlea is a novel finding. We have previously reported sensory innervation between the trigeminal ganglion and the cochlea (Vass et al., Neuroscience 79:605-615, 1997; Neuroscience 84:559-567, 1998). The triple labeling of SP, TrkA and VR1 supports the hypothesis that sensory c-type fibers innervate the cochlea.
Conclusion: Our results provide an anatomical basis for a relationship between the vertebro-basilar type of headache and inner ear vascular disturbances. It is possible that vertigo, tinnitus, and hearing deficits associated with migraine could arise by excitation (as hypersensitivity) of cochlear directed trigeminal ganglion C-type sensory neurons. (Acknowledgments: The present work was supported by

NIH Grants, R01 DC00105, R01 DC03573, Fogarty International Research Collaboration Award R03 TW00502, R21 DC03955, OTKA T022363, T026025, Hungary and by Soros Foundation, Hungary.)

Traumatology and Tissue Repair

PP59

Promotive Effects of Far-infra Red Ray on Full-Thickness Skin Wound Healing

H. Toyokawa, Y. Masui, H. Tsuchiya, S. Teshima, H. Nakanishi, A.H. Kwon, Y. Azuma, T. Nagaoka**, Y. Ogawa**, Y. Kamiyama*

First Department of Surgery, Kansai Medical University, Moriguchi City, Osaka, Japan. Sagano Co., Ltd.*, Kobe City, Hyogo, Japan. Kyodo Byori**, Kobe City, Hyogo, Japan.

Introduction: Far-infrared ray (FIR) is one of the electromagnetic waves from the sun. Accumulated evidence indicates that FIR is biologically active. However, the biological effects of FIR on whole organisms remain poorly understood. We examined the effect of FIR irradiation on full-thickness skin wounds.
Materials and Methods: A full-thickness skin wound (diameter, 15 mm) was prepared on the dorsal wall of Sprague-Dawley rats. To evaluate the effect of irradiation of FIR, the speed of wound healing was compared among 3 groups of animals. The Control Group was kept until the end of the experiment on a normal rack in the absence of FIR (24~25 °C), while Experimental Group A was constantly exposed to FIR at an ambient temperature (26.5~27.5 °C). Experimental Group B was kept on the rack in the absence of FIR but at the same temperature as Experimental Group A. Skin blood flow was measured using a contact laser flowmeter before and during FIR irradiation at ambient temperature. Ten rats in each group were sacrificed on days 1, 3, 5, and 7, respectively, and histologic inspections of the skin wound performed. Sections of wound tissue were stained with hematoxylin-eosin (H&E) and toluidine blue. Furthermore, we performed Mallory's collagen fiber staining and immunohistochemical staining for transforming growth factor (TGF)-ß1.
Results: The wound rapidly healed on day 7 in Experimental group A, compared with the control group and Experimental group B. However, there was no significant difference in the speed of healing between the Control Group and Experimental Group B. There was no significant change in skin blood flow and no elevation of skin temperature before and during FIR irradiation. Histologic findings revealed greater collagen regeneration, fibroblast infiltration, and production of TGF- ß1 in wounds of Experimental Group A than in the other groups.
Discussion and Conclusion: FIR irradiation can increase fibroblast activity and the topical production of TGF-ß1, a cytokine that is known accelerate wound healing. These results suggest that FIR might have promotive effects on skin wound healing. Therefore, FIR irradiation may be clinically useful for wound treatment.

PP60

Therapeutic and Prophylactic Management of Silicone Gel Sheeting (Epiderm) in Hypertrophic and Keloid Scarring

O. Kelemen, L. Kollár, K. Szilágyi

Baranya County Hospital, Surgical Department of Medical School, Pécs, Hungary

Introduction: The silicone gel sheeting (SGS) was first reported to be an effective treatment for pathologic scars in 1982.
Materials and Methods: The authors summarize the experimental and clinical results of previous studies: research on the mode of action (e.g. pressure, temperature, oxygen tension, hydration, occlusion, etc.). They relate own experiences of prophylactic and therapeutic effects in a 3-year period (January 1999 to December 2001). After analyzing the aetiology and location of scarring, as well as the age and sex of patients, they classified the 30 treated patients depending on treatment period and results. The assessment of results was based on subjective complaint, appearances of scars, and comparing photography.
Results: Improvement was observed in two-thirds of cases, the rest was completed by intra-laesional Triamcinolon-injection therapy. 20 of the 30 patients underwent operation: excision with skin single advancement, 'Z'-, and 'W'-plasty, and splitting skin transplantation.
Conclusion: Pathologic scars require complex therapy generally, so that a detailed analysis of aetiology is essential. The SGS therapy is effective as an adjuvant treatment; to achieve state of rest and reduce complaints it can be sufficient in rare cases only. For preventing primary pathologic scar formation it is suggested after aesthetic surgery.

PP61

Prospective Trial Comparing the Prolene and Dacron Mesh in the Lichtenstein Tension-Free Inguinal Hernia Repair

G. Antsaklis, I. Karanikas, A. Fotopoulos, A. Karkaletsis, S. Lamprou, E. Konstantinidou, I. Sahin, C. Alexiou, D. Zogas

Department of Surgery, "Sismanoglion" General Hospital, Athens, Greece

Introduction: The Lichtenstein tension free repair has gained widespread acceptance for repairing inguinal hernia. The aim of this prospective non-randomized study is to compare two different types of mesh that we used in this surgical procedure.
Methods: During an 8-month period 68 patients underwent unilateral primary inguinal hernia repair with the Lichtenstein technique, under epidural or general anaesthesia. The mean age was 65.6 (range 23-91) years. In 37 patients we used the Prolene mash (Group A) and in 31 the Dacron (Group B).
Results: There was no significant difference in the operation time between Group A (mean 39, range 24-71 min) and Group B (mean 37, range 26-74 min). Postoperatively 2 patients from group A and 1 from Group B had minor complications ($p > 0.05$), while no mesh infection was noted in either group. Analgetic requirements were

similar for patients from both groups. During a follow up period of 0.5-8 months no recurrences occurred in either group, and palpation showed a more soft periprosthetic area in patients of Group B compared to those of Group A.
Conclusion: The results of our study suggest that in the Lichtenstein tension-free inguinal hernia repair the Prolene and the Dacron mesh have the same effectiveness in the short term. The Dacron mesh compared to the Prolene, seems to produce a minor tissue reaction.

PP62

Vascular Tunnel Concept in the Acute Surgical Treatment of Severe T-L1 Fractures

A. Csókay, L. Együd, L. Nagy

National Institute of Traumatology, Budapest, Hungary

Purpose: Authors' opinions worldwide are controversial in the route of acute surgery for severe Th-L injuries. Most of them prefer posterior approach as emergency operation. They say it is possible to remove or drive back the broken anterior part without touching spinal cord if they cut two neighbouring nerve roots. By cutting two thoracic nerve roots we can release spinal cord, we can avoid the intraoperative trauma of spinal medulla. The thoracal nerve roots are not important in motor function. The posterior approach is easier for the surgeon and less dangerous than the anterior, for the patients especially in polytraumatized cases - as they said.
Methods: By cutting nerve roots we have to cut the radicular arteries and veins as well. As we know, from the segmental vessels originated radicular veins and arteries (for example art. Adamkiewich) the vascular supply of pyramidal tract and contused medulla can depend on the two neighbouring segmental arteries because of damaging of anterior spinal vascular structures caused by ventral encroachment. For this reason we improve a new anterior plate called Nazareth tunnel plate which protects by a vascular tunnel the segmental vessels against compression. So that we can avoid the occlusion of segmental vessels of two neighbouring vertebral bodies which participate on ventral fixation.
Results: From points of view of both primary neuro- and secondary neurovascular protection, the acute anterior approach gives better result than posterior.
Conclusions: By protecting the segmental and radicular arteries we can avoid the further secondary vascular damage of injured spinal cord on Th-L1 part. (Ref.: A. Csókay et al: Treatment of severe double spinal cord injuries. Spinal Cord (2001) 39, 492-497)

PP63

The Treatment of Polytraumatic Patient's Diaphragm Injuries

C. Oláh, K. Kovács, P. Frölich, M. Svébis, G. Boross, A. Száz

Department of Surgery and Department of Traumatology, County Teaching Hospital, Kecskemét, Hungary

Introduction: The traumatic indirect diaphragm injury is a rare injury. It occurs in 3-5 % of polytraumatic patients. The prognosis of diaphragm injury decisively depends on the accompanying injuries. In our paper we are going to give an account of our experiences gained by diagnostics and the treatments of injured patients.
Methods: This is a retrospective analysis over a period of 10 years. We have analysed the frequency of polytraumatic patient's diaphragm injuries, the method of treatments, the influence of diaphragm injury on the patient's recovery.
Results: We have treated 238 polytraumatic patients. (171 male, 67 female) We treated 21 patients with diaphragm injuries (15 male, 6 female). Their average age was 46. The left-side diaphragm injury was more frequent similarly to the literary data. (12:2) The accompanying injuries most frequently were the injuries of abdominal organs. We treated diaphragm injuries from laparotomy in 10 cases, from thoracolaparotomy in 6 cases, from thoracotomy in 5 cases. The recovery chances of diaphragm injured patients were decisively influenced by the severity of other injuries. 4 patients died of our 21 patients. The causes were the following: 3 patients died of brain failure, and 1 died in multi-organ failure.
Discussion: A high diaphragm or the obscuring of a hemidiaphragm should raise the suspicion of a diaphragmatic injury. Drainage of a hemothorax, if present, may clarify the diagnosis. Presence of the tip of nasogastric tube in an abnormal location lateral and above the diaphragm is diagnostic. Contrast studies of the gastrointestinal tract are useful in a stable trauma patient or in the chronic setting. Use of CT scanning has been reported: however, it has only limited value in the diagnosis of diaphragmatic hernias. USG and radionuclide scanning have been suggested as being useful in making the diagnosis, particularly of right-sided hernias. The operative approach for patients with suspected diaphragmatic injuries must be tailored to the patient. It is dependent upon the stability of the presence of associated injuries.
Conclusion: It is often difficult to identify diaphragm failures of polytraumatic patients. The primary treatment of the injury is necessary in all cases. If the failure of other organs (in the chest or abdominal cavity) require an operation, the diaphragm injury should be treated at the same time. The diaphragm injury in itself is also an operative indication for polytraumatic patients, because the swelling of abdominal organs can cause an acute emergency.

PP64

Surgical Security by Limb Replantation: an Experimental Amputat Model

M. Szokoly, G. Ács, E. Bráth, N. Németh, T. Lesznyák, I. Mikó, I. Furka*

Department of Traumatology*, Hungarian National Ambulance/Emergency Service, Budapest, Department of Operative Techniques and Surgical Research Medical and Health Science Center, University of Debrecen, Debrecen, Hungary

Introduction: The possibility of replantation after traumatic amputation of a limb depends on the time factor and preservation of the amputats from the field to the operating theatre. Traditional method for organ preservation is the cooling but in the emergency praxis it is a time spending method and difficult to perform and the benefit is not certainly proved. The aim of this study was to make an amputat model for analysis of local and systemic hematological, hemorheological and hemostatic changes during cold and warm ischemia-reperfusion circumstances.

Methods: With the permission of the Committee of Animal Research of the University of Debrecen we used 12 mongrel dogs for the development of the amputat model. We divided the dogs into 4 groups: warm sham operated (wS), cold sham operated (cS), warm ischemia-reperfusion operated (wI) and cold ischemia-reperfusion operated (cI). The operation technique was: on the hindlimb of the dogs was prepared the right femoral artery and vein 2 centimeter distal from the inguinal ligament. With a steel loop were excluded the muscles, nerves and small vessels. The femoral artery and vein were closed for 3 h ischemia period and were checked during the 4-hr reperfusion period. For taking of blood samples the right jugular vein was prepared. Laser-Doppler blood flow measurements and hematological, hemorheological and hemostaseological analysis were made from the "amputat" and systemic blood.
Results: There were 3 fatal outcomes: one in group warm sham (wS) and two in cold ischemic (cI) group. Nine dogs survived to the 5th postoperative day. Only one wound infection occurred with separation. All surviving dogs had a good postoperative movement function in the hindlimb. The analysis of the blood samples is in process. Preliminary we detected characteristic changes in A-V granulocyte sequestration, in erythrocyte deformability and in hemostatic parameters in particular on the 4th postoperative day.
Discussion: The amputat model is useable for the examination of the ischemia-reperfusion injury and its systemic effect. Cooling is a traditional method of organ preservation but in the case of limbs we should consider the advantages and disadvantages. We continue this experiment to make clear the effects of all circumstances giving a higher security of limb replantation for the clinical practice.
Conclusion: These data suggest that we have to continue the experimental series exploring the unanswered questions and the optimal method.
This study was supported by The Ministry of Welfare Research Grant Nr. 6003/1/2000/ETT.

PP65

Evaluation of Monopolar and Bipolar Electrocoagulation in Normal and Abnormal Coagulation Status

M. Kontos[1], T. Diamantis[1], A. Arvelakis[1], D. Koronarchis[1], S. Syroukis[1], E. Agapitos[2], E. Felekouras[1], E. Bastounis[1]

1st Dept. of Surgery, University of Athens, "Laiko" Hospital[1], Athens, Greece and Dept. of Pathology[2], University of Athens, Athens, Greece

Introduction: Monopolar (ME) and bipolar (BE) electrocoagulation are often used during operations to achieve haemostasis in patients whose coagulation status is not always ideal. The aim of this study is to investigate the efficacy and the complications of the use of ME and BE in normal and abnormal coagulation status.
Methods: 24 white New Zealand rabbits equally separated in 2 groups (A and B) were used. The animals of the 2nd group received 0.5 mg acenocoumarol each for three consequent days preoperatively and postoperatively until sacrifice. All animals underwent laparotomy during which 3 to 5 major branches of the gastrepiploic vessels close to the gastric wall were divided. Groups A and B were equally divided in A1, A2, B1 and B2 depending on whether ME (A1, B1) or BE (A2, B2) was used. Number of times ME or BE was used in order to achieve haemostasis on each vessel and blood loss intraoperatively was estimated. After 3 days of close observation the animals were reoperated and sacrificed. Signs of intraperitoneal bleeding, gastric perforation or other complications were sought.
Results: One animal from group B1 died on the 1st postoperative day due to intraperitoneal bleeding. Mean number of efforts in order to achieve haemostasis was 2.58 and 3.88 in groups A and B respectively. 23,6% more blood was lost in the cases in group B compared to A. 2 cases of concealed gastric perforation was found in group A1, 1 in A2, 2 in B1 and 2 in B2. Free gastric perforation and weight loss was found in 1 case in the B1 group.
Discussion: ME and BE are commonly used at operations in order to achieve haemostasis sometimes in patients without normal coagulation status. Perforation of the gastric wall occurred due to efforts of the surgeon to achieve coagulation by applying ME or BE to the vessel very close to the gastric wall when the previous efforts had failed and thus reflects the efficacy of the method.
Conclusion: Although no difference was seen in normal haemostatic status, when coagulation system is not normal, complications of the ME were more common as compared with BE.

New Techniques

PP66

Minimal Invasive Adrenal Gland Surgery - Chance and Option

T. Jacobi, U. Wehrmann, T. Zimmermann, H.D. Saeger

Department of Surgery, Technical University Dresden, Dresden, Germany

Introduction: Since 1992, the beginning of minimal invasive adrenalectomy, this method has become a standard in surgery of the endocrinium. The smaller access and the about 15% lower rate complications are the advantages to former operation methods.
Methods: From 1.10.1995 to 31.12.2001 we performed 33 minimal invasive compared to 32 conventional adrenalectomies in 60 patients with benign illness.
Results: Adenomata of the adrenal gland and incidentalomata were the reasons for operation. For minimal invasive surgery we used both, the transperitoneal-laparoscopic (20 operations) and the retroperitoneoscopic (13 operations) access. The conversion rate was 18%.
Conclusion: We report about advantage and problems of both operation methods, the morbidity in connection with the method and the long-term curation. Special indications like phaeochromocytoma and cancer of the adrenal gland are discussed.

PP67

Anaesthesiological Management for Swine Laparoscopic Experimental Surgery

*O. Toma, C. Balasa, C. Plavat, M. Papurica, D. Sandesc, M. Ionac**

Clinical Department of Anaesthesiology and Intensive Care, *Center for Laparoscopic Surgery and Microsurgery, "Victor Babes" University of Medicine and Pharmacy, Timisoara, Romania

Introduction: The anaesthesiological protocol employed in pigs underwent experimental laparoscopic procedures is here reported.
Methods: With approval of the local ethics committee the study included 25 pigs (weighing 35-65 kg) and it was a part of a larger course concerning biliary laparoscopic procedures in swine. Midazolam (0.15-0.20 mg/kg) and ketamine (8-10 mg/kg) was first administered intramuscularly. After venous cannulation (VC) we administered intravenously penthotal (7-9 mg/kg) and the trachea was intubated within the next 3 to 5 minutes and connected to a calibrated ventilator. The anaesthesia was maintained with halothane in pure oxygen. Pulse rate and oxygen saturations were measured shortly on the pig's snout shortly after penthotal was administered. At the end of the procedure inspired anaesthetics were discontinued and the pigs were extubated when they were able to breath for oxygen saturations over 90% with room air. They recovered and they were in awake state few hours later (all but not three pigs, see below).
Results: The satisfaction of the anaesthesia team with VC was better with greater doses of midazolam and there are some anecdotal reports showing that midazolam is far better than diazepam (i.m. 0.2 mg/kg). Three pigs died in the operation theatre (one because of massive intraabdominal haemorrhage, one because of a preexisting diaphragmatic malformation with lung collapse after pneumoperitoneum, and one because of overweight and subsequent difficult, late endotracheal intubation). No muscle relaxants were necessary if the laparoscopic cholecystectomy was performed in less than 90 minutes.
Conclusion: We found the presented technique satisfactory and we conclude that an adequate drug dosage combined with good anaesthesiological skills provides good anaesthesiologial management for swine experimental surgery.

PP68

First Results of the Inguinal Hernia Repair with the Prolene Hernia System

G. Antsaklis, N. Economou, C. Alexiou, A. Karkaletsis, E. Kefalogiannis, N. Fotopoulos, P. Karydakis, E. Bobotis, I. Karanikas

Department of Surgery, "Sismanoglion" General Hospital, Athens, Greece

Introduction: This study was undertaken to determine the efficacy of the Prolene Hernia System (PHS) in the inguinal hernia repair.
Methods: During an 8-month period 120 patients were operated under epidural or general anaesthesia for unilateral primary inguinal hernia. In 52 of them the PHS technique was used (Group A), and in 68 the Lichtenstein tension free repair (Group B).
Results: The mean operative time was 39 (range 22-68) and 38 (range 24-74) minutes for the PHS and Lichtenstein's procedures. Postoperatively 2 patients from group A and 3 from Group B had minor complications ($p > 0.05$), while no mesh infection was noted in either group. Analgetic requirements were similar for patients from both groups. The mean hospital stay following operation, was 1.5 (range 0-2) and 2.5 (range 1-6) days for patients from Group A and B, respectively. During a follow up period of 0.5-8 months no recurrences occurred in either group.
Conclusion: The results of our study suggest that the PHS and the Lichtenstein technique in the inguinal hernia repair have the same effectiveness in the short term. The PHS technique seems to provide certain advantage in terms of hospital stay.

PP69

The Electric Oscillating Brush Dissection Instrument: Evaluation of Vascular Trauma and Clinical Applications for Laparoscopic Cholecystecomy and Colectomy

M. Kakihara[1], Z. Szabó[3], Y. Kagata[2], K. Hatsuse[1], T. Aihara[1], H. Mochizuki[1]

The First Department of Surgery[1], The Second Department of Pathology[2], National Defense Medical College, Saitama, Japan, Moet Institute[3], San Francisco, California, USA

Introduction: To minimize acquisition costs in laparoscopic surgery, we developed an electric oscillating brush dissection instrument. We present a porcine model evaluation of its effects on vascular trauma, compared to traditional electrosurgical dissection. In addition we present the results of its clinical applications in laparoscopic cholecystectomy and colectomy.
Methods: The instrument is comprised of a long thin shaft, with a detachable and disposable brush tip; oscillating in circular motion (50 times per second) and powered by an electric motor. This high-speed oscillation has the ability to liquefy fatty tissue easily and safely.
Results: Histological examination: in porcine model, complete exposure of the common bile duct, portal vein, mesenteric artery, iliac artery and inferior vena cava was performed using both brush and traditional dissection. Specimens were collected 24 hours later and tissue trauma was evaluated microscopically. Minor inflammation and hemorrhage was observed in both groups, but there was no significant difference between the dissection methods.
Discussion: Clinical Applications: 1) Cholecystectomy - the oscillating brush motion has the ability to liquefy fatty tissue in Calot's triangle, while gently exposing the cystic duct and artery without laceration. The mean operative time and blood loss were statistically significantly decreased compared with the traditional technique. 2) Colectomy - the instrument also liquefied fatty tissue to expose mesenteric vessels easily and safely.
Conclusion: The procedure was successfully completed in all cases. Our electric oscillating brush technique is faster and results in less blood loss than traditional electrosurgical dissection, without any evidence of trauma increase. In addition, compared with modern high-tech dissection applications, its less expensive and easier to perform, while approaching the capabilities of these high-tech instruments.

PP70

Comparison of Different Anastomotic Techniques in Tracheal Replacement

Z. Szántó[1], A. Ferencz[1], G. Jancsó[1], Á. Boronkai[1], E. Rőth[1], Ö.P. Horváth[2], T.F. Molnár[2]

Department of Experimental Surgery[1], Department of Thoracic Surgery[2], University of Pécs, Hungary

Introduction: Long segmental tracheal defects are rare, but they often represent life threatening clinical conditions. There is still no generally accepted surgical method to cure these lesions. The aim of our study was the investigation of the proper surgical technique and the healing process after long segmental tracheal replacement with politetrafluoroethylene (ptfe) grafts using different anastomotic techniques in a rabbit model.
Methods: We resected a 2-cm long circumferential segment of the cervical trachea in 20 adult albino rabbits. For the replacement we used ptfe graft (Gore-Tex) regularly applied in vascular surgery. Four groups were formed according to the position of the graft to the cranial and caudal stumps of the trachea (external-external-group I, n=5; internal-internal-group II, n=5; external-internal-group III, n=5; internal-external-group IV, n=5;). All of the anastomoses were completed using interrupted sutures (PDS 6.0). Laser-Doppler measurements were performed intraoperatively for measuring the possible changes in the local microcirculation. We noted the length of survival, the complication rate. Signs of graft neoepithelization was proved by *post-mortem* histological examinations.
Results: There was no significant difference in the microcirculation after the replacement compared to the preoperative state. The length of survival differed from 13 days to 89 days (mean 48 days), with longest survivals in group II (mean 58 days). The *post mortem* histological examinations showed granulation tissue formation in 18 cases causing luminal narrowing of different degree. Process of neoepithelization was seen in 14 cases, which completely covered the inner surface of the grafts in 6 animals. Fatal infection developed in 4 cases.
Discussion and Conclusion: The use of interrupted sutures helped to avoid acute ischaemia of the anastomosis in every group. The postoperative complications were less common in the animals with internal telescopic anastomosis, which resulted in longer survival.

PP71

Experiences with the Retrograde Percutaneous Translaryngeal Tracheotomy (Fantoni) on a Surgical Intensive Care Unit

R. Konopke, T. Zimmermann, S. Kersting, H. Schikore, G. von Gagern, D. Ockert, H.D. Saeger

Clinic for Visceral, Thoracic and Vascular Surgery, Technical University Dresden, Dresden, Germany

Introduction: In the early nineties the retrograde percutaneous translaryngeal tracheotomy was developed by Prof. Fantoni in Italy and introduced in Germany in 1998. The indications for application of this method do not differ from the indications for the conventional surgical tracheotomy.
Methods: The innovative aspect of the "Fantoni method" comprises in a retrograde dilatation of the trachea by means of a specially designed tracheostomy cannula. The cannula is introduced translaryngeally, serving at the same time as a dilatator for the tracheostomy. In this way the cannula fits the tracheostomy perfectly, reducing tissue trauma and danger of bleeding. After removal of the cannula the stoma closes soon with an amazing cosmetic result. The procedure is easy to learn and can be performed by intern under supervision in the ICU under continuous monitoring.
Results: Since the introduction of the Fantoni tracheotomy on our ICU this method was used in 124 patients in the period from 02/2000 to 12/2001. The indications were: expected long term ventilation, ARDS, pneumonia, extensive injuries of the face or the base of the scull and inflammatory changes of the larynx.
All Fantoni tracheotomies were performed on the ICU. In one case local bleeding occurred which ceased spontaneously by local compression. In one adipose patient wound infection was observed. Thus the overall complication rate was only 1.6%.
Conclusion: In our experience Fantoni's retrograde percutaneous translaryngeal tracheotomy is an easy and safely practicable technique causing only few complications and little trauma.

PP72

Validation of a Skills Course Using Objective Measures of Technical Ability

M.S. Khan, S.D. Bann, A. Darzi, P.E.M. Butler

Academic Surgical Unit, St. Mary's Hospital, London, UK

Introduction: With the acquisition of surgical skills seen as being one of the essentials of good surgical practice, there is increasing pressure on surgeons to prove their competency. We present a method of objectively assessing and teaching surgical skill, whilst validating a core skills course in plastic surgery.
Method: Fourteen junior trainees were asked to attend a "core skills in Plastic Surgery" course. They were assessed on essential Plastic surgical skills, namely suturing skin, harvesting a split skin graft and repair of a tendon. Prosthetic, specially designed models were used for the tasks. The candidates were assessed at the beginning of the course, prior to any instruction, and then again at the end of the course after they had received two days instruction on these skills. The tasks were videoed, and then assessed by three independent observers using modified scoring sheets based on the OSATS scheme.
Results: All candidates improved their scores post instruction. Mean percentage increase in score was 12% for skin suturing, 25% for skin grafting and 18% for tendon repair. Candidates who scored higher pre-instruction had a smaller percentage increase post instruction, mean 3%. As the data was parametric, two tailed t-test were performed, showing $p< 0.001$ when comparing pre- against post-instruction scores throughout all tasks. Inter-rater reliability of 92% was obtained using Cronbach's Alpha test of reliability.
Discussion: Using validated methods of technical assessment we have shown that we can give objective measures of technical performance pre and post instruction. This allows us to provide feedback to the candidates. This has also validated the skills course, allowing the commencement of a specific core skills course. Candidates will take these skills away and use them immediately in the clinical environment. The tasks showed face, construct and concurrent validity. This therefore validates the course itself.

Conclusion: Using valid measures of technical competence we have validated the skills course as an important method of assessing and teaching surgical skill.

Molecular Biology and Immunology

PP73

Bioluminometric TC-Assay in Cases of Gynaecological Malignancies - Useful as Pretherapeutical Factor?

S. Albrecht[1], T. Zimmermann[2]; T. Köppen[1], B. Richter[1]; W. Distler[1]

Dept. of Gynaecology[1], Dept. of Surgery[2], Technical University Dresden, Fetscherstraße 74, 01307 Dresden, Germany

Introduction: Individualized chemotherapy in cancer patients is still not widely applied. In order to determine the *in vitro* efficacy of cytostatic drugs, it is necessary to obtain tissue samples representative for the tumor. These samples allow prediction of the *in vivo* responses towards chemotherapy.
Methods: 21 samples obtained from patients suffering from two different gynaecological malignancies (ovary 13, breast 8) were sent for chemosensitivity testing. The samples were classified in 3 stages. 4 of the patients with ovarian carcinoma were classified as stage I, 3 as stage II, 5 as stage III and 2 as stage IV. All patients with breast cancer belong to the stage II. The reaction of the cells to the chemotherapy was defined at the beginning of the evaluation.
Results: A tumor growth inhibition >70% at 25% test concentration was defined as sensitive, while inhibition 50%-<70% as partial sensitiveness and inhibition <50% as resistant. Navelbine and 5-Fluorouracil appeared to be the combination with the highest effect *in vitro* on breast cancer (73.94%; SD 0.13%) followed by Onkotrone which showed partial effects (67.34%; SD 17.67%). On the other hand the combination of Taxol and 5-Fluorouracil (3.8%; SD 10.21%) and Cisplatin (11.91%; SD 12.28%) pointed out a strong resistance. In 4 cases of ovarian carcinoma Taxol and Carboplatin were prescribed, *in vitro* the ATP-TCA measured a tumor growth inhibition of 25.13% (SD 15.66%) which demonstrated the strong resistance. In 3 additional cases the combination Carboplatin and Cyclophosphamid was used, which showed *in vitro* and ATP inhibition of 14.89% (SD 15.83%) only. Other drugs such as Novantron demonstrated higher ATP inhibitions (58.12%; SD 13.21%). For example on ovarian carcinoma patient at stage III was treated with the combination Carboplatin and Cyclophosphamid, which appeared *in vitro* with an inhibition of 40.07%, while other tested drugs like Taxol showed a higher effect on the tumor cells (75.29%).
Conclusions: The chemosensitivity profiles of the tested tumors revealed a big heterogeneity of chemosensitivity results for single drugs and drug combinations. The findings demonstrate that the ATP-TCA is able to determine the fraction of surviving cells and has proved to be an effective tool to measure cytotoxicity.

PP74

Suppression of Proliferative Cholangitis by E2F Decoy Oligodeoxynucleotide

M. Yoshida, N. Yamamoto, T. Nitta, T. Uehara, R. Terao, E. Hatano, Y. Iimuro, Y. Yamaoka

Department of Gastroenterological Surgery, Kyoto University, Graduate School of Medicine, Kyoto, Japan

Introduction: Proliferative cholangitis (PC) associated with hepatolithiasis results in stricture of the main bile ducts, and is a major cause of residual and/or recurrent stones after repeated treatment for hepatolithiasis. The transcription factor E2F controls the expression of several genes involved in cell proliferation. The aim of this study was to inhibit PC using the cytostatic gene therapy by transferring fusigenic anionic liposome-hemagglutinating virus of Japan (HVJ-anionic liposome) complexes containing a synthetic double-stranded oligodeoxynucleotide (ODN) with high affinity for E2F (E2F decoy).
Methods: PC was induced by introducing a fine nylon thread into the bile duct in a rat model. HVJ-anionic liposomes containing the E2F decoy were administered directly into the biliary tract. HVJ-anionic liposomes containing a missense oligodeoxynucleotide (scramble decoy) were also given as a control. The count of peribiliary glands in the bile duct, 5I-bromodeoxyuridine (BrdU) labeling index and immunohistochemical staining for proliferating cell nuclear antigen (PCNA) in the bile duct were compared among untransfected, scramble decoy-transfected and E2F decoy-transfected rats.
Results: E2F decoy-transfected bile ducts showed inhibition of the papillary proliferation of the biliary epithelium and the peribiliary gland hyperplasia. BrdU incorporation and PCNA expression in the bile ducts were inhibited in the E2F decoy-transfected rats.
Discussion: We previously reported that the proliferative changes in the bile duct were successfully inhibited by adenovirus-mediated retinoblastoma (Rb) gene transfer to the bile duct in the rat PC model. A decoy strategy targeting E2F was recently reported to be quite effective in inhibiting proliferation *in vitro*, *in vivo* and *ex vivo*. We applied this strategy to the rat PC model to suppress the proliferation of the biliary epithelium. In this report, HVJ-liposomes were injected directly into the biliary tract. This treatment modality will be clinically applicable because it is feasible to administer the vector directly into the bile duct using an endoscope and the inhibitory effect of the E2F decoy could have been enhanced and prolonged by repetitive endoscopic administration, which is impossible when using adenovirus-mediated vector due to its immunogenicity.
Conclusion: Our cytostatic gene therapy approach using direct E2F decoy transfer into the biliary tract suppressed PC in a rat model and may offer an effective therapeutic option for reducing recurrence following treatment for hepatolithiasis.

PP75

Participation of ERCC1 in Resistance against Cisplatin for Human Esophageal Cancer Cell Lines

T. Miyahara[1], K. Yanagibashi[1], T. Kajiwara[1], M. Akaboshi[2], A. Kawabe[3], J-I. Kaganoi[3]

Department of Surgery, Kobe City General Hospital[1], Kyoto University Research Reactor[2], Department of Surgery and Surgical Basic Science, Graduate School of Medicine, Kyoto University[3], Japan

Introduction: We have reported that it is difficult to explain the variation of Cisplatin sensitivities in human esophageal cancer cell lines solely by reference to platinum-DNA adduct levels, so far. Cisplatin sensitivity of KYSE-220 human esophageal cancer cell line was 4 times sensitive in D0 value than that of KYSE-170. But the level of platinum-DNA of KYSE-170 was 2.5 times higher than that of KYSE-220. Nucleotide excision repair (NER) is responsible for the repair of Cisplatin-DNA adduct. We studied the participation of ERCC1, a critical DNA repair enzyme in the NER pathway, in resistance of human esophageal cancer cells to Cisplatin-induced cytotoxicity.

Methods: We measured the incorporation of 195mPt-Cisplatin into DNA and the rate of disappearance of DNA-bound 195mPt-Cisplatin of each KYSE-170 and KYSE-220 cell. ERCC1 protein was assayed by Western blotting method. Quantification was by densitometry of the film obtained using the NIH Imaging Program. 195mPt-Cisplatin was synthesized at Kyoto University Research Reactor, and the radioactivity was 7.4 x 106 Bq/mg and the half-life was 4.02 days. Sensitivity of esophageal cancer cell lines to Cisplatin was determined by colony-forming assay. DNA was extracted by Schneider's method, and measured by fluorospectrometer using diaminobenzoic acid.

Results: The disappearance of adduct from DNA was biphasic; with a rapid phase of removal during the first 6 hours, followed by a relatively flat plateau. The disappearance velocity of DNA-bound 195mPt-Cisplatin during the first 6 hours was 7.5 and 17.3 cpm/ugDNA/hr in KYSE-220 and KYSE-170 respectively. Cisplatin resistant KYSE-170 cells showed an increased expression of ERCC1 protein by Western blotting.

Conclusion: These findings suggest that ERCC1 participates in Cisplatin resistance of KYSE-170 human esophageal cancer cells.

Acknowledgement: This study was supported by Medical Research Fund of Hyogo Medical Association.

PP76

Severe Tissue Injury Alters Self-Regulation of Neutrophil Phagocytosis

G. Pap[1], J. Fűrész[2], L. Nagy[3], J. Hamar[1]

National Institute of Traumatology and Rehabilitation[1], Budapest, Hungarian Defense Forces, Institute of Health[2], Central Military Hospital, Central Intensive Care Unit[3], Budapest, Hungary

Introduction: As a result of previous investigations carried out on the yeast phagocytosis of neutrophils (PMNL) separated from blood of patients with multiple trauma or acute pancreatitis, the absence of increase in phagocytic activity while increasing cell density was found, which increase is characteristic to healthy PMNLs.

Materials and Methods: In our present experiment naive control PMNLs (nc) and cells activated by the trauma of the patient (tc) were treated with supernatants of phagocytosis assays of PMNLs from control healthy subjects (cs=control supernatant) or patients with polytrauma (ISS>18), (ts=trauma supernatant) in the following setting: cs-nc, ts-nc, cs-tc. Internalized yeast cells were differentiated by methylen blue, Phagocytosis Index (FI) was determined by counting the internalized yeast per 100 PMNLs.

Results: The ts (n=25) in most cases inhibited (-29±27%, mean±SD), while the cs (n=10) mostly increased (+22±43%) the phagocytosis of nc. The cs significantly increased the phagocytosis of tc (+71±110%) ($p<0.05$, Student test).

Discussion and Conclusion: Our results reinforce the theory that in the presence of pathogens "primed" neutrophils produce and release factors, which inhibit some of the cells' anti-microbial functions, but at the same time these cells still keep their capability of increasing anti-microbial activity. Naive PMNLs were found to release factors, which enhance anti-microbial function. The above phenomenon may contribute to the probable immune dysfunction in severe tissue injury.

PP77

Enhancement of Circulating Dendritic Cell Activity by Immunomodulators (OK432 and KP-40)

H. Yanagimoto, H. Toyokawa, M. Inaba[1,2,3], S. Takai, S. Satoi, J. Beuth[4]

First Department of Surgery[1], First Department of Pathology[2], Transplantation Center[3] and Regeneration Research Center for Intractable Diseases[4], Kansai Medical University, Moriguchi City, Osaka, Japan.

Introduction: The effects of biological response modifiers (BRMs) on the functions of two type-dendritic cells (DCs) were examined to apply to anti-tumor therapy.

Methods: The two BRMs studied in our assay system were OK432 (a streptococcal preparation) and KP-40 (Propionibacterium avidum: a heat-killed bacterial vaccine). Recently, techniques have been developed for isolating human DCs from peripheral blood, and DCs can be divided into two subsets: CD11c+ DCs (myeloid DC population) and CD11c- DCs (lymphoid DC population).

Results: Both OK432 and KP-40 were found to up-regulate the stimulatory activity of myeloid-lineage DCs: The expression of MHC class II molecules and adhesion/costimulatory molecules increased and the production of IL-12 showed significantly higher levels.
Conclusion: Therefore, DCs pulsed with OK432 and KP-40 will be applied to vaccination as a new adjuvant for specific immunotherapies.

PP78

Activation of RET Tyrosine Kinase Modulates IL-8 Production

N. Iwahashi, M. Takahashi, Y. Nimura

Nagoya University School of Medicine, Nagoya, Japan

Introduction: Interleukin-8 (IL-8) is known to contribute to human cancer progression through its potential functions as a mitogenic, angiogenic, and motogenic factor. We found that the IL-8 proteins are produced in TT human medullary thyroid carcinoma cell line and TPC-1 human papillary thyroid carcinoma cell line that express activated RET tyrosine kinase. Accordingly, we dissected the mechanism of IL-8 production that is induced by RET activation. Glial cell line-derived neurotrophic factor (GDNF) signals through a multicomponent receptor consisting of RET and GDNF family receptor alpha 1 (GFRalpha1). It is known that phosphorylation of tyrosine 1015 of RET is crucial for activation of the PLC gamma pathway and phosphorylation of tyrosine 1062 is essential for activation of Akt, ERK1/2 and p38MAPK. SK-N-MC human primitive neuroectodermal tumor cell line endogenously expresses GFRalpha1 but not RET.
Methods: The IL-8 protein levels in supernatants from SK-N-MC cells that were transfected wild-type RET (MC+wRET) or RET with the Y1015F mutation (MC+Y1015F) or with Y1062F mutation (MC+Y1062F) were quantified by ELISA.
Results: The IL-8 protein levels in supernatants from MC+Y1015F and MC+Y1062F cells stimulated with GDNF for 24 hours were significantly reduced than that from MC+wRET cells, suggesting that RET activation induces the IL-8 production. Consistently, SK-N-MC cells expressing RET with a multiple endocrine neoplasia (MEN) 2A mutation produced a high level of IL-8. Treatment with ERK1/2 inhibitor, PD98059, p38MAPK inhibitor, SB202190, or protein kinase C (PKC) inhibitor, Calphostin C decreased the IL-8 secretion in the supernatants from GDNF-treated MC+wRET cells. In contrast, treatment with Akt inhibitors, LY294002 and Wortmannin increased the IL-8 secretion.
Conclusions: These results suggest that the IL-8 production is down-regulated through MEK1/ERK pathway and p38MAPK pathway and is up-regulated through PI3K/Akt pathway in MC+wRET cells. The modulation of the IL-8 production through RET tyrosine kinase may play a role in biological properties of RET-expressing cells.

PP79

Modification of the Endotoxin-Induced Inflammatory Cell Response by Glucocorticoids

J. Szakács[1], G. Lázár[1], G. Lázár Jr.[2], E. Husztik[1]

Institute of Pathophysiology[1], Department of Surgery[2], University of Szeged, Szeged, Hungary

Introduction: Bacterial endotoxin or lipopolysaccharide (LPS) from Gram-negative bacteria plays a pivotal role in the inflammatory processes induced by different stimuli (infection, trauma, surgical intervention, burst). This response is characterised by the activation of different cascade systems, recruitment of leukocytes and release of inflammatory mediators. Glucocorticoids exert profound effects on the inflammatory and immune processes antagonising several effects of the bacterial endotoxin. They inhibit the recruitment of leukocytes by interfering with inflammatory processes such as generation of cytokines and inflammatory mediators or upregulation of adhesion molecules. In the present study we investigated the effect of the glucocorticoid Oradexon and the glucocorticoid antagonist RU 38486 on the endotoxin-induced inflammatory cell response.
Materials and Methods: Male CFLP mice (20-25 g, n=5 per group) were injected i.p. with 10 µg (10 g body weight)$^{-1}$ endotoxin (*E. coli* 026:B6 LPS, Difco Lab, Detroit, lot 110273JB). Dexamethasone (Oradexon, N.V, Organon Oss, The Netherlands) was administered i.p., i.v. or s.c. in a dose of 0.1 mg (10 g body weight)$^{-1}$, alone or concomitantly with endotoxin. Other groups were given 0.5 mg (10 g body weight)$^{-1}$ RU 38486 (Russel Uclaf, France) i.p. or s.c., either alone or concomitantly with LPS.
Results: Bacterial endotoxin increased the total cell count at 24, 48 and 72 h, due to neutrophilia at 24 h and, due to increases in the number of macrophages and lymphocytes 48 and 72 h after treatment, respectively. The i.p., s.c. and i.v. injection of Oradexon, concomitantly with endotoxin, reduced the total cell count and the macrophage count at 48 and 72 hours. The number of lymphocytes and neutrophils decreased at 24 and 72 hours. The i.p. and s.c. injection of RU 38486 increased the total cell count, due to increases in the number of macrophages, lymphocytes and neutrophils - at 24, 48 and 72 hours. Endotoxin at 24 hours decreased, but at 48 and 72 hours increased the WBC count and the lymphocyte count. Oradexon decreased the WBC count, the number of lymphocytes and monocytes at 48 and 72 hours. The i.p. and s.c. injection of RU 38486 increased the WBC count, the number of lymphocytes and neutrophils at 48 and 72 hours.
Discussion: Despite advances in critical care medicine, mortality from sepsis in ICU patients remains high. The role of glucocorticoids during clinical and experimental sepsis constitutes a subject of debate.
Conclusions: Our studies suggest that both glucocorticoids and glucocorticoid antagonists are capable of modifying the immune cell reactions induced by endotoxin and may contribute to the elucidation of their effects in the pathogenesis of various forms of stress and shock.

European Surgical Research

Author Index Vol. 34, Suppl. 1, 2002

Numbers refer to pages

Ábrahám, S. 53
Ács, G. 24, 30, 47, 83, 84, 93
Adawi, D. 33, 62
Agapitos, E. 94
Ahrné, S. 33
Aihara, T. 95
Akaboshi, M. 98
Akashi, K. 65, 71
Akbar, S. 12
Albrecht, S. 25, 34, 55, 60, 81, 82, 97
Alexiou, C. 92, 95
Alfaro, V. 17, 31
Alldinger, I. 34, 45
Alonso, A. 39
Alptekin, H. 78
Ami, K. 54, 66, 67
Ancona, E. 3, 52, 87
Andrási, T. 57
Aneman, A. 16
Antoniadis, A. 71
Antoniadis, I. 71
Antsaklis, G. 92, 95
Anurov, M. 63
Aoyama, H. 69
Araki, H. 78
Aronson, D.C. 58
Arvelakis, A. 94
Avsar, F. 64, 78
Avunduk, M. 56, 78
Azuma, Y. 92

Bach, B. 46
Bahrami, S. 31, 82
Bajory, Z. 84, 89
Balasa, C. 95
Balázs, L. 2
Baldan, N. 3, 52, 87
Balibrea, J.L. 35
Balogh, Á. 17, 52, 53, 58, 80
Banafsche, R. 28
Bann, S.D. 61, 96
Baracs, J. 60
Barker, J.H. 4, 20, 49
Barna, T. 49, 53
Barros D'Sa, A.A.B. 85
Bastounis, E. 59, 94
Beierlein, W. 88
Bella, Z. 47
Belviranli, M. 42, 78
Benner, R. 51
Beuth, J. 98
Biberthaler, P. 46
Bijlsma, P.B. 28, 29, 58
Bilbao, J. 29
Blanco, J.I. 2
Bland, K.I. 32
Blázovics, A. 59
Blomberg, B.M.E. 62
Bobotis, E. 95
Bodoky, G. 45
Boelens, P.G. 62
Bognár, G. 72
Boland, M.G. 75
Boldrin, M. 52
Bordos, D. 32, 68, 90
Borel Rinkes, I.H.M. 8, 40, 74
Boronkai, Á. 96
Boros, M. 2, 5, 7, 17, 53, 58, 80, 84, 91
Boross, G. 54, 93
Borsiczky, B. 16, 22
Bosse, M. 21
Boterberg, T. 63
Bráth, E. 30, 49, 53, 77, 83, 84, 87, 93
Brouha, P.C.R. 20, 49
Brzózka, M. 47, 48
Budny, T. 12
Buhr, H.J. 6
Burdío, F. 40
Burzaco, O. 40
Busetto, R. 3
Butler, P.E.M. 61, 96

Cadrobbi, R. 3, 52, 87
Caínzos, M. 35
Calabrese, F. 3, 52
Camoutsis, C. 59
Campbell, F.C. 85
Cancellotti, F.M. 52
Caramés, J. 29, 39
Carbajo, M.A. 2
Carraro, P. 52
Castagnaro, M. 3, 52
Castiella, T. 40
Castro, B. 39
Ceelen, W. 63
Ceepil, G.A. 51
Chaber, A. 35
Charlaftis, N. 79
Chaudry, I.H. 32
Cheholskiy, A.S. 59
Chmiel, B. 81
Chondros, K. 46
Chondroudaki, I. 46
Cierpka, L. 81
Claeys, G. 63
Conze, J. 63
Cozzi, E. 3, 52
Cruz, I. 40
Culebras, J. 35
Cuverlier, C. 88
Cuverlier, C.A. 13
Cybulska, E. 50
Czigner, J. 47, 48
Csanády, J. 14
Csapó, Z. 42
Cserni, T. 30, 77, 87
Csízy, I. 77
Csókay, A. 24, 93
Csonka, E. 91
Csuka, O. 45

Dahnken, S. 21
Dall'Olmo, L. 87
Dán, A. 84
Darzi, A. 61, 96
Darzi, A.W. 44, 65
Davies, B. 33
Dávil, D. 35
de Bruijn, E. 55
de Haan, P. 1
de Hemptinne, B. 15, 63, 88
de Neve, W. 63
de Oca, J. 17
de Roose, J. 15
de Vos, M. 88
Dedja, A. 3, 52
DeFaria, W. 3, 66
Delacuesta, M. 2
Demetter, P. 13
Deszczynski, J. 23
Dezső, B. 77
Diamantis, T. 94
Dietl, K.H. 12
Dimakakos, P. 37
Dindelegan, G. 16
Distler, W. 82, 97
Dluzniewska, J. 73, 76
Dobozy, A. 80
Drixler, T.A. 40, 74
Dubecz, S. 45
Duda, E. 52
Dudás, J. 45
Durlik, M. 11
Duta, C. 68

Economou, N. 95
Együd, L. 93
Ehrnström, R. 33
Eibl, G. 6
Eklund, M. 33
Eleftheriadis, E. 79, 80
El-Malt, M. 63
Erős, G. 7
Eszlári, E. 91
Ewerbeck, V. 5

Fante, F. 52
Farima, M. 66
Farkas, G. 14, 42, 67
Farkas, I. 42
Fehér, E. 59
Fejős, J. 42
Felekouras, E. 94
Ferencz, A. 16, 96
Filipiuk, E. 64
Fischer, J.H. 20, 21
Flautner, L. 45
Fodor, B. 22
Foerder, M. 45
Foitzik, T. 6
Fonaryova-Key, A. 4
Fonk, J.C.M. 62
Forgács, B. 6
Foster, M.E. 70
Fotopoulos, A. 46, 92
Fotopoulos, N. 95
Francois, C. 20
Francois, C.G. 49
Frangou, M. 46
Franke, J. 6
Frerichmann, U. 25
Friedel, G. 55
Frölich, P. 93
Fruhstorfer, B. 47
Fujikura, M. 74
Fujimori, K. 13
Fujio, Y. 74
Fujiwara, Y. 69
Fukao, K. 12, 76
Fukuhara, K. 69
Furák, J. 52
Furka, A. 24, 77
Furka, I. 24, 30, 47, 48, 77, 83, 84, 87, 93
Fűrész, J. 98
Fürst, W. 82

Gagern, G.v. 25, 34, 55, 80, 96
Gál, I. 61
Gál, P. 2
Galkowska, H. 18, 64
Gandia, C. 3, 66
Gapanovich, V.N. 59
García-Alonso, I. 29, 39
García-Caballero, M. 2, 10
Gasser, H. 82
Gebbink, M.F.B.G. 8, 40

Gebhard, H. 90
Gebhard, M.M. 5, 28
Gellér, L. 57
Gelpí, E. 31
Genesca, M. 17
Giorgion, G.M. 60
Glatzel, U. 34
Glinavou, A. 9, 73
Goebel, M. 23
Goebel, S. 7
Goicoechea, I. 29
Gomez, A.A. 35
Gondos, T. 28
Gorantla, V.S. 20, 49
Gorea, A. 66
Gölcük, M. 78
Grabowska-Bochenek, R. 81
Groza, M. 68
Gründel, M. 90
Grützmann, R. 45, 60
Guetens , G. 55
Güemes, A. 40
Gürbilek, M. 78
Gyáni, K. 49, 53
Győrimolnár, I. 89

Haarman, H.J.T.M. 62
Haas, J. 88
Habazettl, H. 7, 90
Hagymási, K. 59
Hahn, O. 76
Hallay, J. 62
Hamada, Y. 37
Hamar, J. 32, 98
Harada, N. 85
Haranomura, H. 74
Harasztosi, C. 48
Harisi, R. 45
Harkin, D.W. 85
Hashida, H. 69
Hashimoto, Y. 69
Hata, K. 26, 27, 44
Hatano, E. 85, 97
Hatsuse, K. 95
Hayashi, I. 87
Heij, H.A. 58
Hejjel, L. 61
Hendriks, J. 55
Herbst, H. 12
Hesse, U.J. 13, 15, 88
Hevesi, Á. 89
Hibino, N. 36
Hijikawa, T. 75
Hirayama, R. 79
Hofmann, G.O. 21
Hoper, M. 85
Horváth, G. 53
Horváth, Ö.P. 16, 96
Horváth, P. 38
Hotter, G. 17, 31
Houdijk, A.P.J. 62
Hölzen, J.P. 12
Hullin, D. 36
Husztik, E. 52, 99
Hutter, J. 89
Hücümenoglu, S. 78

Iimuro, Y. 97
Ikeda, F. 6
Ikeda, H. 36
Imdahl, A. 72
Imvrios, G. 71
Inaba, M. 98
Inoau, T. 72
Interewicz, B. 19, 73
Ionac, M. 19, 32, 68, 90, 95
Ishibashi, H. 36
Ishiguro, S. 12
Ishizaka, M. 69
Isogai, A. 65, 71
István, G. 72
Itabashi, K. 85
Ito, H. 27, 39
Ito, Y. 85
Iturburo, I. 35
Ivanova, S.T. 44
Iwahashi, N. 99
Iwai, T. 54
Iwashiro, N. 69

Jaberansari, M.T. 82
Jacobi, T. 94
Jacobs, B. 15
Jacobs, M.J. 1
Jafarmadar, M. 82
Jancsó, G. 22, 82, 96
Jánossy, T. 51
Jármai, K. 42
Jeekel, J. 8, 9
Jeppsson, B. 4, 33, 62
Jeschkeit, S. 20
Jesenofsky, R. 45
Jiga, P.L. 19
Jiménez, A. 31
Jochum, M. 46
Joist, A. 25
Jóri, J. 48
Jost, D. 88
Józsa, T. 77
Juhász-Nagy, A. 38, 56, 57

Kaai, K. 79
Kaganoi, J-I. 98
Kagata, Y. 95
Kaibori, M. 43, 75, 79
Kajiwara, T. 98
Kakihara, M. 95
Kakita, A. 85, 87
Kalkman, C.J. 1
Kalmár-Nagy, K. 16
Kamigaito, T. 10
Kamiyama, Y. 43, 75, 78, 79, 92
Karamanakos, P. 59
Karanikas, I. 92, 95
Karasavidou, F. 71
Karatzas, G. 9, 73
Karatzas, T. 3, 66
Karkaletsis, A. 92, 95
Karpinski, J. 23
Kartal, A. 41
Karydakis, P. 95
Kashiwagi, J. 36
Kaszaki, J. 2, 7, 17, 53, 58, 80, 91
Kato, A. 27
Kato, H. 10
Katsenis, K. 37
Kawabe, A. 98
Kawada, K. 54, 66, 67
Kawagishi, N. 13, 86
Kawamoto, T. 12
Kawano, T. 54, 66, 67
Kefalogiannis, E. 95
Kékesi, V. 56, 57
Kelemen, O. 92
Kelly, S. 4
Kemény, L. 80
Kerekes, L. 77
Kersting, S. 25, 34, 55, 81, 96
Khadem, A. 82
Khan, M.S. 61, 96
Kimura, F. 27, 39
Kinoshita, H. 69
Kirschner, M.H. 21, 23
Kiss, K. 16
Kiss, S. Sz. 62
Kitade, H. 75
Kiyota, Y. 36
Klar, E. 28
Klenke, F. 5
Koffeman, G.I. 58
Koide, Y. 70
Koike, Y. 78
Koizumi, N. 85
Kojima, N. 72
Kokudo, N. 72
Kollár, L. 92
Kon, M. 4, 20, 49
Konishi, T. 72
Konopke, R. 96
Konstantinidou, E. 92
Kontos, M. 59, 94
Konuma, T. 36
Koronarchis, D. 94
Kotsis, T. 37, 46
Kotsovolou, S. 46
Kotzampassi, K. 79, 80
Kotzsch, M. 80
Kouraklis, G. 9, 73
Kourti, K. 80
Koutselinis, A. 9
Kovács, G. 62
Kovács, GY. 62
Kovács, K. 54, 93
Koyamada, N. 86
Kozlov, A. 31
Köppen, T. 97
Köves, I. 45
Krasnodebski, I.W. 35
Kremenevskiy, I.V. 59
Krishnan, V. 2
Krombach, F. 89
Kröpfl, A. 25
Kuba, A. 22
Kubota, S. 65, 71
Kucsa, K. 5
Kuebler, J.F. 32
Kuebler, W.M. 7, 90
Kuhn-Régnier, F. 20
Kume, M. 28
Kupcsulik, P. 76
Kuppe, H. 7, 90
Kurlberg, G. 16
Kuroki, Y. 72
Kurosawa, H. 36
Kuzuk, O.K. 59
Kwon, A.H. 43, 75, 78, 79, 92

Lakos, G. 62
Lameire, N. 15, 88
Lamprou, S. 92
Láng, I. 45
Lantos, J. 22, 82
László Jr., F. 42
Laurentin-Perez, L.A. 49
Laurinyecz, M. 51
Lázár Jr, G. 14, 52, 99
Lazar, F. 68
Lázár, G. 14, 52, 53, 80, 99
Ledniczky, G. 72
Lee, S. 69
Leindler, L. 42, 67
Lesznyák, T. 24, 30, 47, 77, 83, 84, 93
Levi, M. 28, 29
Lewis, A. 85
Lewis, M.H. 36
Liden, H. 16
Lips, J. 1
Liu, Q. 4
López-Martí, J. 31
Losonczi, L. 57
Lozano, F. 35
Lozano, R. 40
Lukomska, B. 76
Lupu, C.M. 19
Lycke, N. 16
Lysson, M. 34

Maeda, K. 69, 70

Mafune, K. 72
Majima, M. 87
Makedou, A. 80
Makino, Y. 74
Maksymowicz, M. 19, 50
Makuuchi, M. 72
Malata, C.M. 47
Maldonado, C. 4, 20, 49
Mándi, Y. 14, 42
Mangell, P. 33
Mantas, D. 9, 73
Marchini, F. 87
Margeli, A. 9
Marquet, R.L. 9
Martin, F. 2
Martin. J.I. 2
Martínez-Lara, E. 31
Martínez-Moreno, J.M. 10
Maruszynski, M. 38
Maruta, M. 69, 70
Masui, Y. 92
Matesz, K. 48
Matsui, Y. 75
Matsuoka, S. 74
May, S. 90
Mayer, V. 46
Meester, D. 15, 88
Meijer, S. 62
Melander, A. 4
Melnova, N.I. 59
Menenakos, C. 59
Menger, M.D. 50
Merkely, B. 38, 57
Merkle, T. 5
Messmer, K. 21, 89, 90
Metaxas, G. 79, 80
Miclaus, M. 68
Miculit, F. 68
Mijal, J. 18, 64
Mikó, I. 24, 30, 47, 48, 49, 53, 77, 83, 84, 87, 93
Militz, M. 23
Minor, T. 12, 27, 34
Misumi, M. 79
Miyagi, S. 1, 11
Miyahara, T. 98
Miyake, T. 36
Miyazaki, M. 27, 39
Mizuochi, T. 72
Mochizuki, H. 95
Molfese, D. 4
Molin, G. 33
Molnár, G. 91
Molnár, T.F. 96
Morales, S. 35
Morishita, Y. 37
Morita, Y. 27
Morschul, Á. 42
Moscicka, M. 18
Mueller, S.A. 63
Murata, A. 36
Mussack, T. 46
Mutschler, W. 46

Nagai, K. 54, 66, 67
Nagaoka, T. 92
Nagaya, M. 65, 71
Nagy, A. 57
Nagy, L. 93, 98
Nakajima, A. 26, 27, 44
Nakajima, K. 36
Nakajima, Y. 54, 66, 67
Nakanishi, H. 43, 92
Nakano, K. 10
Nakashima, I. 10
Nakata, M. 72
Nation, Y. 36
Navarro, A.C. 40
Németh, N. 30, 47, 83, 84, 87, 93
Nikolopoulou, F. 46
Nikolopoulou, M. 59
Nilsson, O. 16
Nimura, Y. 99
Nishikage, T. 54, 66, 67
Nishizawa, F. 10
Nishizawa, S. 69
Nitta, T. 85, 97
Nozaki, H. 72
Nuttall, A.L. 91
Nyárády, J. 22

Ockert, D. 25, 45, 81, 96
Ocsovszki, I. 51
Oettinger, A.P. 63
Ogata, T. 37
Ogawa, K. 74
Ogawa, Y. 92
Ohara, M. 69
Ohkohchi, N. 1, 11, 13, 86
Ohtsuka, M. 27, 39
Oikawa, K. 1, 11
Ojha, M. 36
Okamoto, S. 10
Okumura, T. 43, 79
Oláh, C. 54, 93
Oláh, V.A. 83
Olausson, M. 16
Ollé, K. 22
Oller, B. 35
Olszewski, W.L. 11, 18, 19, 22, 35, 38, 50, 64
Ondrejka, P. 59, 72
Ortmann, C. 25
Osugi, H. 69
Otaki, A. 37
Otero, B. 29
Otsuka, M. 12, 76

Pafiti, A. 37, 46
Pajor, L. 84
Pákáski, M. 84
Pál, A. 14
Palacios, L. 17
Palásthy, Z. 58
Palmes, D. 12
Palomares, T. 39
Pantea, S. 68
Pap, Á. 42
Pap, G. 98
Papadimitriou, J. 46
Papaemanouil, S. 71
Papp Szekeres, J. 30, 77, 87
Papp, L. 89
Papurica, M. 95
Paramythiotis, D. 79, 80
Pasaoglu, H. 78
Paszt, A. 14, 53
Patsiaoura, K. 71
Pattyn, P. 63, 88
Pauwels, B. 55
Peck, D.H. 44, 65
Peinado, M.A. 31
Peiper, M. 45
Péley, G. 45
Perez-Abadia, G. 20, 49
Perez-Laurentin, L. 20
Perner, F. 28
Pető, K. 30, 77, 83, 84
Petrov, P.T. 59
Pi, F. 17, 31
Pidwell, D. 49
Pilarsky, C. 45
Pineda, A. 39
Plavat, C. 95
Polanski, J. 73, 76
Potel, J. 35
Pries, A.R. 7

Ratayczak, D. 25
Redl, H. 25, 31, 82
Refior, H.J. 90
Riaz, A.A. 30
Richter, B. 97
Ridgway, P.F. 44, 65
Rigotti, P. 3, 52, 87
Rizos, D. 46
Romijn, S. 55
Roossink, E.H.P. 28, 29
Rosenthal, A. 45
Rovó, L. 47, 48
Rőth, E. 16, 22, 82, 96
Rudowska, A. 11
Rusvai, M. 57

Saban, V. 66
Saeger, H.D. 25, 34, 45, 55, 60, 80, 81, 82, 94, 96
Sahin, I. 92
Sahin, M. 41, 56, 64, 78
Saito, K. 69
Sajjadi, S.G. 60
Sakamoto, I. 87
Salgar, S. 3, 66
Sánchez-Ortega, L.M. 35
Sandesc, D. 95
Santiago, S. 3, 66
Sápy, P. 62, 75, 77
Sárkány, A. 5
Sato, H. 64, 65
Sato, K. 79
Sato, M. 1
Sato, W. 10
Satoh, M. 11
Satoi, S. 75, 78, 98
Satomi, S. 1, 11, 13, 86
Scapin, S. 87
Schaefer, T. 50
Schauerte, P. 38
Scheule, A.M. 88
Schikore, H. 34, 55, 96
Schoots, I.G. 28, 29, 58
Schramm, R. 50
Schumpelick, V. 63
Schwab, R. 42
Schwacha, M. 32
Sckell, A. 5
Seino, K. 12
Sekiguchi , S. 86
Serdengecti, M. 56
Shimamura, F. 39
Shimizu, H. 27, 39
Shimizu, Y. 27, 39
Shimoda, M. 10
Shinohara, H. 41
Shinoka, T. 36
Shoji, M. 13
Sikas, N. 71
Simahara, Y. 6
Sipka Jr, S. 77
Sipka, S. 62
Sipos, P. 59
Sitkiewicz, D. 76
Sitzia, M. 12
Slodkowski, M. 35
Slotwinski, R. 35
Smyrniotis, B. 46
Sola, A. 17, 31
Soós, P. 38, 57
Sousa, R. 40
Spiegel, H.U. 12, 25
Stanczyk, M. 38
Stanislawska, J. 19, 73
Steyger, P.S. 91
Stolarczyk, A. 23
Strassmann, S. 40
Suess, L. 21
Sulyma, V. 70
Suzuki, H. 10
Svébis, M. 54, 87, 93

Switkowski, R. 20
Syroukis, S. 94
Szabó, A. 5, 91
Szabó, G. 30, 84
Szabó, Z. 95
Szakács, J. 99
Szalai, L. 51
Szalay, L. 17, 31, 58, 82
Szántó, Z. 16, 96
Szász, Z. 14
Száz, A. 93
Szczesny, G. 22, 23
Szeberényi, J. 16
Széll, M. 80
Szentkereszty, Z. 62
Szentpáli, K. 7, 53, 80
Szijártó, A. 76
Sziklai, I. 48
Szilágyi, K. 92
Szokoly, M. 93
Szőke, T. 52
Szűcs, A. 48, 57
Szűcs, G. 49, 53, 57
Szyper, E. 19
Szyter, E. 73

Taglioni, A. 3
Takács, I. 60, 75
Takács, T. 42
Takada, N. 69
Takada, Y. 12, 76
Takagawa, Y. 10
Takahashi, M. 99
Takahashi, T. 79, 85, 87
Takai, S. 75, 78, 98
Takano, T. 72
Takemura, M. 69
Takeuchi, D. 27, 39
Taminiau, J.A.J.M. 58
Tanaka, A. 41
Tanaka, Y. 69
Tang, W. 72
Taniguchi, H. 12
Taura, K. 26, 27, 44
Tavli, L. 41, 42
te Velde, E.A. 8, 40
Tekin, S. 56, 78
Tellado, J.M. 35
ten Kate, M. 9
Terada, M. 74
Terajima, H. 6
Terakawa, N. 75
Terao, R. 97
Teshima, S. 43, 92
Theoharis, S. 9, 73
Thoman, A. 5
Thorlacius, H. 4, 33, 50
Tietze, L. 63
Tihanyi, B. 42
Tihanyi, T. 42
Tinelli, M. 34
Tiszlavicz, L. 47, 52
Todoroki, T. 12, 76
Togawa, A. 27, 39
Tolba, R.H. 12, 27, 34
Toledano, M. 2
Toma, I. 57
Toma, O. 95
Toprak, S. 41, 42
Torcal, J. 40
Tóth, A. 48
Toth, B. 32
Tóth, I. 49, 53
Tóth, K. 45
Tóth, Z. 89
Toyokawa, H. 43, 78, 92, 98
Trably, C. 33
Trafalis, D. 59
Treutner, K.H. 63
Troisi, R. 13, 15, 88
Troján, I. 52
Trune, D.R. 91
Tsamandas, A. 3
Tsarenkov, V.M. 59
Tsiakiri, E. 79
Tsuchiya, H. 43, 79, 92
Tsuji, Y. 79
Tsukamoto, S. 1, 11, 13, 86
Tumpek, J. 84
Tzakis, A.G. 3, 66

Uchinami, H. 26, 27, 28, 44
Uehara, T. 97
Ueno, M. 69
Ueno, N. 74
Umar, F. 31, 82
Uss, A.L. 59
Usuda, M. 72
Utsumi, T. 69, 70
Utsunomiya, H. 10
Uyama, S. 10

Vagianos, C. 66, 73
Vágó, H. 57
Vágvölgyi, A. 75
Vajda, K. 5
Vajda, M. 55
Valente, M.L. 87
van den Broecke, C. 13
van der Bracht, H. 15
van Eijck, C.H.J. 8, 9
van Gemert, W.C. 58
van Grevenstein, W.M.U. 8, 9
van Gulik, T.M. 1, 28, 29, 58
van Holder, R. 15
van Leeuwen, P.A.M. 62
van Putte, B. 55
van Schil, P. 55
van Vlem, B. 15
van Vlierberghe, H. 88
Varagnolo, M.C. 3
Varga, E. 22
Varga, R. 84
Varga, S. 2, 17
Vascu, S. 68
Vass, Z. 91
Vatansev, C. 42, 56
Vatansev, H. 46
Végh, P. 51
Veihelmann, A. 90
Veress, B. 33
Vermassen, F. 15
Vinanzi, C. 3
Vizler, C. 51
Voest, E.E. 8, 40
Vogel, A. 90
Vogten, J.M. 8, 40, 74
von Gagern, G. 25, 34, 80, 96
Voor, M.J. 20
Vossen, M. 4, 20, 49

Wanders, A. 21
Wang, M. 33
Wang, P. 32
Wang, Y. 4
Warsi, A.A. 36, 70
Watanabe, M. 36
Weber, C. 82
Wéber, G. 60
Wehrmann, U. 94
Weltner, J. 45
Wendel, H.P. 88
Wentzensen, A. 34
Wesolowska, A. 38
Winternitz, T. 45
Wojewodzka, U. 64
Wolfárd, A. 17, 53
Woodward, A. 70
Wudel, E. 6

Xaus, C. 17

Yagi, S. 10
Yamada, H. 75
Yamamoto, N. 85, 97
Yamamoto, Y. 26, 27, 44
Yamaoka, Y. 6, 26, 27, 41, 44, 85, 97
Yamashina, S. 87
Yanagibashi, K. 98
Yanagimoto, H. 78, 98
Yokoigawa, N. 79
Yokoyama, S. 10
Yol, S. 41, 42
Yonezawa, K. 26, 27, 44
Yoshida, M. 85, 97
Yoshidome, H. 27, 39
Yuzawa, K. 12

Záborszky, Z. 24
Zagalski, K. 81
Zajac, L. 73, 76
Zaleska, M. 22, 35
Zaránd, A. 28
Zatagias, A. 79
Zawadzki, A. 4
Ziemer, G. 88
Zima, E. 38, 57
Zimmermann, T. 25, 34, 55, 60, 80, 81, 82, 94, 96, 97
Ziólkowski, M. 23
Ziprin, P. 44, 65
Zogas, D. 92
Zoica, B.S. 19
Zolich, D. 18
Zwipp, H. 55, 80